Key Topics in Public Health

ospital

For Elsevier:

Commissioning Editor: Susan Young
Development Editor: Catherine Jackson
Project Manager: Ailsa Laing/Emma Riley
Designer: Judith Wright
Illustrator: Jonathan Haste

Key Topics in Public Health

Essential briefings on prevention and health promotion

Edited by

Linda Ewles BSc MSc MA RD

Public Health Specialist and Writer

Foreword by

David J Hunter MA PhD HonMFPH FRCP

Chair, UK Public Health Association; Professor of Health Policy and Management, University of Durham, UK

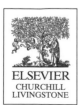

ELSEVIER
CHURCHILL
LIVINGSTONE

EDINBURGH   LONDON   NEW YORK   OXFORD   PHILADELPHIA   ST LOUIS   SYDNEY   TORONTO   2005

ELSEVIER
CHURCHILL
LIVINGSTONE

An imprint of Elsevier Limited

First published 2005
ISBN 0-443-10026-8

British Library Cataloguing in Publication Data
A catalogue record for this book is available from the British Library

Library of Congress Cataloging in Publication Data
A catalog record for this book is available from the Library of Congress

Notice
Knowledge and best practice in this field are constantly changing. As new research and experience broaden our knowledge, changes in practice, treatment and drug therapy may become necessary or appropriate. Readers are advised to check the most current information provided (i) on procedures featured or (ii) by the manufacturer of each product to be administered, to verify the recommended dose or formula, the method and duration of administration, and contraindications. It is the responsibility of the practitioner, relying on their own experience and knowledge of the patient, to make diagnoses, to determine dosages and the best treatment for each individual patient, and to take all appropriate safety precautions. To the fullest extent of the law, neither the publisher nor the author assumes any liability for any injury and/or damage.

The Publisher

Printed in China

Contents

About the editor and contributors

Catherine Dennison PhD BSc is Research Manager for the Sexual Health and Substance Misuse Business Area, Department of Health. Her background is in adolescent health research. From 2000 to 2004 Catherine provided research support to the Teenage Pregnancy Unit, now in the Department for Education and Skills. As part of this role Catherine instigated a large programme of research and evaluation to inform implementation of the government's Teenage Pregnancy Strategy for England. Before joining government Catherine was involved in research on a wide range of issues relating to young people including mental health, youth justice and teenage parenthood.

Gail Errington BSc is a Research Associate in the Centre for Health Services Research at the University of Newcastle-Upon-Tyne and a collaborator on the Health Development Agency's Evidence and Guidance Collaborating Centre on the Prevention and Reduction of Accidental Injury in Children and Young People aged 0–24 years. She has a background in health promotion and education, developing an interest in injury prevention whilst working as coordinator on a local accident prevention programme. Gail joined the University in 1994 and was Evaluation Officer on the Safer Primary Schools Project, a 5-year randomized controlled trial. Her research interests include the evaluation of intervention programmes, engaging target groups and consolidating the evidence base.

David Evans MA BA DFPH is Reader in Applied Health Policy Research at the University of the West of England, Bristol. His background is in social science, health promotion and nursing, and from 2002 to 2003 David was Director of Public Health for Bristol North Primary Care Trust. His research interests include the evaluation of initiatives to tackle inequalities in health, user involvement and the development of multidisciplinary public health. He is also a Non-Executive Member of the Board of NHS Direct, the telephone and internet-based clinical advice and health information service.

Linda Ewles BSc MSc MA RD is a public health specialist, writer, editor and trainer. She has particular interests in nutrition and obesity, and in promoting plain English. After initial training and practice in nutrition and dietetics, she worked for over 30 years in broader fields of health education, health promotion and public health, within the NHS and in higher education. She is co-author (with Ina Simnett) of *Promoting Health – a practical guide*, first published in 1984 and now in its fifth edition and translated into five languages.

Elizabeth Gale BA is the Chief Executive of **mentality**, the national mental health promotion charity. Elizabeth is one of the founding members of the organization, established in 2000. Elizabeth has worked in mental health for over 12 years and for 8 of those she has concentrated on the promotion of mental health and well-being and the broader public mental health agenda. She has worked in the statutory, voluntary and commercial sectors and is an experienced presenter, trainer, writer, broadcaster and advocate. Her academic background is in law and sociology and she has a keen interest in the human rights and civil liberties agenda.

Selena Gray MBChB MD FFPH FRCPCH is currently Reader in Public Health and Director of the Centre for Applied Health and Social Care at the University of the West of England, Bristol. After qualifying in medicine in Leeds, she worked in paediatrics in the UK and Saudi Arabia before training in public health medicine in the south-west. She worked for almost 10 years as Clinical Adviser for the Regional NHS R&D programme, and was a founding Director of the South West Public Health Observatory before taking up an academic post. She has had a longstanding involvement in public health training, and has published research on a variety of public health issues.

Alison Hadley SRN HV works in the government's Teenage Pregnancy Unit as Programme Manager of the 10-year Teenage Pregnancy Strategy for England. Alison joined the Teenage Pregnancy Unit in 2000 after working for 13 years at Brook – the young people's sexual health charity – initially as a nurse in the London Centre and then for Brook Central as manager of the policy and media work. She has also worked as a pregnancy counsellor for Pregnancy Advisory Service. Alison believes passionately in young people's rights to the information, skills and support they need to develop safe and fulfilling relationships. She has edited a book for teenagers about young women's experiences of pregnancy, called *Tough Choices*, published by the Women's Press.

Christine Hine MB ChB MRCP FFPH is Consultant in Public Health Medicine for Bristol and South Gloucestershire Primary Care Trusts. Following junior doctor posts in hospital medicine and public health, she has worked as a consultant for health authorities in Bath, Bristol and Avon and as Director of Public Health for Bristol South and West Primary Care Trust 2002–2003. She was public health lead for diabetes in Bristol and Avon,

and a member of the National Project Advisory Group on Diabetic Retinopathy Screening. She now specializes in public health aspects of acute service commissioning across the Bristol area.

Susan Laverty MB ChB MPH MFPH MRCGP is a consultant in public health medicine in the Black Country and a general practitioner. Prior to training in medicine Susan was a lecturer in special needs and communication skills. Her main interests are in chronic disease management, primary care and organizational development issues.

Pip Mason RGN BSc(Econ) MSocSc is Director of a training consultancy company and Honorary Lecturer at the Centre for Forensic and Family Psychology at the University of Birmingham. She has a background in nursing and counselling in the addictions field with 25 years' experience of services in the community, primary care, prisons and residential rehabilitation. Pip has a special interest in counselling around motivation and change, is a member of the international Motivational Interviewing Network of Trainers and co-author (with Stephen Rollnick and Chris Butler) of *Health Behavior Change, a guide for practitioners* (1999).

Doreen McIntyre MA MPH PGCE is Director of the International Non Governmental Coalition Against Tobacco. After a short spell in the UK civil service, Doreen has worked in tobacco control since 1988, first at city level in her native Glasgow then at UK national level as Director of the No Smoking Day charity. Her work involves the creation of national and international alliances that can mobilize resources and implement best practice in tobacco control, and her particular interest is in the use of mass media for health communications.

Klim McPherson PhD FFPH FMedSci is a Visiting Professor of Public Health Epidemiology in the Nuffield Department of Obstetrics and Gynaecology at the University of Oxford. He works mainly on women's diseases, their causes and treatment from an epidemiological perspective. His main interest is enhancing a strong and rigorous public health structure in the UK that can influence positively the occurrence of avoidable disease in the future. He is Vice Chair of the National Heart Forum, a non-governmental organization dedicated to preventing coronary heart disease.

Dympna Pearson RD works as a freelance trainer and consultant dietitian. She has extensive experience of working in different clinical settings and providing training for healthcare professionals. Dympna has developed behaviour change skills training for healthcare professionals and she now runs multidisciplinary courses at national and local level. This training focuses on the development of interpersonal skills as well as the more advanced motivational and cognitive behavioural approaches. Her interest in obesity management is reflected through her work as chair of 'Dietitians working in Obesity Management (UK)' [DOM (UK)] and vice-chair of the National Obesity Forum (NOF).

R. Nicholas Pugh MA MD FRCP FFPHM DTM&H is a public health consultant at Walsall Teaching Primary Care Trust and the Black Country Health Protection Agency, and Visiting Professor at Staffordshire University. Nick's current research interests are in drug misuse and sexual health. He was previously a Clinical Lecturer at the Liverpool School of Tropical Medicine, spending 12 years in Africa, and a clinical epidemiologist and Associate Professor in Public Health for 8 years at a new medical school in the United Arab Emirates. He has published especially in the fields of communicable disease, snake bite poisoning, and public health.

Chris Riddoch CertEd BA MEd PhD is Professor of Exercise Science and Head of the London Institute for Sport and Exercise at Middlesex University. Originally trained as a physical education teacher, he taught in London schools for 10 years. He then moved to Queen's University of Belfast to lecture in sports science and then to the University of Bristol to lecture in exercise and health science. During his time at Bristol he spent 3 years as Dean of Graduate Studies for the Social Science Faculty. He is an active researcher, focusing predominantly on children's physical activity and health. He has directed a number of large multinational epidemiological studies of children's health.

Linda Seymour BA MA is Research and Policy Development Manager at **mentality**, the national mental health promotion charity. She has worked in health promotion for more than 20 years, initially in tobacco control at Action on Smoking and Health (ASH). Subsequently she worked on the national evaluation team for Health at Work in the NHS. She has been a Board Level Director in the NHS at a health authority (1993–1996) and then at a community, mental health and learning disability trust (1998–2002). She is an experienced trainer, writer and broadcaster and was a Research Fellow in Health and Social Policy at Brighton University.

Lorna Templeton BSc MSc is a Senior Researcher at the Mental Health Research and Development Unit in Bath (Avon & Wiltshire Mental Health Partnership NHS Trust and the University of Bath), managing the Alcohol, Drugs and the Family Research Programme. She has worked in this area for over 7 years. Lorna is also the current Chair of the New Directions in the Study of Alcohol Group, a committee member of the Addictions Forum, a member of Alcohol Concern's Children and Families Forum and a member of the Encare network, an EU-wide collaboration to develop resources for professionals who come into contact or work with children living in families where there are parental alcohol problems.

Elizabeth Towner BSc MA PhD PGCE is Professor of Child Health at the University of the West of England, Bristol. Her background is in teaching, educational research, health promotion and in particular injury prevention. Her research interests include inequalities in childhood injury, school-based interventions, involving children and young people in research and developing the evidence base in the field of injury. She was a member of England's National Task Force on Accidental Injury and is the principal investigator of the Health Development Agency's Evidence and Guidance Collaborating Centre on the Prevention and Reduction of Accidental Injury in Children and Young People aged 0–24 years.

Richard Velleman BSc MSc PhD FBPsS FRSS CPsychol is Professor of Mental Health Research at the University of Bath, where he directs the Mental Health Research and Development Unit (Avon & Wiltshire Mental Health Partnership NHS Trust and the University of Bath). He is also Visiting Professor of Psychology at the University of Naples, Italy. He trained originally as a clinical psychologist, and since then has headed up statu-tory addictions services, worked as an NHS Trust Board Director, undertaken many research projects and published widely. Richard is also a member of the Encare network, an EU-wide collaboration to develop resources for professionals who come into contact or work with children living in families where there are parental alcohol problems.

Foreword

Public health has risen rapidly, if somewhat unexpectedly, up the policy and political agendas in the UK in recent months. There are several reasons for this, including a growing recognition that many of the deep-seated health problems like obesity are not amenable to solution by secondary acute-care interventions – or if they are, the cost is likely to bankrupt the NHS – which means looking afresh at how demand on the Service can be managed and at different ways of tackling ill health. In particular, more attention needs to be given to what keeps people healthy, rather than what makes them ill. Most research into health inequalities in the UK, for example, has been about causation rather than intervention.

A persuasive social and economic case for investing 'upstream' to keep people healthy was made in two influential reports produced by Derek Wanless, the Treasury's special adviser.[1,2] His first report, which looked at the future demands on the NHS until 2022, made the case for investing in public health while saving the NHS some £30 billion, if progress was made in implementing what he termed the 'fully engaged scenario'. In this, people's health status and their level of health literacy would be high and surpass present targets.

His second report reviewed the weaknesses in public health capacity and infrastructure, which serve as serious obstacles to making progress in realizing the fully engaged scenario. He was critical of the government for having made lamentable progress in implementing the scenario, which requires a step change in political leadership and management action. As Wanless concluded, the need was not for more policy pronouncements – there had been a plethora of these stretching back over 30 years – but for action and sustained political commitment.

As a result of the renewed interest in public health, the government is impatient for those engaged in its delivery to be more adept at achieving change and, as Wanless put it, for making the business case for investing in public health measures as opposed to curative healthcare interventions. This book's appearance, therefore, could not be more timely. If ever there was a need for a text which reviews the evidence base in order to establish what we know and do not know in respect of key topics like cancer, stroke, diabetes and obesity, and does so in an accessible way, it is surely now. Linda Ewles and her contributors are to be congratulated.

Public health practitioners are sometimes criticized for an unhealthy preoccupation with acquiring evidence rather than acting upon it, and with seeking perfection rather than settling for good-enough knowledge of what works or might be effective. In short, they optimize rather than satisfice. Nobody disputes the importance of knowledge and evidence when it comes to public health action, but a widely held perception is that often the weakness of the evidence base, or its absence, becomes a pretext for delay and inaction. In fact, as the World Health Organization (among others) often reminds us, quite a lot is already known about the causes of ill health and about many of the actions needed to tackle them. The barriers to acting on the evidence are often political, organizational or professional rather than technical or the consequence of a total knowledge deficit. Many of the chapters in this book lend support to this view.

Yet, despite the wealth of evidence and sources of information available, there remains a hunger for clear and straightforward guidance on what is known about a topic, what can be done to improve health, and the limits of our knowledge. This book goes a long way to meeting this need and should fill a gap in the armoury of the public health workforce.

Public health problems invariably fall into the category of 'wicked issues' where the causes are complex and multiple. The solutions may be equally complex and multiple and we do often lack evidence concerning their effectiveness. Importantly, in seeking to support both practitioners and students of public health, the book resists being reductionist and simplistic in its approach. Instead, the complexity, messiness and political nature of public health are acknowledged and embraced, and run through the chapters as crosscutting themes. Weighing and assessing the value of evidence is largely a matter of judgement – a political as much as a technical process.

Adding to the complexity of applying the evidence in public health is the need for action across a range of professions and organizations, each with its own particular priorities, culture and accountability arrangements. In being everybody's business, public health risks being nobody's responsibility. While the NHS has formally been accorded the lead role on public health matters, until now it has been preoccupied with clinical care and evidence-based medicine. How far it will (or can) shift its focus 'upstream', and whether it is appropriate for the NHS to assume such a leadership role in the first place, remain contested issues.

However these issues are resolved, in its forthcoming policy statement on public health the government will be aiming both to strengthen the evidence base, particularly in respect of establishing the cost-effectiveness of interventions, and to ensure that the evidence is acted upon. In meeting these objectives, the collection of topics reviewed in this book, and the practical advice offered on how they might be tackled and where we lack evidence, should prove indispensable.

As the contributions to this book amply demonstrate there is much that can be done now, even allowing for the uncertainties which exist and the incompleteness of the evidence, to make inroads into many of the public health challenges we confront. Indeed, notwithstanding the need to close gaps in our knowledge, there is also an important development agenda aimed at equipping the public health workforce with the skills to interpret research findings and be able to apply them to their particular situations.

Finally, although it is an issue that goes beyond the scope of this book, the public health academic community needs to consider carefully how it can best engage with practitioners and services, both to help close evidence gaps and to translate evidence into practice. This issue has a direct bearing on the incentive structure for applied research within universities, and the workings and impact of the research assessment exercise in particular. Unless we get these arrangements aligned with the needs of public health practice, then many of the knowledge gaps identified in this book will remain.

Durham, 2004   David J Hunter

REFERENCES

1. Wanless D. Securing our future health: taking a long term view. London: HM Treasury; 2002.
2. Wanless D. Securing good health for the whole population: final report. London: The Stationery Office; 2004.

Editor's preface

My aim in producing *Key Topics in Public Health: essential briefings on prevention and health promotion* was to provide an easy-to-read, succinct reference and guide, setting out:

- essential background information on 12 major public health topics: cancer, heart disease and strokes, diabetes, smoking, obesity, physical activity, injury prevention, teenage pregnancy, sexually transmitted infections, alcohol, drugs and mental health;
- what we know (and don't know) from research evidence about the most effective ways to approach prevention and health promotion in each topic;
- briefings on the two key themes of tackling inequalities in health and helping individuals to change health-related behaviour.

Each chapter is written by an expert in the topic, using a set of sub-headings, often in the form of questions. These vary according to subject matter but all 'topic' chapters cover core issues:

- Definition (what is cancer? what is 'problem' drinking? what is mental health?)
- What causes the problem? (why is the prevalence of diabetes rising so fast? why are people obese?)
- Why is this topic an important public health issue? (why is teenage pregnancy a 'bad thing' – or is it?)
- How is it addressed in national policy? (National Service Frameworks, national health strategy targets, Cancer Plan and so on)
- What's the current picture – who is at risk? (ages, social groups, ethnic groups)
- Is the problem getting better or worse? (trends and epidemiology)
- Do health inequalities feature in this topic? (e.g. social class differences in prevalence of cancer or heart disease)
- What can we do about prevention and health promotion at a community level? (evidence-based approaches)
- How can we best help individuals? (evidence-based approaches to helping people change health-related behaviour, e.g. stopping smoking)
- Are there controversial issues? (current debates and dilemmas)
- Are there common myths and questions about this topic? (e.g. do teenagers get pregnant to get a council flat? is obesity inherited?)
- What don't we know enough about yet? What questions still need answers? (e.g. how can we stop teenagers from smoking?)
- Where to find further information and help (a selection of the most important and helpful resources including the Health Development Agency's online reviews and effectiveness guides, national strategy documents, National Service Frameworks, books, websites and organizations such as Diabetes UK and Alcohol Concern).

WHO IS THIS BOOK FOR?

This book was written with five groups of readers in mind.

● Students on basic training in health and allied professions, who are part of the wider multiprofessional public health workforce. This includes nurses (including primary care nurses, midwives, school nurses and health visitors), doctors and dentists, other health professionals such as dietitians, community development and community health workers, social workers and youth workers.

● Professionals in post-basic training or professional development courses in public health, such as those studying for the many Masters degree and postgraduate diploma courses in health promotion and public health.

● Front-line practitioners in public health, health services and related fields who would like to look at health issues as part of their professional development and to help with their day-to-day work.

● Health and social services managers who need a basic understanding of health issues in order to plan and manage services.

● Lay people who may be active in, for example, voluntary, community or patient groups, and who seek to be more informed about important health topics.

Because readers may not be familiar with public health and medical 'jargon' and acronyms, I have kept them to a minimum, with explanations in the text and a glossary at the end of the book.

WHY WAS IT WRITTEN?

The idea for this book came to me on a train journey. I was reviewing a health promotion textbook written for the American market; it was a massive 600-page tome, but amongst other things it contained a lot of information on health promotion topics. It made me think that I knew of no UK book that provided basic, easy-to-read information on essential *topics* in public health: topics such as teenage pregnancy, drug misuse, heart disease or diabetes. Other books tended to focus on *population groups* such as older people, young people, or black and minority ethnic communities; or on *settings* such as schools, communities and workplaces; or on *processes* such as counselling, health education, urban regeneration and community development. But often *topics* were the focus of day-to-day work in public health.

I thought of the times when, as a health promotion manager, I had been responsible for developing interventions and strategies for issues such as sexual health and alcohol – and had struggled to get clued-up about the topic quickly so that I would not make crass mistakes or appear woefully ignorant in planning meetings. I thought of front-line workers who want to see themselves and their work in the context of a bigger picture. I considered the public health strategists and health service managers who need to grasp the basic epidemiology and the potential for prevention and amelioration of the major health problems currently causing so much ill health in the population.

It is of course possible to get information on health topics from sources such as medical and nursing textbooks, professional journals and websites. But these may be too technical and detailed, and are time-consuming to access. And how, as a non-expert, do you discriminate between sound websites and those disseminating extreme views or downright quackery? Where do you start if, for example, you put 'obesity' into Google and come up with three and a half million references?

So the idea of a starting-from-square-one 'topics' public health book was born. I discussed it with public health practitioners and academics, and with my publisher, gleaning helpful suggestions along the way. And now, 2 years after the first seed of an idea was planted on that train journey, I am writing this Preface to *Key Topics in Public Health* (books have a longer gestation period than elephants!).

MAKING THE CHAPTERS HANG TOGETHER

When this book was at the ideas stage, a shrewd public health colleague commented that it would be a great shame if the book simplified public health into a number of disease-related topics, and became a kind of 'painting public health by numbers'. She also hoped it would not ignore the wide range of complex and political issues surrounding the topics.

I have been mindful of these two issues throughout the editing process. I thought about how to 'join the dots' so that the topics would be seen as part of a wider picture. At one point I tried to create a diagram showing the links between topics, but there were so many that what I produced resembled a piece of inexpert knitting. I toyed with matrices and three-dimensional cubes but they merely demonstrated that the interrelationships are far too complex to be set down in a diagram. However, crucially, these relationships are explained and cross-referenced throughout the book. I hope this means that readers will readily see themes that cut across topics and the connections between chapters.

Figure 1 is a well known and helpful depiction of the main determinants of health. It is a useful reminder that consideration of any topic involves many factors at many levels from an individual's age, sex and genetic make-up to the general socio-economic, cultural and physical environment in which they live. In other words, health is determined by things we cannot change as well as our ways of living and conditions of living which we may be able to change. Each chapter reflects this complexity.

We have also not ignored other difficulties and political issues. Chapters have highlighted debates, dilemmas and controversies, about, for example, 'nanny-state-ism' in relation to lifestyle issues such as obesity and the media minefields surrounding teenage pregnancy. Many chapters also highlight the paucity of the evidence base for effective interventions in numerous areas, posing choices about what to do (or whether to do nothing) when there is no clear evidence to point the way.

DECISIONS AND DILEMMAS

Editing this book was not always straightforward. The first dilemma I encountered was which topics to include and which to leave out. 'Why not dental health?' 'Why not breast feeding?' 'Why not domestic violence?' asked colleagues involved in those areas. In the end it was a personal and pragmatic decision: I had to draw the line somewhere, and I included topics which have a high national profile and which, in my experience in health promotion and public health, are the ones that public health practitioners most need to know about. They are the 'must-dos' of public health, arguably those that could make the most difference to the health of the population in the UK.

Many of the topics in this book were included in the government's consultation on public health *Choosing Health?* in 2004 (www.dh.gov.uk). We go to press before the subsequent White Paper on public health is published, but it is evident that the topics in this book will feature in the future development of national and local public health strategy.

Another 'where to draw the line' dilemma concerned the book's focus on prevention and health promotion. Initially I thought that we would look

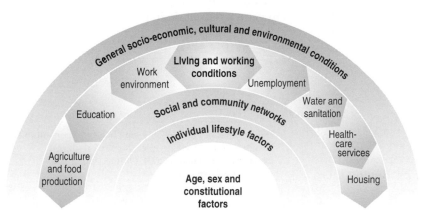

Figure 1   The main determinants of health. (From Dahlgren G, Whitehead M (1991) Policies and strategies to promote social equity in health. Reproduced with permission from Institute of Future Studies.)

at primary prevention and only cover secondary and tertiary prevention, and treatment, in the briefest way to complete a picture. But screening (for cancer, for example) is secondary prevention, and was far too important to be omitted. Treatment of obesity could mean primary prevention of type 2 diabetes and coronary heart disease. Treatment of drug addiction could mean prevention of serious mental health problems for misusers and their families. In the end, decisions were made chapter by chapter, bearing in mind the author's preferred emphasis and the likely overall usefulness for readers. So, for example, there is almost nothing about cardiac rehabilitation ('tertiary prevention') in the chapter on heart disease and stroke, but quite a lot about helping people to lose weight ('treatment') in the chapter on obesity.

Then, as I edited my way through the 14 chapters, there was the question of consistency of style. Contributors wrote in their own unique way; I did not seek to iron this out completely. So although all chapters conform to being easy-to-read and jargon-free and cover the core aspects, readers will find some diversity as well, reflecting the creative individuality of the authors.

Neither did I edit out the diversity of individual views: it adds to the richness of the book that the expert contributors have emphasized aspects of their topic which are closest to their hearts. Thus Klim McPherson stresses the importance of addressing heart disease risk factors in childhood; Richard Velleman and Lorna Templeton emphasize the impact of alcohol and drug misuse on the families of misusers; and Linda Seymour and Elizabeth Gale take issue with the view that randomized controlled trials should be at the top of a hierarchy of evidence of effectiveness of mental health promotion initiatives.

ACKNOWLEDGEMENTS

In editing this book, I have had the privilege of working with 18 contributors, all experts in their fields, in a stimulating and creative process. I am hugely indebted to them all for producing their chapters, and additionally to Christine Hine and Selena Gray for help with the Glossary. Many contributors struggled hard to find the time and meet the deadlines, but all did so willingly and knowledgeably, responding to my numerous requests and progress-chases with good grace and a spirit of cooperation. Many thanks, too, to David Hunter for readily agreeing to write the Foreword.

Many people also helped in the 'ideas' stage of developing the book proposal: I am especially grateful to Judy Orme and Pat Taylor (who discussed it with me over fish and chips, and whose invitation to help edit a book in 2002 gave me the confidence to tackle this one), and to Mary Hart, Angela Scriven and Gill Velleman for helpful constructive comments on the original proposal.

I am also grateful to my commissioning editor Susan Young and my development editor Catherine Jackson at Elsevier for unfailing help and encouragement along the way. Finally, my thanks go my husband Jim Pimpernell, for providing patient technical support and guidance, for trouble-shooting whenever a gremlin got into my computer, and for reminding me that there was never really any need to panic – I would get there in the end.

FINALLY...

It is my hope that this book will help readers in the public health workforce towards a better understanding of prevention and health promotion in key topic areas, and will help them to make their contribution towards improved health and well-being and a reduction in inequalities in health.

Bristol, 2004   Linda Ewles

REFERENCES

1. Department of Health. Choosing health? A consultation on action to improve people's health. London: Department of Health; 2004. Online. Available: http://www.dh.gov.uk

Update 2005

While the text of this book was being prepared for publication, there were important developments in public health. Rather than delay publication, we would like to draw readers' attention to them here.

The Health Development Agency

Throughout this book, the Health Development Agency (HDA) has been cited as a key source of information on the effectiveness of interventions to address major public health issues. In August 2004 it was announced that the HDA and the National Institute for Clinical Excellence (NICE) will become a single NHS organization with the remit to provide guidance covering the full spectrum of interventions (prevention as well as treatment) needed to tackle health and healthcare issues, including the public health issues addressed in this book. In April 2005, HDA functions transfer to NICE, which then becomes the National Institute for Health and Clinical Excellence. See websites for up-to-date information: www.hda-online.org.uk and www.nice.org.uk.

The Children's NSF: The National Service Framework for Children, Young People and Maternity Services[1]

This NSF was published in September 2004. It is a 10 year programme which sets standards for health and social services for children, young people and pregnant women. Its implementation is part of the government's *Every child matters: change for children* programme, arising from the 2003 Green Paper *Every child matters* and the legislative framework of the Children Act 2004. The NSF is especially relevant to the topics of teenage pregnancy, sexual health, mental health and unintentional injury. See websites: www.everychildmatters.gov.uk, www.dh.gov.uk and www.dfes.gov.uk.

The Public Health White Paper *Choosing Health*

In November 2004 the Department of Health published the long-awaited White Paper on public health: *Choosing health: making healthier choices easier.*[2] It sets out 'a starting point for national renewal of practical and acceptable action to make a difference to the health of people in England' (p. 6) and includes action on many of the topics addressed in this book, such as health inequalities, smoking, obesity, physical exercise, sensible drinking, sexual health and mental health. See website: www.dh.gov.uk.

References

1. Department of Health, Department for Education and Skills. National Service Framework for children, young people and maternity services. London: Department of Health; 2004. Online: www.dh.gov.uk.
2. Department of Health. Choosing Health: making healthier choices easier. Public Health White Paper. London: Department of Health; 2004. Online: www.dh.gov.uk.

Chapter 1

Cancer

Selena Gray

SUMMARY OVERVIEW AND LINKS TO OTHER TOPICS

Cancer is the biggest single cause of death in the UK: one in four people die of it (one in three of those dying under 65), and one in three will be diagnosed with it in their lifetime. The number of people newly diagnosed with cancer is increasing, but there are strikingly different trends in incidence rates and death rates for different types of cancer. With improvements in treatment and better survival rates there are also more people living who have been cured, are in remission or are living with cancer.

With some exceptions (notably breast and skin cancer) cancer is more common in more disadvantaged groups.

Cancer services, screening and prevention feature prominently in national and local strategies and plans, including *The NHS Cancer Plan*.[1] Cancer is a key topic in UK national health strategies such as *Saving Lives: Our Healthier Nation*.[2]

Much cancer is preventable, with smoking being the most significant factor. Other important risk factors to address in primary prevention strategies are diet and obesity, excessive alcohol consumption, over exposure to ultraviolet (UV) light and unprotected sex with multiple partners. Although the contribution of screening is debated, screening, along with early diagnosis and treatment, are important elements of health promotion and secondary prevention.

Because of their importance in cancer prevention, the following chapters are highly relevant: Chapter 4 'Smoking'; Chapter 5 'Obesity'; Chapter 6 'Physical activity'; Chapter 9 'Sexually transmitted infections'; Chapter 10 'Alcohol'.

As health inequalities feature in cancer, and lifestyle changes are crucial for primary prevention, the following chapters are also important: Chapter 13 'Tackling inequalities in health' and Chapter 14 'Helping individuals to change behaviour'.

WHAT IS CANCER?

Cancer is not a single disease; rather, it is a process that can affect cells in any part of the body. Cancer cells grow faster than other cells; they start to spread and invade other parts of the body, losing their original function. Cancer can occur in almost all types of cells or organs within the body, but does so much more commonly in some than others. There are about 200 different types of cancer.

Initially, as the cells grow faster than those they surround, they form a lump or *primary tumour*, but as they get bigger, small parts can break off and spread around the body in the bloodstream (*metastasize*). These lodge in other parts of the body and start growing; they are usually referred to as *secondaries*. They can occur anywhere, but most often in the lymph nodes, liver and brain. The cancer may be referred to as a *tumour* (lump) or *neoplasm*.

Cancers arising in different parts of the body and from different types of cells tend to behave differently. Some cancers (*benign tumours*) grow slowly and do not usually invade other cells or cause many problems unless they get too big. Other cancers (*malignant tumours* or *neoplasms*) tend to grow quickly and invade other tissues; they are often referred to as aggressive or invasive tumours.

Treatment of cancer generally aims to remove the primary tumour through surgical means, and then to stop further spread by using radiotherapy or chemotherapy. Some types of cancer are very sensitive to hormones within the body, and treatment with hormone blocking drugs can be helpful to prevent relapse.

Whilst the majority of cancers occur in older people, some specific types also occur in children and young adults, such as childhood leukaemia and cancer of the testicle respectively. (For further discussion, see the Cancer Research UK and Macmillan Cancer Relief websites.[3,4])

WHAT CAUSES CANCER?

CANCER RISK FACTORS

Changes in cells which lead them to grow too fast and invade other parts of the body are complex and not fully understood. However, it is clear that a number of factors make this process much more likely to happen and that different types of cancer have different causes. For some cancers there is an obvious cause, but for most a number of different factors come into play – they are *multifactorial*.

Age

This is the major risk factor for cancer. As our bodies age, cells are more likely to become damaged and to develop genetic changes that predispose them to become cancerous (see Fig. 1.1).[3] The normal rules controlling how they grow and function cease to operate properly.

Environment

A number of substances or chemicals – *carcinogens* – have the potential to produce cancer. We may be exposed to carcinogens through the environment in which we live or work, through direct contact with skin, through the air we breathe, or substances we eat or drink. These may damage cells and lead to an increased likelihood that cancers will develop. A few chemicals are extremely *carcinogenic* – that is, likely to cause cancer in those who are exposed to them – such as asbestos, which produces a rare cancer of the lung known as mesothelioma. Cigarette smoke contains over 4000 chemicals, many of which are highly carcinogenic (see Ch. 4 'Smoking'). However, most other chemicals only cause cancer in conjunction with other factors.

Radiation

Exposure to high levels of radiation increases the risk of certain cancers. This includes:

- ionizing radiation such as that used in X-rays and computerized tomography (CT scans);
- ultraviolet radiation such as sunlight and sunbeds;
- radon gas, which is emitted naturally from underlying rocks in the ground in some areas.

Figure 1.1   Number and incidence of new cases of cancer per 100 000 population (excluding non-malignant skin cancer) by age and sex UK 2000. (Reproduced with permission from Cancer Research UK.[3])

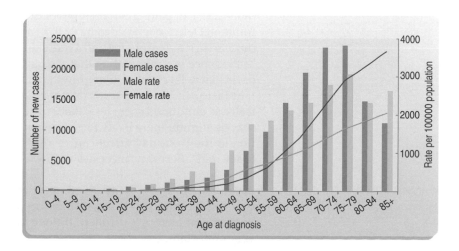

One study estimates that around 6% of cases of cancer diagnosed annually in the UK could be attributable to exposure to diagnostic X-rays.[5]

Genetic factors

Some types of cancer are more common with a certain genetic make-up. This may have been inherited, or sometimes genetic changes that predispose to cancer may occur spontaneously. There is a complex interaction between genes and exposure to carcinogenic substances, so that individuals with different genetic make-up may be more or less likely to develop cancer if exposed to certain carcinogens. In breast cancer two high risk genes (BRCA1 and BRCA2) have been identified, but they account for less than 1 in 20 breast cancer cases.[3]

Infections

The role that infections play in the development of cancer is increasingly being recognized. For some types of cancer, infections (particularly viral infections) occurring many years earlier and remaining within the body are the forerunner of the disease, probably through ongoing damage to cells. Examples include:

- the association of stomach cancer and infection with *Helicobacter pylori;*
- the link between cervical cancer and *papillomavirus* (the genital wart virus – see Ch. 9 'Sexually transmitted infections');
- the link between primary liver cancer and hepatitis B infection;
- the emerging link between Hodgkin's disease and the Epstein–Barr virus (EBV), which causes glandular fever.

This is not to say that everyone who gets infected with these viruses will get cancer, but the infection is a major predisposing factor.

Diet

Diets low in fruit and vegetables and high in meat and processed foods are associated with an increased risk of cancer.[6] Being overweight or obese also carries an increased risk of certain types of cancer, particularly breast and uterine (womb) cancer in women, prostate cancer in men, and colon (bowel) or rectal cancer in both sexes.[6] Physical activity is a key part of the management of obesity. (See Ch. 5 'Obesity'.) High alcohol intake is also associated with an increased risk of a number of cancers.

Other factors

Individuals who have weakened immune systems from whatever cause are more at risk of getting certain types of cancer. Thus patients with Acquired Immune Deficiency Syndrome (AIDS) are more likely to develop certain cancers such as lymphoma and a rare skin cancer called Kaposi's sarcoma.

Evidence is accumulating that the pattern of growth in childhood, and particularly levels of insulin growth promoting factor, may be an important factor in the long term risk of cancer. Children who have grown faster in childhood seem less likely to suffer from heart disease but they may be slightly more likely to get cancer as adults. Thus childhood nutrition in the past may affect cancer risk today, and childhood nutrition today may affect the cancer risk of future generations.[7]

WHAT ARE THE MOST IMPORTANT RISK FACTORS?

Because there are so many different types of cancer, and most are caused by a combination of factors, estimating the proportion of cancer caused by different factors is difficult. But we know that smoking and diet are very important.

| Smoking | It is clear that the biggest single preventable factor is smoking. Smoking is associated with an increase not only in lung cancer, but of all other cancers of the respiratory tract such as the trachea (windpipe), larynx, pharynx, and also of the oesophagus, pancreas, stomach, bladder and cervix.[8] It is estimated that 30% of all cancers are attributable to tobacco smoking in the UK.[9] (See Ch. 4 'Smoking'.) |

Smoking

It is clear that the biggest single preventable factor is smoking. Smoking is associated with an increase not only in lung cancer, but of all other cancers of the respiratory tract such as the trachea (windpipe), larynx, pharynx, and also of the oesophagus, pancreas, stomach, bladder and cervix.[8] It is estimated that 30% of all cancers are attributable to tobacco smoking in the UK.[9] (See Ch. 4 'Smoking'.)

Diet

There is debate about the extent to which diet is responsible for cancer. Some estimates suggest that one in three cases may be due to diet, both directly because of the content of the diet, and indirectly through the increased risk of cancers associated with increasing degrees of overweight.[8]

The Department of Health Committee on the Medical Aspects (COMA)[6] of Food and Nutrition policy working group on diet and cancer in 1998 reviewed the links between various dietary factors and cancers at 15 sites in the body. This report recommended that in order to reduce the risk of cancer at a population level we need to:

- increase the consumption of a wide variety of fruits and vegetables;
- increase intakes of dietary fibre from bread and other cereals (particularly wholegrain varieties), potatoes, fruit and vegetables;
- maintain a healthy body weight (within the body mass index [BMI] range 20–25) and avoid an increase during adult life;
- avoid an increase in the average consumption of red and processed meat, current intakes of which are about 90g a day;
- avoid the use of beta-carotene supplements to protect against cancer and be cautious in using high doses of purified supplements of other nutrients.

(Chapter 5 'Obesity' discusses guidelines for healthy eating which take account of these recommendations.)

WHY IS CANCER AN IMPORTANT PUBLIC HEALTH ISSUE?

Cancer is now the biggest single cause of death in the UK, having overtaken coronary heart disease and stroke in recent years. Approximately one in four people are likely to die of it, and one in three will have a diagnosis of cancer during their lifetime.[1] In the UK in 2000, there were approximately 134 000 new cases of cancer in women and 136 000 in men, a total of 270 000 altogether.[3] In 2001 there were approximately 80 000 deaths in women and 74 000 in men, a total of 154 000.[3] With improvements in treatment and better survival rates there are also many more people living who have been cured, are in remission or are living with cancer.

As cancer is a general term for a great many diseases, to understand it we need to look at different types of cancers arising in different parts of the body, as they have different causative factors, different treatments, and different epidemiological patterns. Although there are over 200 different types of cancer, lung, breast, colorectal and prostate cancer are the most common, and account for over half of all cases diagnosed. These four cancers are all more common as people get older.

In younger age groups there is a different pattern. In children, leukaemia is the most common cancer and accounts for over a third of cases; in young men, testicular cancer is the most commonly occurring cancer.

Overall, lung cancer, because it has such a poor survival rate even with treatment, is the biggest single cause of cancer deaths, accounting for about one fifth of all cancer deaths. About a quarter of cancer deaths are from the other three most common cancers, breast, colorectal and prostate. In those under 65 years of age, just over one in three of all deaths is caused by cancer.[3]

HOW IS IT ADDRESSED IN NATIONAL POLICY?

Current national strategies for health in UK countries feature cancer and its risk factors prominently.[2,10–13] The 1999 White Paper *Saving Lives: Our Healthier Nation*,[2] a comprehensive strategy for health in England, set an explicit target for cancer: 'to reduce the death rate from cancer in people under 75 years by at least a fifth by 2010 – saving up to 100 000 lives in total'. Comparable national policies in Scotland, Wales and Northern Ireland also address cancer.[10–13]

Cancer is addressed in many other key national policy documents, and policy approaches can be thought of in three categories:

- cancer services;
- preventive services such as screening;
- key determinants of general health and exposure to specific carcinogens.

CANCER SERVICES

The landmark Calman-Hine report in 1995[14] was a key report with respect to the organization and delivery of cancer services. The report examined variations in the pattern and outcomes of care to cancer patients. It made sweeping recommendations about how cancer services should be organized. This was followed by further strategies for cancer care set out in *The NHS Plan*[15] and more detailed recommendations in *The NHS Cancer Plan*.[1] These covered not only the delivery of cancer services, but also primary prevention and screening.

Progress towards the initial recommendations was reported in 2001.[16] This showed that smoking cessation services and the school fruit programme had been established, and that the breast screening programme was being extended to older women. Improvements had been made in waiting times for urgent referrals and access to services had been streamlined.

SCREENING

The other area where national policy is critical is in establishing and monitoring screening programmes for specific cancers. This is now managed through the UK National Screening Committee[17] which issues guidance on what screening programmes should be supported, and detailed advice on how they should be implemented and monitored.

There are currently two nationally coordinated screening programmes running in the UK for breast and cervical cancer. The NHS Breast

Screening Programme provides free breast screening every 3 years for all women in the UK aged between 50 and 64 and is being extended to women up to and including the age of 70 by 2004. Women aged between 25 and 64 are eligible for a free cervical smear test every 3–5 years.

There is considerable interest in other cancer screening programmes (see section on 'Controversial issues' below).

KEY DETERMINANTS OF GENERAL HEALTH

Smoking, diet and alcohol intake

Given the importance of smoking, the White Paper *Smoking Kills*,[18] which set out a tobacco control programme and included detailed targets for a reduction in smoking, is of enormous importance for cancer prevention. Similarly, with respect to diet and nutrition the COMA report[6] of 1998 was highly significant. Other aspects of primary prevention of relevance to cancer run through the National Service Frameworks, particularly those for coronary heart disease and diabetes.[19,20]

Exposure to specific carcinogens

As we have already discussed, tobacco is one of the most potent carcinogens known, and is addressed in the White Paper *Smoking Kills*.[18]

In terms of exposure to other carcinogenic substances, such as asbestos and other carcinogenic and toxic chemicals used in industry and manufacturing, various agencies have key roles:

- The Health and Safety Executive has a critical role in setting and working with local authorities and environmental agencies on monitoring standards in the workplace.[21]
- The National Radiological Protection Board (to be incorporated into the Health Protection Agency in England) sets and monitors standards for radiation exposure from all sources.[22]
- The Food Standards Agency (created in 2000) in England has a key role to play in monitoring food quality, ensuring that food is safe and free from contaminants or additives that might be carcinogenic.[23]

Guidance is usually based on international standards developed by the World Health Organization (WHO) or by the European Union (EU). Increasingly, environmental standards for air and water and food quality are being set at EU level.

WHAT ARE THE KEY TRENDS IN CANCER?

The number of people being newly diagnosed with cancer is increasing. Cancer statistics for 2000[24] show that the absolute numbers of people diagnosed with cancer in the UK has increased to 270 000 cases, 3000 more than in 1999 and 14 800 more than 5 years previously. In contrast, Scotland has actually had a fall in cases, reflecting success in reducing tobacco-related cancers with falls in smoking rates.

There are a number of reasons why more cancer is being diagnosed:

- people are living longer, so there are more years of older life during which cancer may develop;
- cases are picked up at an early stage through screening programmes;
- there are better diagnostic tests and opportunistic testing.[24]

In contrast, overall the number and proportion of people dying from cancer in the population is starting to fall, and has decreased by 12% in the last 30 years despite an ageing population.[25]

There are strikingly different patterns for different types of cancer. For some both the incidence (the number and rate of new cases) and death rates continue to rise. In contrast, for some cancers, treatment has improved so much that even where the incidence is increasing the death rates are stable or even falling. For others, both the incidence and death rates are beginning to fall. A summary of recent major changes is shown in Table 1.1.

In some cases it is very clear why these changes are occurring.

- Lung cancer death rates are now falling in men, reflecting the decline in smoking in men 20–30 years ago, but are still rising in women who started smoking later and have stopped more slowly.

- In breast cancer, death rates have fallen, despite an increase in new cases, because of early detection through screening and substantial improvements in treatment with the drug tamoxifen.

- Better treatments have led to dramatic improvements in survival for children with leukaemia, and those with cancer of the testicle.

DO HEALTH INEQUALITIES FEATURE IN CANCER?

Cancer affects all ages and all parts of society but health inequalities run throughout the cancer field.

Table 1.1   Recent trends in new cases of cancer and death rates[3]

	Trend in new cases	Trend in death rates	Comments
Breast cancer	↑	↓	Early diagnosis with screening, and improvements in therapy
Smoking-related cancers – men	↓	↓	Reflects historical decline in smoking rates
Smoking-related cancers – women	↑	→	Reflects later start and slower decline in smoking in women
Bowel cancer	↑ →	↓	Increasing rates of new cases are now stabilizing; better treatment
Prostate cancer	↑	→	Increased use of testing with Prostate Specific Antigen (PSA) is probably identifying cases earlier, creating apparent rise
Malignant melanoma	↑	↓	Rapid increase of cases in last 5 years. Increased past and current sun exposure, sun beds. However, earlier treatment is improving survival
Stomach cancer	↓	↓	Decline of *Helicobacter pylori* infection
Cervical cancer	↓	↓	Falling
Uterine cancer	↑	↑	Increase may be due to rising rates of obesity
Childhood cancers	→	↓	Dramatically improved treatment and survival
Cancer of the testicle	→	↓	Dramatically improved treatment and survival

Age and gender

As indicated earlier, the biggest single risk factor for cancer is age, and most of the more common cancers become more frequent with age.

Certain types of cancer, specifically those relating to the reproductive system, are only associated with men or women, and some like breast cancer are very much more common in women (although rare cases can occur in men).

Social class

As smoking is the single most common cause of cancer, there are, as expected, strong social class differences in the rates of lung cancer and other smoking-related cancers such as those of other parts of the respiratory system like the trachea and larynx.[26] As variations in patterns of smoking between social classes become ever wider, with smoking becoming more concentrated in manual classes, this will extend the differences in mortality rates even further. (See also Ch. 4 'Smoking'.) Table 1.2 shows the huge difference between lung cancer rates in different social classes in the early 1970s and 1990s.

There is evidence from many studies that people living in deprived areas who are diagnosed with cancer have poorer 5 and 10 yearly survival rates than people from better off areas.[1] The reasons for this are complex and not entirely clear. Poorer access to treatment and delay in going to the doctor with symptoms account for some of the difference, but it may be that factors such as having other illness at the same time and less psychosocial support are also important. Within screening programmes, there is a tendency for those from less advantaged groups, and some ethnic groups, to be less likely to attend, which may also result in delayed treatment.[1]

In general, exposure to environmental carcinogens is socially determined. More disadvantaged groups are more likely to work in dangerous or poorly regulated industries, where exposure to potentially harmful chemicals is more likely. Mesothelioma, a rare and very aggressive cancer of the tissues surrounding the lungs, which reflects past exposure to asbestos, is more common in manual workers in the building and naval industries.[27]

Bowel cancer has a strong social class gradient, likely to be related to a smaller amount of fruit and vegetables in the diet. Stomach cancer is also more common in more disadvantaged groups, and this may reflect poorer living conditions in childhood and greater infection with *Helicobacter pylori* in childhood. Cervical cancer is more common in those from manual social classes.[28]

Table 1.2 UK lung cancer rates by social class per 100 000 men[26]

Social class	1970–1972	1991–1993
I	41	17
II	52	24
III Non-manual	63	34
III Manual	90	54
IV	93	52
V	109	82

In contrast, for a number of common cancers there is a social class gradient running in the other direction. Notable ones are:

- Breast cancer: more common in the highest social classes compared to the lowest social classes.[28] Possible reasons for this include the pattern of childbirth, with fewer children and a later age of first baby generally in professional classes, and higher levels of alcohol consumption, both factors which are associated with an increased risk.

- Malignant melanoma: more common in those from higher social classes, and is likely to reflect increased past exposure to ultraviolet light through travelling abroad and summer holidays. This pattern may change in future with the increased availability of package holidays and increased sun exposure in all groups.

WHAT CAN WE DO ABOUT PREVENTION AND HEALTH PROMOTION AT A COMMUNITY LEVEL?

Saving Lives: Our Healthier Nation set a target for a reduction of 20% in cancer deaths.[2] An analysis of how that target might be met concluded that:

- one fifth of the reduction could come from improvements in treatment of cancer;
- one fifth from improvements in screening and early diagnosis;
- three fifths from primary prevention;
- almost a third could come from a reduction in tobacco consumption alone.[29]

A summary is shown in Figure 1.2.

Although many cancers relate to exposure to carcinogens many years previously it is clear that there is enormous potential for current local action.[30] We also need action or policy change at national level to prevent cancer, such as control of hazardous chemicals, banning tobacco advertising, and providing a helpful policy framework for action at local level (such as the school fruit programme).

Action can be considered under the three broad categories already identified in relation to national policy: improving treatment, improving screening and early diagnosis, and primary prevention. The first is outside the remit of this book, but is covered well in *The NHS Cancer Plan*.[1] The other two are discussed in more detail below.

Critically, work at local level needs to be underpinned by robust systems of surveillance recording all new cases of cancer, so that if necessary, epidemiological investigations can look at possible clusters of disease.

SCREENING AND EARLY DIAGNOSIS

Local action is needed to:

- Ensure high quality, well organized and accessible breast and cervical screening services, with culturally sensitive approaches that will

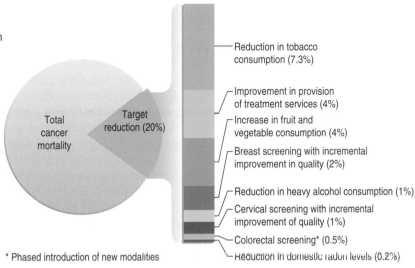

Figure 1.2   Improvements in cancer mortality from specific interventions. (Source: Adapted from DoH (2001) NHS Plan. Technical supplement on target setting for health improvement. Reproduced with permission from Prof. Nick Day, Institute of Public Health, Cambridge.)

Total cancer mortality

Target reduction (20%)

Reduction in tobacco consumption (7.3%)

Improvement in provision of treatment services (4%)

Increase in fruit and vegetable consumption (4%)

Breast screening with incremental improvement in quality (2%)

Reduction in heavy alcohol consumption (1%)

Cervical screening with incremental improvement of quality (1%)

Colorectal screening* (0.5%)

Reduction in domestic radon levels (0.2%)

* Phased introduction of new modalities

improve population coverage and hence increase early detection rates in the local population.

- Ensure comprehensive and timely access to high quality primary care services, so that individuals are encouraged to go to their doctor with early symptoms at a stage when they can be treated.
- Develop properly resourced and accessible sexual health services to ensure that sexually transmitted infections are treated that would otherwise predispose to cancer. (See Ch. 9 'Sexually transmitted infections'.)
- Mount awareness raising campaigns of early signs and symptoms of key cancers. Colorectal, testicular, breast and skin cancer are all examples of cancers where treatment at an early stage has a very much better outcome than at a later stage. For example, raising awareness of the signs and symptoms of suspicious moles or skin changes can help promote early diagnosis of skin cancer (melanoma).
- Provide advice on genetic issues in a primary care setting.

PRIMARY PREVENTION
Smoking

As already emphasized, the single most critical area for action at local level to reduce cancer is smoking. Most smoking-related cancers are entirely preventable, and this is the area that contributes most to inequalities in health in this field. (See Ch. 4 'Smoking'.)

Food, alcohol and physical activity

Other key lifestyle issues that are highly significant in cancer prevention include diet and nutrition, obesity, alcohol and physical activity. (See Ch. 5 'Obesity', Ch. 10 'Alcohol use and misuse', and Ch. 6 'Physical activity'.)

It is estimated that increased fruit and vegetable consumption could contribute to a fifth of the 20% target for a reduction in cancer death rates, and reduction in heavy alcohol consumption 5%.[29]

Exposure to UV light and carcinogens

Other areas at local level where action is needed to prevent cancer include:

- promoting avoidance of excessive exposure to ultraviolet light, and promoting the importance of sun avoidance at midday, shade in schools and parks, wearing hats and appropriate clothes, and using sunscreen;[30,31]
- local authorities and other statutory bodies ensuring that beauty and tanning salons with sun beds are properly licensed and used, and that there are clear guidelines and advice about the inadvisability of frequent use particularly for certain skin types;[30]
- regulation and monitoring of industrial processes dealing with potential carcinogenic chemicals or radiation by local authorities, the Environment Agency or relevant regulatory body. Regular occupational health checks may be needed by some groups. Asbestos, a very carcinogenic substance, is now highly regulated and its removal from old buildings must be scrupulously monitored and supervised;
- providing advice and support about how to reduce radon levels in the limited areas of the country where levels are high and local communities live in the type of housing where high levels may build up.[30,32,33]

HOW CAN WE BEST HELP INDIVIDUALS?

Lifestyle

At an individual level, people need to be able to live their lives in a healthy environment that is supportive of a lifestyle associated with health. Again, probably the single most important action any individual can take to prevent cancer is not to smoke, or if they do so, to stop immediately. Benefits continue to accrue from stopping smoking at any age, and quitting in middle age can lead to reduction in risk almost back to that of non-smokers within a few years.[34]

Other lifestyle patterns likely (but not of course guaranteed) to be associated with a reduction in risk of getting cancer include:

- eating fruit, vegetables and other fibrous foods as a substantial part of the diet, and not eating red meat every day;
- avoiding unprotected sex with multiple partners;
- not drinking to excess on a regular basis;
- not indulging in excessive sunbathing or use of sun lamps.[3]

(See Ch. 5 for more about a 'healthy' diet, Chs 8 and 9 on sexual behaviour, Ch. 10 on alcohol and Ch. 14 on helping individuals to change behaviour.)

Early diagnosis and screening

The other area where individuals need support is firstly to be able to recognize signs and secondly to consult a doctor early if, for example, they notice a lump anywhere or a change in bowel habit. There is good evidence of delay between people identifying a sign or symptom and then seeking treatment. For some this is because they do not recognize the importance of the sign or symptom; for others it may be anxiety, a lack of willingness to acknowledge something is wrong, or a fear of losing control.

Individuals should participate in national screening programmes on a regular basis, giving due consideration to their personal circumstances. If they have a strong family history of one particular type of cancer, it is worth seeking advice from their family doctor, as some types of cancer do have a strong genetic component.

CONTROVERSIAL ISSUES

Controversial issues include screening, the relative survival rates between Europe and the UK, and the contribution of genetics.

SCREENING

There is debate in three main areas.

How effective is breast cancer screening?

The substantial declines in mortality from breast cancer have already been noted and attributed to earlier diagnosis through screening programmes and better treatment, in particular tamoxifen. However, there is controversy about the relative contribution of the breast screening programme, in comparison to the widespread use of tamoxifen, to this significant reduction in death rates. Evidence from the early randomized controlled trials of breast cancer screening has been interpreted as indicating the efficacy of the programmes, but other experts, notably the Cochrane Collaboration,[35] have interpreted data to show that there is little evidence for efficacy. However, it is clear that breast cancer screening is here to stay, and there are not likely to be further opportunities to investigate this by starting again from scratch.

Should we introduce screening for prostate cancer using Prostate Specific Antigen (PSA) testing?

Advocates claim that routine screening will save lives; others that it will merely bring forward diagnosis and increase the number of men having surgery and other treatments without benefit but with possible harm. Certainly until more robust evidence of the effectiveness of early intervention can be demonstrated (and trials are underway to assess this), there is no merit in introducing a screening programme.[17] Evidence shows that similar falls in death rates from prostate cancer have occurred both in areas where PSA testing has not been introduced and in areas where it has been widely used, such as the USA.[36]

Should we introduce other screening procedures?

For almost every major cancer, be it bowel cancer, prostate cancer or ovarian cancer, there is interest in the feasibility and effectiveness of introducing a screening programme. Pilot screening programmes for bowel cancer using fecal occult blood screening (looking for tiny amounts of hidden blood in the feces) are already well established in the UK. The important point is that we need to be very clear that any new screening procedure is effective and does more good than harm before it is introduced.

RELATIVE SURVIVAL RATES BETWEEN EUROPE AND THE UK

The demonstration of apparently poorer 5 and 10 year survival rates and subsequent higher mortality rates in the UK[1] compared to mainland Europe was a key driver in the Calman-Hine reforms[14] and *The NHS Cancer Plan*.[1] It is debatable whether these apparent differences reflected real differences in outcomes, or more comprehensive and accurate data collection systems within the UK where the national cancer registration system is very much more complete than in other parts of Europe.

However, what *is* clear is that there have been substantial increases in 5 year survival rates almost without exception for most cancers in the UK since 1999.[37]

THE CONTRIBUTION OF GENETIC FACTORS

As already noted, there is a complex interplay between the genetic make-up of individuals, their exposure to potential carcinogens, and their subsequent risk of developing cancer.

For a few types of cancer, there is a strong genetic component; in these cases, there is usually a strong family history of the condition. But more commonly, genetic make-up predisposes individuals to an increased risk of developing some types of cancer if they are exposed to certain carcinogens. However, it is clear that major changes in the incidence and mortality rates of the common cancers are dependent on and amenable to changes in environmental factors.

COMMON MYTHS AND QUESTIONS

There are many myths around cancer. Some are addressed below.

Is cancer associated with living near to certain environmental hazards?

Despite concerns that living near a nuclear power station, waste incinerator, landfill site, incinerator chimney, or under a high voltage power line may lead to an increase in cancer, there is little conclusive evidence to support these concerns. This is despite numerous studies that have attempted to look at exposure and quantify if there is an increase in risk of cancer in those living in close proximity to such sites.[38–41] This is in contrast with conclusive, easily demonstrated links between, for example, smoking and lung cancer,[34] or exposure to radon and lung cancer.[33]

Do mobile phones cause brain cancer?

There is currently no biological or epidemiological evidence that mobile telephones or mobile base stations cause cancer. However, there are limitations to the research carried out so far, and mobile phones have only been in widespread use for a relatively short time. It is recommended as a precautionary principle that children in particular should refrain from using mobile phones for prolonged periods.[42]

Does cancer run in families?

Some types of cancer with a very strong genetic component do run in families and can be inherited; this includes the rare childhood eye cancer, retinoblastoma.

The most important cancer with a genetic component is breast cancer, where it is estimated that approximately 1 in 20 of all breast cancers are attributable to the BRCA1 and BRCA2 gene. For bowel cancer, fewer than 1 in 10 cases are due to inherited gene defects, but there are some families with an increased risk of developing the condition due to a variety of conditions.[3]

WHAT DON'T WE KNOW ENOUGH ABOUT YET?

We do not yet know enough about the complex mechanisms by which genes and predisposing factors such as chemical carcinogens, infection and radiation interact to cause cancer. The long term impact of changes in diet, nutrition and obesity levels in children today on their cancer risk as adults is not clear, but gives rise for concern. Given the long lead time for cancer, changes in exposure in the past can be felt many years into the future, and changes today can have unforeseen effects 20 or 30 years hence.

On a more practical level, we need to understand better how best to support individuals in making healthier lifestyle choices, and how society can best support communities and those within them in doing this. (See Chs 13 and 14 on 'Tackling inequalities in health' and 'Helping individuals to change behaviour'.) We need to understand better the most effective ways of doing this, for example, in the debate around food and health, what should the balance of activity be in terms of regulating the promotion and advertising of food versus promoting individual choice, and how can action at local and national level be most effective?

Key sources of further information and help

- **Action on Smoking and Health (ASH):** www.ash.org.uk. A registered charity providing up-to-date, authoritative information, news and educational resources on tobacco issues.
- **BACUP:** www.cancerbacup.org.uk. A service offering cancer information, practical advice and support for cancer patients, their families and carers.
- **Cancer Research UK:** www.cancerresearchuk. org.uk. A website with information on cancer and cancer research. Includes a free information service for people with cancer and their families.
- **Cancer section of the Department of Health website:** www.publications.doh.gov.uk/cancer/. Information on *The NHS Cancer Plan*[1] and other cancer information.
- **Health Development Agency:** www.hda-online. org.uk. The national authority on what works to improve people's health and reduce health inequalities. It gathers evidence and produces advice for policy makers, professionals and practitioners, working alongside them to get evidence into practice. Useful in the cancer field is the Health Development Agency's *'Cancer Prevention. A Resource to Support Local Action in*

Delivering the NHS Cancer Plan.[43] This is aimed at people working in primary care trusts, cancer networks, strategic health authorities, local authorities and partner agencies, to assist them in their local strategic planning and delivery of initiatives to prevent cancer. It makes recommendations for action based on the evidence of what works best in tackling the key cancer risk factors highlighted in *The NHS Cancer Plan.*[1]
- **Macmillan Cancer Relief:** www.macmillan. org.uk. Helps people living with cancer with expert information, advice and services.
- **National Radiological Protection Board:** www.nrpb.org. Works in partnership with the Health Protection Agency; sets and monitors standards for radiation exposure from all sources.
- **National Screening Committee:** www.nsc.nhs.uk. Assesses proposed new screening programmes against a set of internationally recognized criteria to ensure that they do more good than harm at a reasonable cost.
- **UK Association of Cancer Registries:** www.ukacr.org.uk. Collates and publishes information on cancer statistics across the UK.

References

1. Department of Health. The NHS cancer plan. London: DOH; 2000.
2. Department of Health. Saving lives: our healthier nation. London: HMSO; 1999.
3. Cancer Research UK. www.cancerresearchuk.org.uk
4. Macmillan Cancer Relief. www.macmillan.org.uk
5. Berrington de Gonzalez A, Darby S. Risk of cancer from diagnostic X-rays: estimates for the UK and 14 other countries. Lancet 2004; 363(9406):345.
6. Department of Health. Nutritional aspects of the development of cancer. Report of the Working Group on Diet and Cancer of the Committee on Medical Aspects of Food and Nutrition Policy. London: HMSO; 1998.
7. Gunnell D, Okasha M, Smith GD, et al. Height, leg length, and cancer risk: a systematic review. Epidemiol Rev 2001; 23(2):313–342.
8. Doll R, Peto R. The causes of cancer: quantitative estimates of avoidable risks of cancer in the United States today. Journal of the National Cancer Institute 1981; 66: 1191–1308.
9. ASH. Fact Sheet No 2. Smoking and Disease. Online. Available: http://www.ash.org.uk January 2004.
10. The Scottish Office. Towards a healthier Scotland: London: The Stationery Office; 1999.
11. The National Assembly for Wales. Improving health in Wales: a summary plan for the NHS with its partners. Cardiff: National Assembly for Wales; 2001.
12. The National Assembly for Wales, Health Promotion Division. Promoting health and wellbeing: implementing the National Health Promotion Strategy. Cardiff: National Assembly for Wales; 2001.
13. Department of Health and Social Services. Health and Wellbeing: into the next millennium. Belfast: DHSS; 1997.
14. Department of Health. Improving the quality of cancer services – a report by the Expert Advisory Group on Cancer to the Chief Medical Officers of England and Wales (the Calman-Hine Report). London: HMSO; 1995.
15. Department of Health. The NHS plan. London: DOH; 2000.
16. Department of Health. The NHS cancer plan – making progress 2001. London: DOH; 2001.
17. National Screening Committee. The remit and terms of reference of the NSC. UK National Screening Committee EL96(110). Online. Available: http://www.nsc.nhs.uk/uk nsc/uk nsc ind.htm
18. Department of Health. Smoking kills. A White Paper on tobacco 1998. London: HMSO; 1998.
19. Department of Health. National Service Framework for coronary heart disease. London: Department of Health; 2000.
20. Department of Health. National Service Framework for diabetes, delivery strategy. London: Department of Health; 2003.
21. Health and Safety Executive. The health and safety system in Great Britain. 3rd edn. Norwich: HMSO; 2002. Online. Available: http://www.hse.gov.uk
22. Radiological Protection Act 1970. National Radiological Protection Board. Online. Available: http://www.nrpb.org
23. Food Standards Act 1990. London: HMSO; Food Standards Agency. Online. Available: http://www.foodstandards.gov.uk
24. Association of UK Cancer Registries and Cancer Research UK. New UK cancer statistics releases for year 2000. Press Release. 7th Jan 2004. Online. Available: http://www.cancerresearchuk.org/news/pressreleases February 2003.
25. Cancer Research UK. Campaign launched to sound an 'All Clear' for future generations. Press Release. 4th February. Online. Available: http://www.cancerresearchuk.org/news/pressreleases February 2003.
26. Department of Health. Independent inquiry into inequalities in health. Report chaired by Sir Donald Acheson. London: HMSO; 1998.
27. Treasure T, Waller D, Swift S, et al. Radical surgery for mesothelioma. BMJ 2004; 328:237–238.
28. Bethune A, Brown J, Harding A, et al. Incidence of Health of the Nation cancers by social class. Population Trends 90. London: Office for National Statistics; 1997.
29. Department of Health. NHS Plan technical supplement on target setting for health improvement. London: Department of Health; 2001.
30. Health Development Agency. Cancer prevention. A resource to support local action in delivering the NHS Cancer Plan. London: Health Development Agency; 2002.
31. Koh H, Geller A, Miller D, et al. Prevention and early detection strategies for melanoma and skin cancer. Archives of Dermatology 1996; 132:436–443.
32. National Radiological Protection Board. Health risks from radon. Joint publication by NRPB, Faculty of Public Health Medicine and Chartered Institute of Environmental Health. Didcot: NRPB; 2000.
33. Darby S, Whitely E, Silcocks P, et al. Risk of lung cancer associated with residential radon exposure in southwest England: a case-control study. British Journal of Cancer 1998; 78:394–408.
34. Doll R, Peto R, Wheatley K, et al. Mortality in relation to smoking: 40 years' observations on male British doctors. BMJ 1994; 309:901–911.
35. Olsen O, Gøtzsche PC. Screening for breast cancer with mammography (Cochrane Review). In: The Cochrane Library, Issue 1. Chichester: John Wiley; 2004.
36. Oliver SE, Gunnell D, Donovan JL. Comparison of trends in prostate-cancer mortality in England and Wales and the USA. Lancet 2000; 355:1788.
37. Office for National Statistics. Cancer survival, England and Wales, 1991–2001. London : ONS; 2003. Online. Available: http://www.statistics.gov.uk Jan 2004.
38. Committee on Medical Aspects of Radiation in the Environment (COMARE). Fourth report. The incidence

of cancer and leukaemia in young people in the vicinity of the Sellafield site, West Cumbria: further studies and an update of the situation since the publication of the report of the Black Advisory Group in 1984. London: Department of Health; March 1996. Online. Available: http://www.comare.org.uk Jan 2004.

39. Department of Health Committee on Carcinogenicity. Cancer incidence near municipal solid waste incinerators in Great Britain. Committee on Carcinogenicity Statement. COC/00/S1. London: Department of Health; 2000. Online. Available: http://www.doh.gov.uk/munipwst.htm Jan 2004.

40. Department of Health. Study by the Small Area Health Statistics Unit (SAHSU) on health outcomes in populations living around landfill sites. Committee on Toxicity COT/2001/04. London: Department of Health; 2001. Online. Available: http://www.doh.gov.uk/landfill.htm Jan 2004.

41. National Radiological Protection Board. ELF Electromagnetic fields and the risk of cancer. Report of an advisory group on non-ionising radiation. Documents of the NRPB, vol 12, no 1. London: NRPB; 2001.

42. National Radiological Protection Board. Health effects from radiofrequency electromagnetic fields. Report of an independent advisory group on non-ionising radiation. Documents of the NRPB, vol 14, no 2. Didcot: NRPB; 2003.

43. Health Development Agency. Cancer prevention. A resource to support local action in delivering the NHS Cancer Plan. London: Health Development Agency; 2002.

Chapter **2**

Coronary heart disease and stroke

Klim McPherson

SUMMARY OVERVIEW AND LINKS TO OTHER TOPICS

Coronary heart disease (CHD) and strokes are caused by blockage to blood vessels supplying the heart and brain. The damage is due to the formation of fatty deposits in a lengthy complex process linked with high fat diets, high blood pressure, obesity, lack of physical activity and smoking.

CHD and stroke are the leading cause of death and premature illness in the UK, but are amenable to prevention. CHD and stroke feature prominently in national public health strategies such as *Saving Lives: Our Healthier Nation*[1] and the *National Service Framework for CHD*[2] published in 2000.

Overall rates of premature death from coronary vascular disease are declining, but the signs are appearing at earlier ages; we are set to witness higher CHD rates among young people in their 40s and 50s than are experienced by their parents in their 60s.

Genetic factors, fetal health, socio-economic status and ethnic group are associated with the risk of CHD and stroke. Important factors in childhood and adolescence which sow the seeds of disease in later life include diet, smoking, reduced stature, overweight and high blood fat levels. Prevention therefore requires action in childhood and adolescence.

Population-based approaches are needed, especially to improve diet and participation in physical activity, particularly in those most at risk such as lower socio-economic groups. We need concerted efforts at national level to make healthier options an easier choice for everyone, whatever their age or socio-economic circumstances. This means understanding the real determinants of making unhealthy choices and, where possible, changing them for more healthy opportunities.

Chapters 3, 4, 5 and 6 are especially relevant, as they cover major risk factors for CHD and stroke: diabetes, smoking, obesity and physical activity. Chapter 13 'Tackling inequalities in health' is highly relevant because CHD and strokes are more common in lower socio-economic groups. Many risk factors are behavioural, so Chapter 14 'Helping individuals to change behaviour' is also important for prevention.

CORONARY HEART DISEASE AND STROKES EXPLAINED

The term *cardiovascular disease* (disease of the heart and the body's entire network of blood vessels) covers both coronary heart disease (CHD) and strokes.

CHD is caused by poor circulation of blood to the heart muscle because the blood vessels have become blocked. This may show up as a heart attack (myocardial infarction) or chest pain (angina). Heart attacks happen when blood supply to the heart muscle is damaged sufficiently to injure or to kill these muscles, thus rendering the heart less able to supply blood to the rest of the body.

A *stroke* is a sudden weakness of the vessels when the blood supply to the brain is similarly damaged, causing the affected part of the brain to function less well or not at all. Or the damage may cause a fracture in the brain's blood vessels, which may itself lead to the formation of a large occlusive clot.

Thus both heart attacks and strokes are the consequence of disordered blood supply to the heart or the brain, both essential for life. The cause is largely attributable to clots forming in arteries and breaking away through the circulatory system to lodge in the heart or the brain and cause the inevitable damage. This whole process is known as *atherosclerosis*. The clots are fatty deposits (*plaque*) formed by a complex process encouraged by high fat diets, high blood pressure, lack of exercise and smoking. Clearly individual susceptibility may also be a factor in the formation and the danger of fatty plaques.

WHY ARE CHD AND STROKES AN IMPORTANT PUBLIC HEALTH ISSUE?

The processes leading to CHD and stroke are important for two fundamental reasons.

● Cardiovascular disease including heart attack and stroke are common and form the major part of premature illness in communities. They are responsible for sudden unexpected deaths and, in the case of stroke particularly, cause major and permanent disability. They are the leading cause of death in the UK (see Fig. 2.1).

● They are amenable to prevention and with proper care even people of high risk can avoid them by modifying those aspects of their life that will affect their risk.

WHAT ARE THE CAUSES, RISK FACTORS AND AT-RISK GROUPS?

Coronary heart disease is eminently preventable, even among individuals who are apparently at high risk due to their family history or genes. The primary reason is that all the major risk factors can be avoided – although possibly with significant difficulty. The major determinants of CHD are:

● high levels of a particular type of fat (low-density lipoprotein [LDL] cholesterol) in the bloodstream
● high blood pressure
● smoking tobacco
● lack of exercise
● obesity.

For strokes the risk factors are similar but there is greater susceptibility to high blood pressure.

Figure 2.1   Deaths by cause in the UK 2002. (Source: British Heart Foundation, with permission.[47])

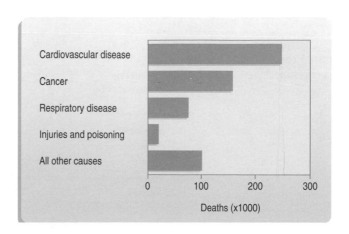

The first two of these are amenable to changes in diet, the next two to changes in lifestyle. Obesity is subject to a combination of diet and lifestyle. All of this is well known and indeed so well known that CHD death rates are decreasing quite fast in almost all developed countries (see section 'What are the current trends' below).

The contribution of the different risk factors to CHD is shown in Figure 2.2 which shows the relative size of the total CHD disease burden in the UK which is preventable by achievable changes in the prevalence of risk factors. Overlapping areas denote changes in risk factors that tend to go together. Of course what is achievable may be more than what is shown, in which case more CHD would be prevented. In many communities, especially in the East and the developing world where CHD is much less common, the levels of some of these risk factors are considerably lower.

People are born with different intrinsic risk (which may come, as we shall see, partly from genes and partly from fetal health) and superimposed on that risk are the exposures to diet and lifestyle factors that give rise to higher risk of CHD. In general, these will be different according to circumstances and particularly age and sex.

The process of the formation of dangerous clots is gradual and only slowly discernable; it may take 30 or more years to produce such a clot. Thus the issues of prevention have to do with having opportunities for a less fatty and salty diet, more exercise and less tobacco throughout life. But crucially these opportunities must represent real choices in the particular contexts in which people live. That means that the healthier options ought to be cheaper, more available, more acceptable and taste better than the riskier options. (See section below 'What can we do about prevention and health promotion?'.)

Much of what follows in this chapter derives from the 'young@heart' strategy for CHD prevention,[3] the strategy of the National Heart Forum, summarized in Box 2.1 at the end of the chapter. But before looking in more detail at what we can do to prevent CHD and strokes, we examine the causes and risk factors that predispose people to have CHD or strokes, under the headings of:

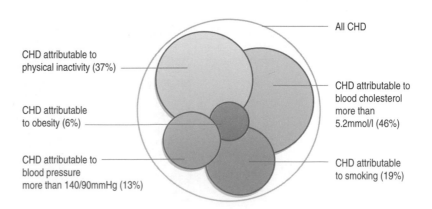

Figure 2.2   Components of CHD. (Source: British Heart Foundation. 2002, with permission.[48])

- genetic factors
- fetal health
- the range of risk factors in childhood and adolescence
- socio-economic status in childhood
- socio-economic status in adults
- ethnic group
- children's diet
- young people's participation in physical activity.

Because cardiovascular risk factors are established in early life, we focus especially on risk factors in childhood and adolescence. (See also later chapters on smoking, obesity and physical activity – Chs 4, 5 and 6 respectively.)

GENETIC FACTORS

Medical family history data are effective in identifying high risk families and individuals; selected genotypes will ultimately provide more specific information about risk and about potent gene/environment interactions. At the moment no known genotype predicts a higher risk among larger population groups, nor any particular susceptibility to particular risk factors.

However, family history is important. A positive family history of CHD in one study[4] represented only 14% of the general population but accounted for 72% with early CHD (men up to 55 years, women up to 65) and 48% of CHD at all ages. Analyses of over 5000 families sampled each year in Utah for 14 years demonstrated a gradual decrease in the frequency of a strong positive family history of CHD (around 25% per decade) that has paralleled a decrease in incidence rates for CHD.[4]

We need genetic tests to predict CHD risk that are more effective at identifying the potential for prevention than either family history or the assessment of risk factors such as blood fat levels, diabetes and blood pressure.[5] But studies so far indicate that the genetic component of CHD risk is complex, interacts with environmental factors and is unlikely to be the major determinant of CHD. The focus for early detection and intervention in people who have not yet developed symptoms will no doubt expand in the near future and will be important for effective prevention and treatment.[6]

FETAL HEALTH

Research shows that fetal development is crucial to many aspects of adult physiology and is determined largely by nutrition in pregnancy.[7] Risk of CHD is associated with low birth weight and high rates of weight gain as babies make up for their lower-weight start in life. The mechanisms responsible for this increased risk appear to be complex and not yet fully understood, but are known to be linked with blood pressure, insulin deficiency and resistance (see also Ch. 3 'Diabetes'), and blood fat levels. It is clear, though, that an important aspect of CHD prevention is implementing effective strategies to promote healthy eating throughout pregnancy, so that women bear healthy offspring.[8]

CHILDHOOD AND ADOLESCENCE

CHD and stroke are conditions with their roots in childhood: there is good evidence from cohort and autopsy studies that patterns of cardiovascular risk factors identified in adults are also seen in children, and that these childhood characteristics are predictive of disease in later life.

Studies suggest that the following factors in childhood and adolescence may play a part in increasing the risk of developing CHD in later life:[9–11]

- eating low amounts of fruit;
- smoking before age 21;
- crowded housing (an indicator of social conditions);
- mildly raised blood pressure in childhood and adolescence; hypertension is rare at these ages but is even more strongly associated with future risk;
- reduced stature;
- overweight, particularly in overweight children who remain overweight as adults or in underweight babies who become overweight in childhood and subsequently as adults;
- adverse blood fat levels;
- high blood levels of other factors: glucose, insulin, C-reactive protein (a protein involved in inflammation of blood vessel walls, linked with plaque formation) and homocysteine (a substance which damages blood vessel walls).

There is a dose–response relationship between the number of risk factors in early life and later CHD risk: the more risk factors, the greater the likelihood of developing CHD.

SOCIO-ECONOMIC STATUS IN CHILDHOOD

As we shall see, in adults, CHD and many of its known determinants show that levels of risk decline with increasing socio-economic advantage. Batty and Leon[12] collated published evidence to assess if these socio-economic differences in adult risk factors are also apparent in children in the UK. They found that there is a surprising paucity of published information on the socio-economic distribution of most CHD risk factors in childhood. However, based on what was available, they found that of 11 CHD risk factors consistent evidence of an association in childhood with socio-economic position was seen for:

- cigarette smoking
- birth weight
- height
- some aspects of diet, particularly fat and fibre consumption.

As in UK adults, the most favourable levels of these risk factors were in children from socially advantaged backgrounds. What was particularly striking is that obesity does not appear to show a socio-economic gradient in children under 16 years, the well documented negative association in adults only emerging in the later teenage years.

Other risk factors in children are: physical inactivity and low cardiorespiratory fitness; blood pressure; blood cholesterol; and the emerging risk factors of C-reactive protein, homocysteine and fibrinogen (which contributes to fibrous plaque formation). For all these risk factors, there is little evidence of any clear association with socio-economic status, although only a limited number of studies have looked at these relationships.

SOCIO-ECONOMIC STATUS IN ADULTS

Premature deaths from both coronary disease and stroke in England and Wales, as already mentioned, are currently becoming less common.

In CHD especially, the decreases are occurring more rapidly in the upper social classes than in the manual occupations, certainly for men (see Fig. 2.3). Treatment is not much more effective for non-manual people and so these changes will be a consequence of changes in lifestyle, probably deliberate, that make risk reduction happen more quickly in wealthier classes. This is probably a consequence of greater awareness and ability to determine aspects of lifestyle such as diet and smoking in the context of external circumstances. The rate of decrease in mortality from CHD under age 65 among social class I and II men is staggering – so much so that a simple extrapolation of the trend suggests that there will be few such deaths in this group in only a few years.[13]

Smoking

Social class differences in cigarette consumption are increasing and, in terms of the proportion of current CHD that can be attributable to smoking, the dividends associated with quitting are profound. In social class V men 24% of CHD is caused by smoking compared with 13% in social class I. If all smokers in the top band cut to less than 10 a day little would change, but if all social class V smokers cut to 10 a day their CHD would decrease by around 8%.[13]

ETHNIC GROUP

Young people

A study on the specific health needs of young people from ethnic minority groups found little information.[14] The younger generation (aged roughly below 30) is very heterogeneous. This group comprises the growing number of youth who are born and raised in Britain; more than 90% of the ethnic minority population aged below 30 were born in Britain.

South Asians

For the period 1988–1992, amongst South Asians the death rate from CHD is 38% higher in men and 43% higher in women compared to the

Figure 2.3   Male standardized CHD and stroke death rates under 65, England and Wales. (Source: British Heart Foundation, with permission.[49])

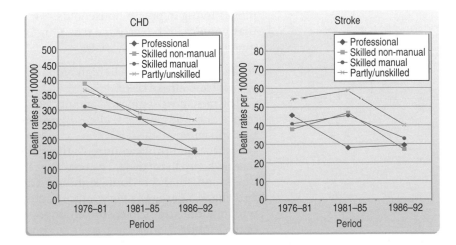

general population of England and Wales. The pattern shows some variations between the groups, with the highest rates being amongst Bangladeshi men (in excess of 47%), followed by Pakistani men (in excess of 42%) and Indian men (in excess of 37%).

In the South Asian groups, the death rate from heart disease of 20–30 year olds is twice as high as in the general population. This is of particular concern when the relatively young age profile of the South Asian population in the UK is considered; unless the relative burden of ill health is addressed, it will have a dramatic effect on South Asian communities in the future.[15] Death rates from CHD amongst South Asians have not declined as fast as in the general population.

Caribbean and Chinese

The Caribbean population has lower CHD death rates than the general population, as do the Chinese.

Better training of health service professionals in developing and communicating a sensitive and positive attitude towards ethnic, cultural or religious differences is vital. Such training should encourage listening and communication skills and affirm the patient's right to be different – in a way that does not assume the dominant culture to be the norm. Similar training is also necessary for staff in schools. Ethnic foods should be included when promoting healthy meals.

CHILDREN'S DIET

Evidence from the *National Diet and Nutrition Survey*[16,17] shows the following for children in the UK aged 4–18:

● Intakes of sodium are twice the recommended level, even although salt added during cooking or at the table was excluded.

● The percentage of energy derived from fat in the overall diet is considerably higher than recommended levels.

● Young people's diets are still too high in saturated fat, sugars and salt.

● Very few young people eat enough fruit and vegetables and a worrying number of children and adolescents do not eat any at all.

● There is considerable cause for concern about the diets of young people living in poorer households. For children and adolescents, particularly males, in households receiving benefits, findings point to inadequate and poorer quality diets.

All this ultimately leads to high blood pressure, which is strongly related to CHD and stroke risk.[18]

The measures of physical activity, coupled with the findings on energy intake and body weight, also suggest that most young people are relatively inactive.

Efforts to improve children's diets should seek to improve the foods that make up these diets. The results of this work provide information on those foods that contribute significant amounts of fat, saturated fat, salt and sugars. There is a very important role for governments in working with manufacturers to ensure an improvement in the nutritional quality of their foods.[19]

YOUNG PEOPLE'S PARTICIPATION IN PHYSICAL ACTIVITY

What are the determinants of young people's participation in physical activity?

A review of the evidence of environmental factors that are consistently associated with greater levels of physical activity among the young[20] showed that for children, boys are more active than girls; and, paradoxically, overweight parents tend to have more active children. Perceived barriers to physical activity are important, as are expressed intentions, healthy diets, previous physical activity and access to facilities.

For adolescents, again male gender predicts activity while increasing age predicts less activity, as does being from an ethnic minority. As might be expected, competence, intention and sensation-seeking tendencies predict activity, as well as activity by family members, particularly support from parents.

Do physically active young people become physically active adults?

The evidence shows that physical activity in childhood and activity in adolescence or adulthood has only a low-to-moderate level of association. Studies show slightly stronger effects for the nature of early life experiences in physical activity as precursors of adult physical activity, but still these effects appear small. These small effects may be real or the result of other factors. For example, it is possible that a third variable, say motor competence or early maturation, is the key influence, with children experiencing early success less likely to quit later on. Further research into tracking must account for the quality and pertinence of childhood experiences in physical activity as well as the changes in activity levels during childhood, adolescence and adulthood.[21]

This finding questions the commonly held view that physical activity interventions among the young should increase the physical activity of adults. It could thus be argued that, if physical activity does not have a strong impact on young people's current health, then attention on physical activity should be turned away from young people as a priority target group. This, however, ignores the evidence regarding the possible influence of the quality and nature of the childhood physical activity experience, which supports efforts to design interventions that aim to maximize the possibility that physical activity in youth may be continued into adulthood.

In addition, there are a number of other compelling reasons to promote quality physical activity among young people, including its influence on psychological well-being, childhood obesity, self-esteem and social and moral development. It does, for example, seem that educational attainment predicts future exercising whether or not exercise was important while young.

What is the relationship between physical activity during childhood and adolescence and risk factors for cardiovascular disease in young adults?

Analysis of major studies on this relationship reveals a complex picture. However, some general findings emerge.

- Physical activity is inversely related to a cluster of CHD factors in childhood and adolescence.[22–24]

- Physical activity tends to decline with age from early teens to late 20s.[25,26]

Current physical activity is what counts in reducing CHD risk.[27] CHD risk is as great for people who exercised in their youth (e.g. played vigorous sport) but then stopped as it is for people who have never done so.[28]

People who become active in later life show a reduced CHD risk similar to that of people who have always been active.[29]

The aim, therefore, should be to increase the proportion of the population at all ages who live a physically active lifestyle.

WHAT ARE THE CURRENT TRENDS IN CHD AND STROKE PREVALENCE?

Overall, rates of death under age 65 from CHD and stroke have been declining (see Fig. 2.4). In young people, favourable trends have been occurring in blood pressure, height and blood fat levels, but increasing proportions of this age group are becoming overweight (see also Ch. 5 'Obesity').

Reduction in death rates in the UK is similar to favourable trends in many other developed countries. Better care of patients with heart problems explains some of the reduction, but the patterns of change clearly

Figure 2.4   Death rates from CHD and stroke for people aged under 65, 1970–2000, England. (Source: British Heart Foundation. 2004, with permission.[50])

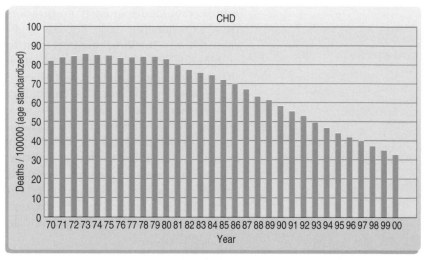

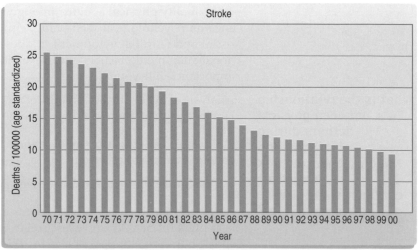

represent changes in the prevalence of risk factors, in turn related to concomitant changes in public acceptance of dietary and other causes. Usually, as has been the case in Australia, the USA and Finland for example, a high level of CHD mortality has given rise to varying publicity campaigns in these countries, which have had an effect on the prevalence of risk factors.

It seems it takes a country to become a world leader in CHD mortality to intervene successfully to bring the death rates down (see Fig. 2.5). Whether that is a consequence of novel and successful strategies or a more receptive population is unclear. But it remains clear that these changes are certainly in large measure a consequence of a greater public awareness and consciousness of a real threat to life. For the most part these changes are thought to have an effect on immediate risk, which is only true for older people. Often the major changes happen among the section of the population, at least in terms of age and gender if not social position, that is at highest current risk of a cardiovascular disease.

INFLUENCING FUTURE TRENDS

To ensure that death rates from cardiovascular disease continue to decline, we need to consider the long term effects – rather than the immediate effects – of the known risk factors. To capture the public imagination we need to stress that we are due to witness higher CHD rates among young people in their 40s and 50s than are experienced by their parents in their 60s. Public awareness has not happened yet, but the signs of CHD and strokes occurring at younger ages are there; when this becomes clearer, the gradual development of coronary disease over decades will be more widely appreciated. No longer will small reductions in the main risk factors by a large number of people be enough to bring the rates down sufficiently – rather, a systematic avoidance of risk factors throughout life by a large number of people will be required. In the end this is likely to be more effective if people simply become accustomed, from birth, to low salt and low fat diets and so do not need to change their preference. Such are the changes that are required in the immediate future.

Figure 2.5 Standardized CHD death rates, males 35–74 by country. (Source: British Heart Foundation. 2003, with permission.[49])

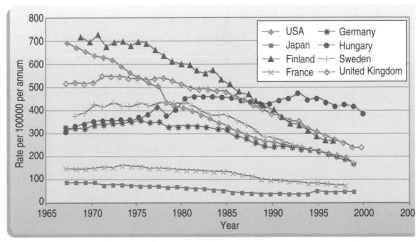

Thus the life course of the development of coronary disease would be understood and the implications carried through to the elimination of avoidable coronary disease. This would not require extreme measures by anyone, merely a greater understanding of the implications of real choices in particular circumstances, and of changing opportunities.

HOW ARE CHD AND STROKES ADDRESSED IN NATIONAL POLICY?

In the UK, national public health strategies have all addressed CHD and stroke.[1,30–33] In England, the White Paper *Saving Lives: Our Healthier Nation*, published in 1999, identified CHD and stroke as one of its four major priorities. It set a target 'to reduce the death rate from CHD and stroke and related diseases in people under 75 by at least two-fifths by 2010', with action on smoking, healthier eating, obesity, physical activity, high blood pressure, sensible drinking, stress and more effective treatments.[1]

Since then, other national policies have emerged on risk factors for CHD and stroke – see the relevant sections in Chapters 3, 4, 5, 6 and 10 on diabetes, smoking, obesity, physical activity and alcohol respectively.

NATIONAL SERVICE FRAMEWORK (NSF) FOR CHD

A major national initiative on CHD was the publication of the *National Service framework for Coronary Heart Disease* in 2000,[2] which the government described as 'our blueprint for tackling heart disease'; it set out the standards and services which should be available throughout England. It established 12 standards: the first four are concerned with reducing heart disease in the population and preventing CHD in high risk populations; the last one is on secondary prevention and rehabilitation; the remaining seven are about treatment.

The five preventive standards are as follows:

● Standard 1 specifies that the NHS and its partner agencies should develop, implement and monitor policies that reduce the prevalence of coronary risk factors in the population, and reduce inequalities in risks of developing heart disease.

● Standard 2 specifies that the NHS and partner agencies should contribute to a reduction in the prevalence of smoking in the local population.

● Standards 3 and 4 specify that GP practices should identify all people in their practice populations with established cardiovascular disease, and all people who have not developed symptoms but who are at significant risk, and offer them comprehensive advice and treatment.

● Standard 12 specifies that NHS trusts should put in place systems of care so that, prior to leaving hospital, people with CHD are invited to a multidisciplinary programme of secondary prevention and cardiac rehabilitation to reduce their risk of further cardiac problems and promote their return to a full and normal life.

The NSF has led to considerable developments in GP practices in identifying and monitoring patients with CHD or at risk of developing it, and the development of cardiac rehabilitation programmes in hospitals. But the CHD NSF tends to treat the burden of disease as a matter for more appropriate treatment once it has happened and concentrates little on preventing it.[34] This may be the major deficiency of national policy when it is estimated that current reductions in risk factors are responsible for most of the observed reductions in mortality.[35]

In 2001 the Health Development Agency published guidance on implementing the preventive aspects of the CHD NSF.[36] It provides evidence-based examples of effective interventions for dealing with all the primary risk factors – smoking, poor nutrition, physical inactivity, overweight and obesity – and makes practical suggestions about how to develop local programmes.

WHAT CAN WE DO ABOUT PREVENTION AND HEALTH PROMOTION?

Later chapters on smoking, obesity and physical activity – Chapters 4, 5 and 6 respectively – look at the evidence for effective interventions in these three risk factors across all age groups, and discuss what we should be doing. Therefore we do not address this again here, but we can usefully focus on looking more closely at effective interventions to reduce cardiovascular risk in children and young people.

The rationale for this is that (as outlined earlier in this chapter) the risk of cardiovascular disease is established in early life, long before preventive therapy is usually implemented. The risk factors are not only doing damage from early days but also laying the ground for more problematic disease prevention, both because of that damage, and because of the lifestyles that are being consolidated. Prevention therefore requires action in childhood and adolescence. Population-based approaches are needed, especially to improve diet and participation in physical activity, particularly in those most at risk such as lower socio-economic groups.

PREVENTION IN CHILDREN AND ADOLESCENTS – THE SOCIAL CONTEXT

First, we look at the social context in which lifestyle patterns conducive to developing cardiovascular disease are set in train.

Researchers in one study argue that socio-economic, cultural and familial circumstances are part of the pathway towards inequalities in CHD risk factors among children.[37] Families with children represent the largest, fastest growing disadvantaged group in the UK[38] and apparently one third of children go without at least one necessity, such as three meals a day, toys, other activity or clothing, but the response of children to these exogenous influences is poorly understood. Research into the mechanisms of acquiring high or low risks tends to ignore the perspective of the child, which is clearly vital.

The research emphasized that children perceived the immediate virtues of a 'healthy body' to be about the attitude of peers, inclusion in pleasurable activities, and avoidance of unwanted stigmatization. Notions of illness as a physical problem to be fixed were alien to children, who were more likely to perceive it as an immediate interruption to everyday routines and important social interactions. Since many of the risk factors carry no immediate consequence of illness, strategies for prevention in the long run need to be based on palpable effects that are important to children.

Other researchers[39] argue from a 'demand–control–support' model,[40] which they have developed to try to explain psychosocial factors in the development of CHD. For mothers with low income the place of work is the home, characterized by high workload for the family, including the children. Often poor control and decision latitude inside and outside the home and an absence of social support give rise to dominant concerns, for example that children should eat what they are given as opposed to a balanced diet. In such circumstances, the children achieve more autonomy and hence are more likely to 'graze'. Advertising of 'junk' food and other hazards on Saturday morning TV was more likely to influence them. Evidence suggests that progression into similar environments when older is associated with a greater inability to change to healthier lifestyles.

This suggests that action could be taken to increase decision latitude by coordinating and developing support given to mothers through statutory and voluntary services. This could:

- ensure time to talk, give the right support, and provide a wider net to detect and 'treat' postnatal depression;
- help parents to access attractive training opportunities;
- develop exercise opportunities tailored to mothers;
- provide better support for shopping and cooking through measures which ensure low cost healthy food supplies and groups to develop cooking skills;
- develop community approaches to smoking cessation which include mentoring and buddy support.

All these measures are relatively underdeveloped.

INTERVENTIONS WITH ADOLESCENTS ON RISK FACTORS

A useful paper by Macfarlane[41] wisely argues that none of the evidence available for effective interventions in the field of adolescent health is particularly strong. In fact, where there is evidence, in broad terms almost all discrete single issue interventions in the field seem not to work. In the field of tobacco use and food intake by young people, what evidence there is would suggest that the most effective interventions involve:

- coherent pricing policies;
- coherent advertising policies;
- simultaneous and coordinated multifactorial inputs at a national, local and individual level.

Smoking

The evidence is limited, at the present time, that school-based programmes for the prevention of smoking uptake by young people are effective. However, programmes which include reinforcement of social norms, and which also include information on the social influences which lead to smoking, seem more effective than the traditional 'knowledge-based' programmes. These need to be combined with training on how to resist pressures to smoke.

Obesity

Obesity in young people is the result of several factors – genetics, diet, and exercise – some of which are themselves controlled by other factors, including the availability of different foods, access to exercise facilities, advertising, parental attitudes and so on. Evidence for the effectiveness of specific interventions concerning diet in young people is limited. Most UK school-based interventions have not yet been proven to have a positive effect. There is, as yet, no evidence of any effective primary care based interventions with young people in relation to diet.

Physical inactivity

For physical inactivity, the conclusions are much the same. In Australia a 'healthy heartbeat' school initiative produced significant gains in fitness in 11–12 year olds, despite the fact that the initiative did not produce any measurable effects on knowledge, attitudes or behaviours. In adults, the evidence on interventions to increase physical activity suggests that personal instruction, continued support, and participation in an activity that does not necessitate attendance at a special fitness centre are all important factors in encouraging continued participation. There are no fully evaluated studies to suggest whether the same factors are pertinent to young people.

The best kind of intervention is to promote health *for* young people rather than *to* them, on a number of different levels from government downwards. Preaching does not work, and health professionals are at their most effective when we are:

- advocates on behalf of the health of young people; and
- providing young people and their carers with the most relevant and up-to-date evidence-based information we can, using the appropriate methods and technologies to make this information available in ways that they can most easily access.

CONCLUSIONS – WHAT WE NEED TO DO

National heart forum young@heart strategy

In 2002, the National Heart Forum (a leading alliance of over 40 national organizations working to reduce the risk of coronary heart disease in the UK) launched its 'young@heart' initiative.[42] Its approach is to tackle the causes of CHD from its beginnings in early life; the initiative is summarized in Box 2.1.

Those with major influence on current national policy fully understand the scientific nature of the risk factors and indeed how to help to prevent cardiovascular disease. But issues of personal choice and what governments can and should do about them complicate the realization of coherent policy. Moreover, commercial interests in smoking and poor diets are very strong indeed and thus represent major barriers to effective policy.

It is very clear that premature stroke and CHD could be prevented by an enormous margin were we able to achieve the blood fat levels and blood pressure of many communities in developing countries – whose diet is low in fat and in salt.

It is also clear that the inexorable rise of these risky parameters of health with age is entirely controllable – but not while choices are more

---

Box 2.1   National Heart Forum's young@heart initiative 2002

The aim of young@heart

The **aim** of the young@heart national plan is that every child born in the UK today should be able to live to at least the age of 65 free from avoidable coronary heart disease.

The scope of young@heart

The young@heart initiative puts forward:

- proposals for a national plan for children's and young people's health and well-being, with a particular focus on coronary heart disease prevention
- recommendations to develop comprehensive national strategies for improving nutrition, increasing physical activity, and tackling smoking among children and young people.

A national plan must address all the different direct and indirect influences on children's and young people's health. It must engage the many opportunities for policy action across all sectors, and seek to build health capacity for families, children and young people, in the home, at school and in the community.

Key areas for policy action

The young@heart proposals for a national plan are grouped into **six key areas for policy action:**

- End child and family poverty.
- Make every school a healthy school.
- Build healthy communities.
- Strengthen and expand public health roles.
- Secure corporate responsibility for health.
- Give a voice to children and young people.

The national plan draws on the recommendations made to develop comprehensive national strategies focused on children and young people to improve nutrition, increase physical activity and tackle smoking. There are recommendations for action at local, national and international levels.

Young@heart also makes recommendations for future research and development, and for how the government could best take forward national plans for children's and young people's health and well-being.

---

easily made in an unhealthy direction and there is nothing obvious to signal consequent risk. Obviously people will continue to eat what is cheap, available and pleasant while no adverse effects are immediately discernible. Relating that properly to what will happen in 30 years' time is the essential dilemma of effective public health. The future health of the current young generation depends on it.

The response must be a coordinated strategy to make healthier options more acceptable – and in the end that cannot be hard. Somehow the short term needs of shareholders in makers of unhealthy products ought to be subsumed by the long term needs of people to enjoy a healthier life. This requires clear government commitment to all of the implications, and particularly to working out a clear and wide reaching strategy with the stakeholders – namely all of us.

Part of this must be a clear and skilled public health workforce with sound leadership. The problem now is that public health practitioners are seen as managers of health services, not as effective enablers of disease prevention who fight the corner of the vulnerable in ways that work.

Many strategies are thus not properly tried. Examples are:

- healthy pricing incentives from the treasury;
- banning advertising which compromises the real choices of young children;
- subsidizing the manufacturing of healthier options;
- incentives for healthier food in hospitals and schools;
- halting the sale of school playing fields;
- better labelling of foods to provide pertinent information;
- removing the cost disincentives of banning tobacco in public places and banning junk food at schools.

Much is already being done, of course, in programmes like Sure Start (see website www.surestart.gov.uk), and it is clear that people welcome that. But turning the corner to really reduce the burden of CHD and stroke in the long term is the next difficult step. That requires first a shock, then a national response. The shock of the effects of higher obesity levels, less exercise and awful diets is sadly imminent. Turning that corner may not now be slow. The 2004 report of the House of Commons Health Committee on obesity[43] signals very clear policy options for government to develop opportunities for reducing obesity levels, starting with the very young. It is precisely this kind of policy initiative that will create the climate for reducing the CHD burden in the longer term.

CONTROVERSIAL ISSUES

The main issues of contention have to do first with the understanding of the aetiology of stroke and CHD, and secondly the acceptability of consequent policy. Many argue that cholesterol, for example, is of less importance than supposed, but combined with a reasonable interpretation of the precautionary principle the evidence is far too strong to ignore. Randomized trials of drugs which lower cholesterol have concomitant effects on subsequent CHD and stroke incidence apparently across the board. There is a putative residual role for aspects of personal control on the causes of cardiovascular disease. The Whitehall study[44] shows a gradient of mortality according to diminishing rank among civil servants even when adjusting for known risk factors.[45] But such results are unlikely to give rise to amenable strategies for prevention, and anyway do not explain much of the variation in incidence not explained by known risk factors.

The issues of controversy in implementing coherent policy are largely political. Firstly how are accusations of 'nanny stateism' coped with when combined with a real threat to the profitability of large commercial interests whose existence depends on maintaining market shares of unhealthy products? This is a complex contemporary problem and relies on an equally strong public health sector, whose understanding of the entire process of unhealthiness is complete, and which has a potent public responsibility. Cleary merely advising individuals and communities subject to such enormous commercial pressures is futile.

WHAT QUESTIONS STILL NEED ANSWERS?

DATA ON CHD RISK FACTORS IN CHILDREN

In spite of a relative paucity of published data on socio-economic gradients in CHD risk factors in childhood, there is considerable scope to undertake analyses of existing databases that would go beyond what is already in the public domain. Although the practice of including samples of children in national health surveys is increasing, *Health in England 1998: Investigating the Links between Social Inequalities and Health*[46] published in 2000 was notable in not collecting information on individuals under the age of 16. The available evidence base could be improved at relatively low cost and this should be considered a priority for future work.

The policy imperatives will never be seen to be sufficient until we have a clearer idea about the influences of these diseases throughout the life course among different social groups, in both sexes. Obviously such uncertainties as still exist are a permanent opportunity for lack of strong action. The role of reasonable precautionary principles across the board of public policy implies the need, however, to put the prevention of CHD and stroke in a broader policy perspective, along with road safety, defence, agricultural policy and much else.

Key sources of further information and help

- **British Heart Foundation (BHF):** www.bhf.org.uk. A national charity for heart disease, providing support to patients, education for the public and professionals, research and equipment.
- **BHF statistics website:** www.heartstats.org. This website provides statistics on the burden, prevention, treatment and causes of heart disease in the UK.
- **Health Development Agency:** See *Coronary Heart Disease – Guidance for Implementing the Preventive Aspects of the National Service Framework.*[36]
- **National Heart Forum (NHF):** www.heartforum. org.uk. A leading alliance of over 40 national organizations working to reduce the risk of coronary heart disease in the UK.
- **National Service Framework for Coronary Heart Disease:** www.dh.gov.uk. National policy setting standards for prevention, diagnosis and treatment of CHD.
- **Young@heart:** a major policy development initiative of the NHF. Its aim is to ensure through effective policy action, that every child born in the UK should be able to live to the age of at least 65 years free from avoidable coronary heart disease. The young@heart policy framework can be downloaded from the NHF website.

References

1. Department of Health. Saving lives: our healthier nation. London: HMSO; 1999.
2. Department of Health. National Service Framework for coronary heart disease. London: DOH; 2000.
3. The National Heart Forum. A lifecourse approach to coronary heart disease prevention. Scientific and policy review. London: The Stationery Office; 2003.
4. Williams RR, Hunt SC, Heiss G, et al. Usefulness of cardiovascular family history data for population-based preventive medicine and medical research (the Health Family Tree Study and the NHLBI Family Heart Study). Am J Cardiol 2001 Jan 15; 87(2):129–135.
5. Hegele RA. Genetic prediction of coronary heart disease: lessons from Canada. Scand J Clin Lab Invest Suppl 1999; 230:153–167.
6. Ellsworth DL, Sholinsky P, Jaquish C, et al. Coronary heart disease. At the interface of molecular genetics and preventive medicine. Am J Prev Med 1999 Feb; 16(2):122–133.
7. Godfrey KM, Barker DJP. Fetal programming and adult health. Public Health Nutrition 2001; 4(2B):611–624.
8. Acheson D. Independent inquiry into inequalities in health. London: The Stationery Office; 1998.
9. Wadsworth M, Hardy R. Coronary heart disease morbidity by age 53 years in relation to childhood risk factors in the 1946 birth cohort. In: The National Heart Forum. A lifecourse approach to coronary heart disease prevention. Scientific and policy review. London: The Stationery Office; 2003: Ch. 2.
10. Davey Smith G, Hart C, Blane D, et al. Adverse socioeconomic conditions in childhood and cause specific adult mortality: prospective observational study. British Medical Journal 1998; 316:1631–1635.
11. McCarron P, Davey Smith G. Physiological measurements in children and young people, and risk of coronary heart disease in adults. In: The National Heart Forum. A lifecourse approach to coronary heart disease prevention. Scientific and policy review. London: The Stationery Office; 2003.
12. Batty D, Leon D. Socio-economic position and coronary heart disease risk factors in children and young people. In: The National Heart Forum. A lifecourse approach to coronary heart disease prevention. Scientific and policy review. London: The Stationery Office; 2003.
13. National Heart Forum. McPherson K, Britton A, Causer L. Coronary heart disease: estimating the impact of changes in risk factors. London: The Stationery Office; 2002.
14. Rehman H, Gervias M-C. Ethnic minority young people and health. In: The National Heart Forum. A lifecourse approach to coronary heart disease prevention. Scientific and policy review. London: The Stationery Office; 2003: Ch. 5.
15. Raleigh V. Diabetes and hypertension in Britain's ethnic minorities: implications for the future of renal services. British Medical Journal 1997; 314:209–213.
16. McColl K. The diets of children and young people; implications for coronary heart disease prevention. In: The National Heart Forum. A lifecourse approach to coronary heart disease prevention. Scientific and policy review. London: The Stationery Office; 2003: Ch. 7.
17. Gregory J et al. National diet and nutritional survey: young people aged 4 to 18 years. 2000. Vol 1. Report of the diet and nutrition survey. London: The Stationery Office; 2001.
18. Prospective Studies Collaboration. Age-specific relevance of usual blood pressure to vascular mortality: a meta-analysis of individual data for one million adults in 61 prospective studies. Lancet 2002; 360:1903–1913.
19. Lang T. Food and nutrition. In: Weil O, McKee M, Brodin M, Oberle D. Priorities for public health action in the European Union. Brussels: European Commission; 1999.
20. Cavill N, Biddle S. The determinants of young people's participation in physical activity, and investigation of tracking of physical activity from youth to adulthood. In: The National Heart Forum. A lifecourse approach to coronary heart disease prevention. Scientific and policy review. London: The Stationery Office; 2003: Ch. 8.
21. Casperson CJ, Pereira MA, Curran KM. Changes in physical activity patterns in the United States, by sex and cross-sectional age. Medicine and Science in Sports and Exercise 2000; 32:1601–1609.
22. Hillsdon M, Foster C. The relationship between physical activity during childhood and adolescence and coronary heart disease risk factors in young adulthood. In: The National Heart Forum. A lifecourse approach to coronary heart disease prevention. Scientific and policy review. London: The Stationery Office; 2003: Ch. 9.
23. Twisk JW, Kemper HC, van Mechelen W. Tracking of activity and fitness and the relationship with cardiovascular disease risk factors. Medicine and Science in Sports and Exercise 2000; 32:1455–1461.
24. Raitakari OT, Porkka KVK, Rasanen L, et al. Clustering and six year cluster tracking of serum cholesterol, HDL-cholesterol and diastolic blood pressure in children and young adults. The cardiovascular risk in young Finns study. Journal of Clinical Epidemiology 1994; 47:1085–1093.
25. Telama R, Yang X. Decline of physical activity from youth to young adulthood. Medicine and Science in Sports and Exercise 2000; 32:1617–1622.
26. van Mechelen W, Twisk JW, Post GB, et al. Physical activity of young people: Amsterdam longitudinal growth and health study. Medicine and Science in Sports and Exercise 2000; 32:1610–1616.
27. Sherman SE, D'Agostino RB, Silbershatz H, et al. Comparison of past versus recent physical activity in the prevention of premature death and coronary artery disease. American Heart Journal 1999; 138:900–907.
28. Morris JN, Clayton DG, Everitt MG, et al. Exercise in leisure time: coronary attack and death rate. British Heart Journal 1990; 63:325–334.

29. Paffenbarger RS, Hyde RT, Wing AL, et al. A natural history of athleticism and cardiovascular health. Journal of the American Medical Association 1984; 252:491–495.

30. The Scottish Office. Towards a healthier Scotland: London: The Stationery Office; 1999.

31. The National Assembly for Wales. Improving health in Wales: a summary plan for the NHS with its partners. Cardiff: National Assembly for Wales; 2001.

32. The National Assembly for Wales, Health Promotion Division. Promoting health and wellbeing: implementing the National Health Promotion Strategy. Cardiff: National Assembly for Wales; 2001.

33. Department of Health and Social Services. Health and wellbeing: into the next millennium. Belfast: DHSS; 1997.

34. Department of Health. National Service Framework for coronary heart disease: winning the war on heart disease. Progress report 2004. London: The Stationery Office; 2004.

35. Unal B, Critchley JA, Capewell S. Explaining the decline in coronary heart disease mortality in England and Wales between 1981 and 2000. Circulation 2004; 109:1101–1107.

36. Health Development Agency. Coronary heart disease – guidance for implementing the preventive aspects of the National Service Framework. London: HDA; 2001. Online. Available: http://www.healthpromis.hda-online.org.uk

37. Backet Milburn K, Davies J, Cunningham-Burley S. Social and cultural circumstances and health related lifestyles – understanding children's experiences and perspectives. In: The National Heart Forum. A lifecourse approach to coronary heart disease prevention. Scientific and policy review. London: The Stationery Office; 2003: Ch. 13.

38. Bradsaw J. Poverty; the outcomes for children. Economic and Social Research Council children 5–16 research briefing no 18. Swindon: ESRC; 2000.

39. Harker P, Hemmingway A. Health related behaviour in low-income families. In: The National Heart Forum. A lifecourse approach to coronary heart disease prevention. Scientific and policy review. London: The Stationery Office; 2003: Ch. 6.

40. Karasek R, Theorell T. Healthy work: stress, productivity and the reconstruction of working life. New York: Basic Books; 1990.

41. Macfarlane A. Health promotion for young people in primary care: what works, and what doesn't work. In: The National Heart Forum. A lifecourse approach to coronary heart disease prevention. Scientific and policy review. London: The Stationery Office; 2003: Ch. 11.

42. National Heart Forum. Young@heart: towards a generation free from coronary heart disease. Policy action for children's and young people's health and well-being. London: NHF; 2002.

43. Commons Select Committee. Obesity. London: The Stationery Office; 2004.

44. Marmot M, Shipley M, Brunner E, Hemingway H. Relative contribution of early life and adult socioeconomic factors to adult morbidity in the Whitehall II study. J Epidemiol Community Health 2001; 55: 301–307.

45. Marmot M. Aetiology of coronary heart disease. BMJ 2001; 323:1261–1262.

46. Mason V. Health in England 1998: investigating the links between social inequalities and health. London: The Stationery Office; 2000.

47. British Heart Foundation. Coronary heart disease statistics. London: BHF; 2004. Online. www.bhf.org.uk.

48. British Heart Foundation. Coronary heart disease statistics. London: BHF; 2002. From: National Heart Forum. McPherson K, Britton A, Causer L. Coronary heart disease: estimating the impact of changes in risk factors. London: The Stationery Office; 2002.

49. British Heart Foundation. Coronary heart disease statistics. London: BHF; 2003.

50. British Heart Foundation. 2004. Statistics website www.heartstats.org.

Chapter 3

Diabetes

Christine Hine

SUMMARY OVERVIEW AND LINKS TO OTHER TOPICS

Diabetes (type 1 diabetes and the far more common type 2 diabetes) is a serious, chronic disease affecting about 3% of the UK population. It affects health and life expectancy and has major financial and social impacts. It can lead to other serious health problems and problems in pregnancy, and can have a great impact on quality of life.

Diabetes is becoming increasingly common; the 1.3 million people with diabetes in the UK are predicted to rise to 3 million by 2010. Both genetic and environmental factors are significant in explaining this rise, with physical inactivity and obesity important factors. Some ethnic groups, older people and lower socio-economic groups are more at risk of developing type 2 diabetes.

The National Service Framework for diabetes[1] was published in 2001, with a national delivery strategy in 2003[2] setting out action to be taken by local services.

We do not yet know how to prevent type 1 diabetes, but it is clear that healthier diets, weight control and physical activity are the main priorities for primary prevention of type 2 diabetes and for preventing complications in both types.

Good diabetes health care helps reduce diabetes complications. Planning good services involves: listening to and planning around the needs of people with diabetes; using evidence on effective interventions, surveillance and service organization; understanding inequalities; and planning to meet growing future needs.

Screening to diagnose diabetes earlier, and balancing resources between treatment and prevention, present uncertainties and dilemmas. Many issues still need addressing, including questions about causes and the best way to tackle primary and secondary prevention.

As promoting physical activity, controlling weight gain and reducing obesity are all important elements of diabetes prevention and treatment, Chapters 5 and 6 on 'Obesity' and 'Physical activity' are highly relevant, alongside Chapter 14 'Helping individuals to change behaviour'. As health inequalities feature in diabetes, Chapter 13 'Tackling inequalities in health' is also relevant.

WHAT IS DIABETES?

Diabetes is the name of a group of disorders sharing the common feature of sustained high blood glucose levels.

Glucose is normally carried in the bloodstream to all parts of the body where it is taken up by body cells and used for energy. The level of glucose in the blood is kept within a limited range by the action of the hormone insulin, produced by the pancreas, which helps glucose to enter body cells. In diabetes, the body fails to produce insulin, or there is insufficient insulin and/or it fails to work effectively (insulin resistance). The result is a sustained high level of glucose in the bloodstream and disruption to the normal ways the body uses carbohydrate and fat.

Diabetes cannot be cured; it is a common, serious, chronic disease. It affects health and life expectancy, has major financial and social impacts, and in its most prevalent form (type 2 diabetes) is a preventable disease. The less prevalent form (type 1 diabetes) is one of the most common chronic diseases of childhood.

DIAGNOSING DIABETES

In populations blood glucose levels vary. Most people have blood glucose levels lying within a defined normal range; a few people have very low levels, and some have the high levels that meet diagnostic criteria for diabetes.

In practice, deciding the exact threshold – in terms of levels of blood glucose – at which a person can be said to have diabetes, and the most appropriate measure to use, is a complex task.[3] Setting the threshold blood glucose level for diabetes too high would exclude too many people with a significant risk of complications. Conversely, a low threshold would include many people whose risk levels might not be high enough to justify a diagnosis of diabetes, given possible psychological, legal, lifestyle and other implications of being told one has diabetes.

International criteria for diagnosing diabetes have been published by the World Health Organization.[3]

TYPES OF DIABETES

There are two common types of diabetes, known as type 1 and type 2, and some other less common forms and related conditions.

Type 1 diabetes

This usually starts in childhood or early adult life, and is estimated to account for about 15% of cases in England.[1] Production of insulin falls because of damage to the cells in the pancreas that produce insulin, in most cases as a result of action by the body's own immune system.

People with type 1 diabetes can develop symptoms very acutely: increased thirst and urine production, weight loss, increased appetite, tiredness and blurred vision. Without treatment they can become so short of insulin that they rapidly develop life threatening imbalances in their body chemistry (diabetic ketoacidosis). Treatment involves attention to diet and physical activity, and insulin injections.

Type 2 diabetes

This is by far the commonest type of diabetes, accounting for about 85% of cases in England.[4] It typically starts in overweight people in mid or later life, but the number of younger people developing type 2 diabetes has increased recently. People with type 2 diabetes do not produce enough insulin, and most also have some insensitivity to it (insulin resistance).

Symptoms usually develop over longer periods compared with type 1 diabetes, with blood glucose levels rising over a number of years without people being aware of it. Improvement can follow dietary changes, weight loss and increased physical activity, but type 2 diabetes is a progressive disease and in time most people will need to take medication and, in some cases, insulin.

Other types of diabetes

Other less common types of diabetes include:

- temporary diabetes during pregnancy (gestational diabetes);
- maturity onset diabetes of the young (MODY) and other rare genetic disorders.

Impaired glucose tolerance

There is another group of people with poor glucose regulation (called impaired glucose tolerance) who have difficulty keeping their blood glucose within the normal range, but not to the extent classified as diabetes. This population group is important because they are at increased risk of developing diabetes and cardiovascular disease. These risks can be reduced through increased physical activity, appropriate diet and achieving a healthy weight.

Metabolic syndrome

When thinking about diabetes, we also need to consider a condition known as metabolic syndrome. Often people with impaired glucose tolerance or diabetes are found to have one or more of the following cardiovascular risk factors:

- central obesity (excessive weight gain with fat particularly around the waistline, often known as being 'apple-shaped');
- high blood pressure;
- abnormal blood lipids (levels of fats in the blood).

This syndrome has been variously labelled metabolic syndrome, insulin resistance syndrome or syndrome X. People with this combination of risk factors are at high risk of cardiovascular disease. People who have features of metabolic syndrome with normal blood glucose are considered to be at very high risk for future diabetes, and early preventive action, through diet and greater physical activity, has the potential to reduce risk and the impact of disease. Further work is needed to define this syndrome: recommendations have been made for a more precise clinical definition.[3]

WHAT CAUSES DIABETES?

Individual risk factors have been identified, but it is not clear how much any one risk factor can explain diabetes.

CAUSE OF TYPE 1 DIABETES

The geographical pattern of incidence and rates of change in incidence suggest that both genetic and environmental factors are important.[4] Children moving from a high risk to a low risk area remain at high risk for at least one generation, demonstrating that genetic factors are significant.

The following environmental factors may trigger diabetes in those who are genetically susceptible, but no single environmental factor can account for the cause of diabetes.

Viruses

There is evidence that some viruses can directly damage the insulin-producing cells in the pancreas, but conflicting evidence leads to an inconclusive picture overall. For example, people with congenital rubella have been shown to have a higher incidence of type 1 diabetes and the virus has been shown to damage the pancreas – but the incidence of type 1 diabetes has continued to rise even though congenital rubella has been largely eradicated in many countries.

Diet

Dietary factors may trigger type 1 diabetes.

● There is conflicting evidence for early introduction of cow's milk protein causing type 1 diabetes.

● Intake of nitrosamines (toxic compounds found in smoked foods, in water supplies and in food produced in areas using fertilizers) has been associated with increased risk of diabetes.

● Vitamin D deficiency: an association has been shown between vitamin D supplementation during infancy and reduced risk of type 1 diabetes.

Maternal factors

There is some evidence that mothers over 40 have up to a threefold risk of having a child who develops type 1 diabetes, compared with mothers in their 20s.

Growth in childhood

Children who develop type 1 diabetes have been shown to be taller and gain more weight compared to their peers. Evidence on perinatal factors is inconclusive for this type of diabetes, and may be more difficult to obtain as weight gain in early life may mask the underlying disease process.

Overall, we lack the conclusive evidence about causation that we need to set up primary prevention programmes for type 1 diabetes.

CAUSE OF TYPE 2 DIABETES

Geographical and ethnic variations combined with rapid changes in prevalence suggest that both genetic and environmental factors are important, but compared with type 1 diabetes, the risk factors and scope for prevention are clearer.

Physical inactivity and diet

Physical inactivity, high calorie intakes and increasing prevalence of obesity are important contributors to the current growth in diabetes worldwide. Associations between type 2 diabetes, urban environments and socio-economic disadvantage may be largely explained by underlying patterns of physical activity and diet.[5] Failure to evolve in response to rapid changes in lifestyle (from highly active hunter-gatherers to relatively sedentary urban dwellers) has been suggested as an explanation for our apparently limited capacity to remain healthy given modern lifestyles involving less physical activity and higher calorie diets. (See also Ch. 6 'Physical activity'.)

Fetal development

Studies of the fetal origins of disease suggest that a mother's inadequate nutrition during critical stages of fetal development leads the unborn child to adapt its metabolism to cope with being undernourished. These metabolic adaptations are disadvantageous in later life if nutrition improves, with unhealthy levels of weight gain being a particular concern.

Other maternal factors may also constrain development and lead to babies being small at birth. Greater postnatal growth in these babies (as they make up for their small birth weight) is associated with higher risk of type 2 diabetes in later life.[6]

WHY IS DIABETES AN IMPORTANT PUBLIC HEALTH ISSUE?

Diabetes is an important public health issue because it affects health and life expectancy and has major financial and social impacts. It can lead to serious complications, problems in pregnancy, and can have a great impact on the quality of life. Not least, it is of concern because it is becoming increasingly common.

IMPACT ON QUALITY OF LIFE

Diabetes has a wide ranging impact on day-to-day life.

● The psychological impact of being diagnosed with a lifelong condition and knowledge of its risks can be profound.

● The challenges of transition from childhood through adolescence to adulthood are that much greater for the child with diabetes, who needs daily medication and a healthy lifestyle.

● The impact of diabetes on day-to-day life includes increased personal costs (relating to diet, treatments and travel to health services) and restricted job opportunities.

The issues that people with diabetes face in their daily lives are described in Box 3.1.

Box 3.1   The impact of diabetes on daily life[7]

Physical issues

- Discomfort (of symptoms not fully controlled, of blood testing, of injecting)
- Symptoms hindering activities (both work and leisure).

Emotional issues

- Anxiety (worsening condition, unable to get control, fear of being alone and having a hypo, perception it weakens the health generally, perceived lack of immediate access to help)
- Difficulty in accepting restrictions to diet and lifestyle
- Stigma (at school where one is 'different', lack of public understanding, misunderstanding leading to negative labelling e.g. 'drug addicts')
- Sense of isolation

- Effects of stress and illness on relationships, personal well-being, education, employment etc
- For carers – guilt that they may have somehow contributed to the development of the condition or that they are not managing the condition effectively; and stress associated with the responsibility of caring for someone with diabetes.

Practical issues

- Day-to-day hassles and restrictions (diet, testing, injections, tablets, getting prescriptions, attending appointments etc)
- Added expense (extra costs of eating the foods advised, of travelling to clinic appointments, of purchasing equipment etc).

LIFE EXPECTANCY

Compared with the non-diabetic population, life expectancy is shorter for people with diabetes.[8] Premature mortality increases with lower socio-economic status, mainly due to cardiovascular disease (coronary heart disease and stroke).[9] A British study has demonstrated reductions in life expectancy of 8 years for people diagnosed with type 2 diabetes by the age of 40.[8] Reductions of an average of 20 years have been reported for type 1 diabetes.[1]

COMPLICATIONS

Individuals with diabetes have an increased risk of a range of serious health problems as a result of their diabetes. Chronic complications are commoner with increasing age; this is demonstrated in Figure 3.1, which shows the prevalence of diabetic complications in patients in GP practices in South Glamorgan, Wales.[10]

Acute blood glucose imbalances

Imbalances in blood glucose can lead to coma and death. Coma can result from high blood glucose accompanied by severe disturbances in body chemistry (diabetic ketoacidosis), and as a complication of treatment where glucose levels fall too low (hypoglycaemia).

Chronic problems

These result from prolonged exposure of body tissues to raised levels of blood glucose. Irreversible damage can be caused in small blood vessels, leading to a risk of *microvascular* complications affecting:

Figure 3.1   Prevalence of diabetic complications with age. (Reproduced with permission from Morgan, Currie, Stott et al 2000.[10])

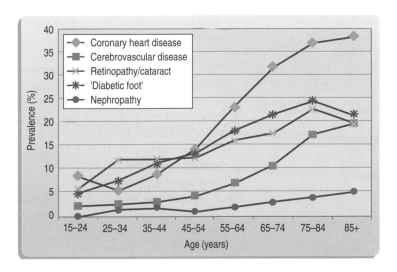

- eyes: damage to the back of the eye (diabetic retinopathy), causing visual loss and blindness;
- kidneys: leading to progressive renal failure and need for dialysis or renal transplant;
- nerves: leading to a variety of problems including impotence and loss of sensation in the feet (which in turn predisposes to development of ulcers and limb-threatening infections).

Damage to large blood vessels (*macrovascular* damage) can result in blocked arteries. Consequently people with diabetes (particularly type 2) are at higher risk of cardiovascular disease affecting:

- heart: angina, heart attack (myocardial infarction) and heart failure;
- brain: stroke and transient ischaemic attacks ('mini-strokes');
- limbs: lower limbs have poor circulation, causing pain when walking and increasing the risk of ulceration, infection and amputation.

Cataracts, infections, certain skin problems and mental health problems are also commoner in people with diabetes.

Multiple complications are common in diabetes, being found in almost one fifth of patients with diabetes in one health authority population.[10]

PROBLEMS IN PREGNANCY AND IN THE NEWBORN

Women with diabetes who become pregnant are at higher risk of miscarriage and death of the fetus in the uterus, and they have an increased risk of fetal abnormalities. Perinatal mortality amongst babies of pregnant mothers is five times higher than in the general UK population, with congenital malformations the commonest causes of death.[1]

COSTS OF DIABETES TO SOCIETY

Although about 3% of the population have diabetes, people with diabetes account for 10% of hospital admissions. For the UK, an estimated 9% of hospital costs (£1.9 billion) has been attributed to diabetes, with additional costs in primary care.[11] A more recent estimate suggests diabetes incurs NHS costs of £1.3 billion, mostly relating to long term complications.[12]

INCREASING POPULATION WITH DIABETES

The current adverse trend of increasing numbers of people with diabetes is a major public health problem.

More children and adolescents are becoming overweight and levels of physical activity are falling. Consequently, we expect the incidence of type 2 diabetes to continue to rise in younger people as well as in the older adult population. Earlier onset of diabetes is a serious problem because the longer people have diabetes, the more likely they are to develop complications.

As diabetes becomes more common, estimates of prevalence can rapidly become out of date, but some key facts to illustrate the size of the problem are set out in Box 3.2.[13,14] Figure 3.2 illustrates the dramatic estimated rise in diabetes prevalence in the UK.[15]

Type 1 diabetes

The incidence of diabetes shows wide variations between populations. In the early 1990s, incidence varied from an age adjusted rate of 0.1 per 100 000 in Zunyi, China, to 49 per 100 000 in Finland. These variations occur even where populations are not genetically diverse, suggesting that genetic susceptibility alone cannot explain the development of type 1 diabetes.

The incidence of type 1 diabetes is increasing in almost all populations for whom data are collected, with a steeper rise in countries with a low incidence than in countries that already have a high incidence. A number of studies suggest higher incidence in males.

Overall 90% of cases of diabetes diagnosed before 30 years of age will be type 1. Relatively greater increases have been reported in younger children, with a steep increase in the under 5s; this has changed the previous age pattern of highest incidence in 10–14 year olds. About half of cases are not diagnosed until after 15 years of age.

There is no clear evidence that type 1 diabetes is more common in less well off socio-economic groups.[4]

Box 3.2   The rising prevalence and incidence of diabetes[13,14]

- The overall global prevalence of diabetes is estimated to double between 1994 and 2010.

- Approximately 8% of people in much of Europe and the USA have diabetes.

- Approximately 3% (1.3 million people) in the UK are known to have diabetes; estimates are that up to 90% have type 2 diabetes.

- This figure of 1.3 million with diabetes in the UK is predicted to rise to 3 million by 2010.

- 1 in 20 people over 65 has diabetes, rising to 1 in 5 people over 85.

- There are also an estimated 1 million people in the UK who have diabetes but do not know it.

- Estimates of prevalence in the UK suggest that 0.3% of the population have type 1 diabetes.

- In many parts of the world, the incidence of childhood diabetes is rising by 2%–5% each year – this translates to a rise of about 50% in the last 10 years.

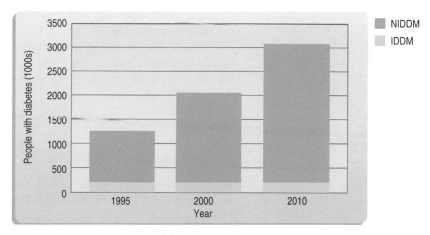

Figure 3.2   Estimated population with diabetes, UK 1995–2010. NIDDM: non insulin dependent diabetes (an older term for type 2 diabetes); IDDM: insulin dependent diabetes (an older term for type 1 diabetes).[15]

Type 2 diabetes

The prevalence of type 2 diabetes is rising worldwide. Rapid increases in incidence suggest that the rise is mainly due to environmental factors rather than genetic susceptibility. Increasing prevalence of obesity (in turn due to insufficient physical activity and inappropriate diet) is a major contributor to this trend, although longer life expectancy also helps explain some of the rise.[5]

Prevalence varies between countries and ethnic groups, ranging from almost 0% in parts of Africa to 50% of American Pima Indians. In the UK, South Asian, African and African-Caribbean populations have higher prevalence than Caucasians.[15] Poverty and deprivation have been cited as contributing to higher prevalence in British inner city areas, affecting all ethnic groups.[16]

Risk of type 2 diabetes increases with age, with highest incidence in the over 60s. However, the age distribution is shifting towards younger age groups, particularly in developing countries. Rising incidence in children is a major current concern.

In the UK, higher prevalence of type 2 diabetes can be expected in relatively disadvantaged urban neighbourhoods with multi-ethnic populations, and in older populations.

HOW IS DIABETES ADDRESSED IN NATIONAL POLICY?

The National Service Framework for Diabetes: Standards[1] was published by the government in 2001. (National Service Frameworks – NSFs – set national standards, with the aim of tackling variable standards and overall raising quality of care in the UK.) Actions required are included in *The NHS Plan*,[17] and there are performance management arrangements to help ensure local implementation.

A national delivery strategy for the diabetes NSF was published in 2003.[2] It sets out action to be taken by local health and social services, with two specific targets on implementing improvements in GP registers of people with diabetes, and implementation of diabetic retinopathy screening programmes.

The prime goal of the NSF for diabetes is to enable people with (or at risk of) diabetes to manage their own lifestyle and diabetes, by providing support, education, drugs and other treatments. The NSF standards are set out in Box 3.3.

WHO IS AT RISK OF DIABETES?

RISK OF TYPE 1 DIABETES

Family members are at risk. There is evidence that genetic susceptibility is inherited, but mode of inheritance is not straightforward. Only 12–15% of people with type 1 diabetes are from families with a history of the disease, the majority of cases arising sporadically. The risk of type 1 diabetes amongst siblings is estimated to be 12–15 times higher than that in the general population. Both genetic susceptibility and exposure to environmental factors are likely to be needed for type 1 diabetes to develop in those at risk.[4]

RISK OF TYPE 2 DIABETES

The following factors are associated with increased risk of type 2 diabetes:

- overweight;
- 'central obesity' where there is excess fat around the waistline (even if the person concerned is not overweight);
- physical inactivity;
- family history of diabetes;
- ethnicity (South Asian, Chinese, African, African-Caribbean and Middle Eastern people are more at risk);
- age: in the UK, prevalence increases from 1 in 20 people over 65 to 1 in 5 people over 85;
- lower socio-economic status;
- low birth weight;
- previous gestational diabetes.

DO HEALTH INEQUALITIES FEATURE FOR DIABETES?

The risk of getting diabetes is greater in people of lower socio-economic status, and in people of South Asian, Middle Eastern, Chinese, African and African-Caribbean ethnicity.

Diabetic retinopathy, cardiovascular complications and kidney disease are commoner amongst people in lower socio-economic groups and people with lower educational attainment.[18,9] Contributory factors include:

- Access to health services. People who have difficulty attending for regular, long term chronic disease management are a concern, e.g. prisoners, homeless people, travellers, people with disabilities. Difficulties in communication with professionals can be a barrier to effective care for those who do attend.

Box 3.3 National Service Framework for Diabetes: Standards (Reproduced with permission from Department of Health 2001[1])

Prevention of type 2 diabetes

The NHS will develop, implement and monitor strategies to reduce the risk of developing type 2 diabetes in the population as a whole and to reduce the inequalities in the risk of developing type 2 diabetes.

Identification of people with diabetes

The NHS will develop, implement and monitor strategies to identify people who do not know they have diabetes

Empowering people with diabetes

All children, young people and adults with diabetes will receive a service which encourages partnership in decision making, supports them in managing their diabetes and helps them to adopt and maintain a healthy lifestyle. This will be reflected in an agreed and shared care plan in an appropriate format and language. Where appropriate, parents and carers should be fully engaged in this process.

Clinical care of people with diabetes

All adults with diabetes will receive high quality care throughout their lifetime, including support to optimize the control of their blood glucose, blood pressure and other risk factors for developing the complications of diabetes.

Clinical care of children and young people with diabetes

All children and young people with diabetes will receive consistently high quality care and they, with their families and others involved in their day-to-day care, will be supported to optimize the control of their blood glucose and their physical, psychological, intellectual, educational and social development.

All young people with diabetes will experience a smooth transition of care from paediatric diabetes services to adult diabetes services, whether hospital or community based, either directly or via a young person's clinic. The transition will be organized in partnership with each individual and at an age appropriate and agreed with them.

Management of diabetic emergencies

The NHS will develop, implement and monitor agreed protocols for rapid and effective treatment of diabetic emergencies by appropriately trained healthcare professionals. Protocols will include the management of acute complications and procedures to minimize the risk of recurrence.

Care of people with diabetes during admission to hospital

All children, young people and adults with diabetes admitted to hospital, for whatever reason, will receive effective care of their diabetes. Wherever possible they will continue to be involved in decisions concerning the management of their diabetes.

Diabetes and pregnancy

The NHS will develop, implement and monitor policies that seek to empower and support women with pre-existing diabetes and those who develop diabetes during pregnancy to optimize the outcomes of their pregnancy.

Detection and management of long term complications

All young people and adults with diabetes will receive regular surveillance for the long term complications of diabetes.

The NHS will develop, implement and monitor agreed protocols and systems of care to ensure that all people who develop long term complications of diabetes receive timely, appropriate and effective investigation and treatment to reduce their risk of disability and premature death.

All people with diabetes requiring multi-agency support will receive integrated health and social care.

- Prevalence of risk factors, e.g. obesity is commoner in lower socio-economic groups, as is smoking (a risk factor for retinopathy and cardiovascular disease).
- Barriers to self care, e.g. financial costs and access to healthier diets.

(See also Ch. 13 'Tackling inequalities in health'.)

WHAT CAN WE DO TO PREVENT DIABETES AND ITS COMPLICATIONS AT COMMUNITY LEVEL?

Given gaps in understanding of the precise causes of diabetes, prevention must address a number of risk factors at national, regional and local levels as well as helping individuals with diabetes to reduce their personal risks.

PRIMARY PREVENTION

As we can deduce from the list of risk factors for diabetes, type 2 diabetes has some preventable risk factors, but there is no current effective strategy to prevent type 1 diabetes.[19]

There is no doubt that the main priorities for primary prevention of type 2 diabetes are:[19]

- healthier diets
- weight control
- physical activity.

Strategies to prevent obesity are highly relevant, including those aimed at children and families.[20,21] Broad strategies for promoting active living are important for both prevention and treatment of diabetes. The priority is to live an active lifestyle; this does not necessarily have to involve sport or formal exercise sessions.

Obesity and promoting physical activity are addressed in detail in Chapters 5 and 6.

Evidence for fetal origins of higher risk of type 2 diabetes indicates the importance of appropriate maternal diet during pregnancy, although what constitutes an appropriate diet in this case is not yet clear.[6]

SECONDARY PREVENTION

Secondary prevention of complications is vital. This means that we need to provide effective health care and help individuals to make changes to their diet, physical activity and lifestyle.

Local services need to ensure high uptake of preventive services, taking account of the higher risk associated with socio-economic disadvantage, lower educational attainment, greater age and minority ethnic groups. Older people in residential or nursing homes may have difficulty accessing diabetes care.

Physical activity

Physical activity is not relevant to prevention of type 1 diabetes, but it is recommended for people already diagnosed to help them reduce their cardiovascular risk.

In adults, dietary changes in conjunction with increased physical activity can prevent progression from impaired glucose tolerance to type

2 diabetes.[22] Diet and activity are also important in reducing the risk of heart disease in people who have already developed diabetes. There is also evidence that physical activity can reduce the risk of diabetes in individuals who remain obese.[23]

Diabetes UK recommend that people with diabetes participate in regular, moderate physical activity, and have set out a 'Care Recommendation' providing supporting evidence, and advice on steps to be taken to promote greater physical activity by individual patients.[23] Most people with diabetes should be encouraged to take 20–30 minutes of physical activity on most days, the activity level being adjusted for age and fitness.[24] There is evidence from prospective studies that people with diabetes are more likely to adhere to programmes offering initial supervised activity, followed by informal home based activity and follow-up assessments.

(See also Ch. 6 'Physical activity'.)

Healthy eating

The principles of a healthy diet and weight control for people with diabetes are broadly similar to those for people without diabetes: low in fat (with most fat being monounsaturated), sugar and salt, with meals based on starchy foods (such as potatoes, pasta, rice or bread) with plenty of fruit and vegetables. General guidance on alcohol consumption is the same as for the rest of the population, but people with diabetes on some medication or on insulin need to be aware that alcohol, particularly heavy drinking, can lead to hypoglycaemia. Diabetic foods are not required. Sugar, sweets and chocolate are not excluded provided they form part of a balanced diet and weight is controlled.

Guidelines have been produced for health professionals on dietary advice for people with diabetes.[24] (For more about healthy eating and tackling overweight, see Ch. 5 'Obesity'.)

Who to target?

To have the greatest benefits to the health of the population as a whole, should preventive programmes be aimed at those with diabetes (who have the highest individual risk of complications), or the whole population? The Rose theorem states 'a large number of people exposed to a small risk may generate many more cases than a small number exposed to a high risk'.[25] To prevent diabetes and its complications, we must aim to shift the population range of blood glucose downwards, so that overall the whole population (with and without diagnosed diabetes) achieves a lower risk of complications. Once again, the main ways to reduce overall blood sugar levels are healthy eating, preventing overweight, and increasing physical activity.

HOW CAN WE BEST HELP INDIVIDUALS WITH DIABETES?

Good diabetes health care helps reduce diabetes complications. Planning good services involves listening and planning around the needs of people with diabetes; using evidence on effective interventions, surveillance and service organization; understanding inequalities; and planning to meet growing future needs.

LISTEN TO PEOPLE WITH DIABETES AND RESPOND TO THEIR NEEDS

People with diabetes need to understand diabetes and learn how to control it, so that they can live life as fully and normally as possible. Listening to people with diabetes is crucial in designing person-centred services that help them to achieve what they want and encourage use of services and treatments. Service users have asked for:[7]

- A holistic approach, where health professionals:
  - see patients as equals;
  - are non-patronizing;
  - are willing to understand the wider impacts of diabetes on their patients' lives;
  - listen, discuss and answer questions;
  - treat patients as individual human beings rather than just focusing on their disease.
- Continuity of care, as seeing the same doctors and nurses can help to build rapport and understanding.
- Good communication between health professionals. Both routine and acute care involve different professions such as doctors, nurses, optometrists, podiatrists and dietitians. Poor liaison and inefficient systems (e.g. for repeat prescribing) cause frustration and are a source of errors and misunderstanding.

PROVIDE WELL ORGANIZED AND CLINICALLY EFFECTIVE SERVICES

Information and education

People with diabetes need to become proficient in managing their condition. The National Institute of Clinical Excellence (NICE) has recommended that structured patient education is made available at diagnosis and on an ongoing basis as required. There is insufficient evidence to indicate the best type of educational method, setting or frequency of sessions, but NICE recommends principles of good practice: the use of adult learning techniques adapted to personal learning needs, delivery by multidisciplinary teams and accessibility (taking account of ethnicity, disability and geography).[26]

Service aims

There is robust evidence that good diabetes care reduces the risk of complications, and delays the rate of progression of complications, thus keeping people with diabetes in better health for as long as possible.

Diabetes services in primary and secondary care aim to:

- optimize blood glucose levels and blood pressure;
- detect and treat complications at an early stage;
- assess and manage cardiovascular risk.

An illustrative case study in Box 3.4 shows how a person with diabetes might be cared for by a range of healthcare professionals in primary and secondary care.

The following interventions have been shown to reduce diabetes-related morbidity and mortality.[27]

- Better **blood pressure control** can reduce the risk of:
  - death from long term complications of diabetes;
  - strokes;
  - serious deterioration of vision.

Box 3.4   Case study: diabetes care

Mrs T is 59 years old. She visits her GP complaining of tiredness, increased thirst and blurred vision. Her GP checks her urine and blood, and tells her she might have diabetes. Further diagnostic tests confirm this. Meanwhile she has been given information on a healthy diet and an appointment with the practice nurse.

The practice nurse discusses diabetes and its implications with Mrs T, checks her physical health and does blood tests. She explains how Mrs T can have annual eye screening, and arrangements for foot care. Mrs T learns how to monitor her diabetes and when to seek advice.

Mrs T has regular reviews every 6–12 months, for which the practice send her reminder letters. Initially, her diabetes is controlled by changes in her diet and increased physical activity, but after some years she needs tablets for diabetes, blood pressure and lipids (levels of fat in the blood). Her GP explains that diabetes is a progressive condition, and that this is not unexpected despite her best efforts with diet and activity.

Mrs T's diabetes gradually becomes more difficult to control, and her GP advises referral to the local Diabetes Centre for specialist advice on whether she should now start insulin.

- Better **blood glucose control** can reduce the risk of:
  - diabetic eye disease;
  - early kidney damage;
  - loss of feeling in the feet;
  - cardiovascular disease.
- **Medication to reduce the risk of blood clot formation and regulate blood fat levels** can reduce the risk of cardiovascular deaths and morbidity.
- **Smoking cessation** is also needed to reduce cardiovascular risk.

Screening and surveillance for complications

As we have said, well organized, systematic care can reduce the risk of diabetes complications.[28]

- Annual review is recommended as a minimum, with more frequent follow-up according to assessed risk of complications.[29–31]

- Diabetic retinopathy screening is being implemented nationally.

- Systematic screening and prevention (including referral of high risk patients to a specialist foot clinic) has been shown to reduce risk of lower limb amputation.[27]

- In type 2 diabetes, urine tests (for raised levels of urinary albumin and/or serum creatinine) indicate increased risk of cardiovascular problems and, more rarely, kidney disease. Annual review is recommended, so that risk can be assessed and preventive action taken to improve blood pressure and blood glucose control.[30]

Service coverage

As well as effective care for individuals, services must achieve high levels of population coverage to reduce the population burden of disease. Checklists for good practice have been produced[11,29] and the NSF includes the following two targets that aim to achieve high coverage by well organized services:[1]

In primary care, update practice based registers so that patients with CHD (coronary heart disease) and diabetes continue to receive appropriate advice and treatment in line with NSF standards and by March 2006, ensure practice based registers and systematic treatment regimes including appropriate advice on diet, physical activity and smoking, also cover the majority of patients at high risk of CHD, particularly those with hypertension, diabetes and a body mass index (BMI) greater than 30.

Primary care services have shown that in the short term they can achieve standards of care as good as, or better than, hospital care alone if they use computerized recall and prompt patients to attend for check-ups. But unstructured community care is associated with worse control of blood glucose levels and mortality.[28]

By 2006, a minimum of 80% of people with diabetes to be offered screening for the early detection (and treatment if needed) of diabetic retinopathy as part of a systematic programme that meets national standards, rising to 100% coverage of those at risk of retinopathy by end of 2007.

Diabetes is the single commonest cause of visual loss in people aged 16–64 years. Many people with retinopathy and maculopathy will not have symptoms until the changes in their eyes are severe. Early detection and laser treatment can reduce the associated risk of visual loss.[27,31] The national programme of annual eye screening aims to:

- detect sight-threatening retinopathy so that it can be treated;
- assess presence of any retinopathy so that the person with diabetes can be aware of changes in the eye, indicating a need to improve blood pressure and blood glucose control.

PLAN TO MEET FUTURE NEEDS

We need to plan sufficient service capacity to meet the needs of the growing population with diabetes. The growing burden of type 2 diabetes will fall disproportionately on lower socio-economic groups and their local health services. As diabetes is so common, needs for diabetes health care cannot be met by specialist services alone; greater capacity will be needed in primary and secondary care.

CONTROVERSIES, DILEMMAS AND MYTHS

SCREENING FOR DIABETES

People can have type 2 diabetes for 9–12 years, with over one third having developed at least one complication, before diagnosis. This has led to calls for a national screening programme.[32] But we do not have sufficient evidence on the most effective screening method. A pilot scheme is under way to assess targeted screening of people with risk factors indicating high risk of diabetes, stroke and heart disease.[1]

PRIORITIES

The Wanless Report *Securing our Future Health: Taking a Long Term View*[12] suggests that following a period of increased investment to achieve national standards of care, cost savings might be made over the next 20 years as diabetes is better prevented, managed, and its adverse consequences reduced.

Rising rates of obesity and gaps in evidence of effectiveness threaten these achievements. Also, identifying the best pattern of investment presents problems: a balance has to be struck between preventing further growth in the population with diabetes, and treatment for those who already have it.

In the immediate future, we will continue to be faced with difficult decisions about the best pattern of investment.

COMMON MYTHS

There are many myths around causes and implications of diabetes. Diabetes UK has published advice on many of these on its website (www.diabetes.org.uk/diabetes/myths.htm) and challenges perceptions of diabetes that can damage opportunities for people with diabetes, such as restrictions on driving.

Common misconceptions include the following:

● 'Eating sugar causes diabetes' – this is untrue. As described earlier, the cause of diabetes is unclear but both genetic and environmental factors are important.

● 'It is possible to have "mild" diabetes' – this does not exist. All diabetes (including type 2 diabetes in older people) involves risks to survival and health, and everyone who has diabetes should be offered advice and effective health care to reduce their risks.

● 'People with diabetes cannot do sport' – this is untrue. However, people on insulin and some drug treatments should get advice on how to avoid their blood glucose levels dropping too low during sport.

WHAT QUESTIONS STILL NEED ANSWERS?

● The cause of type 1 diabetes needs to be better understood, and preventive strategies identified and tested.

● In type 2 diabetes, we need greater understanding of fetal origins of diabetes, and ways of intervening to prevent later onset of diabetes.

● We know that physical activity and appropriate diet can reduce progression to type 2 diabetes in later life. The main question here is how best to encourage individuals to make these changes. (See also Chs 5 and 6 on 'Obesity' and 'Physical activity'; and Ch. 14 'Helping individuals to change behaviour'.)

● Screening for diabetes has potential to secure earlier diagnosis but there are important gaps in our knowledge of the most effective screening test, and in evidence that screening benefits will outweigh costs.

● In treatment and surveillance of diabetes, the development of new drugs and therapies continues to provide a substantial research agenda, for example about transplanting pancreas cells that produce insulin.

Key sources of further information and help

- **Diabetes National Service Framework:** www.dh.gov.uk; follow links via A–Z index to NSF.
- **Diabetes UK:** www.diabetes.org.uk Diabetes UK is the largest organization in the UK working for people with diabetes, funding research, campaigning and helping people live with the condition. The website has a section for healthcare professionals providing information on research, training and policy development.
- **Diabetic retinopathy:** www.diabetic-retinopathy. screening.nhs.uk/recommendations.html.

Advisory Panel Final Report to the UK National Screening Committee.
- **Nutritional advice for people with diabetes:** www.diabetes.org.uk. Nutrition subcommittee of the Diabetes Care Advisory Committee of Diabetes UK 2003.[24]
- **Update for healthcare professionals:** www.bma.org.uk. British Medical Association, Board of Science and Education 2004.[13]

References

1. Department of Health. National Service Framework for diabetes: standards. London: Department of Health; 2001. Online. Available: www.dh.gov.uk; follow links via A–Z index to NSF.
2. Department of Health. National Service Framework for diabetes. Delivery strategy. London: Department of Health; 2003. Online. Available: http://www.dh.gov.uk/PolicyAndGuidance/HealthAndSocialCareTopics/Diabetes/fs/en
3. World Health Organization, Department of Non-Communicable Disease Surveillance. Definition, diagnosis and classification of diabetes mellitus and its complications. Report of a WHO consultation. Part 1 Diagnosis and classification of diabetes mellitus. Geneva: WHO; 1999.
4. Karvoonen M, Tuomilehto J, Podar T. Section 1 Epidemiology of type 1 diabetes. In: Pickup JC, Williams G, eds. Textbook of diabetes, vol 1, 3rd edn. Oxford: Blackwell; 2003.
5. Tong PCY, Cockram CS. Section 1 The epidemiology of type 2 diabetes. In: Pickup JC, Williams G, eds. Textbook of diabetes, vol 1, 3rd edn. Oxford: Blackwell; 2003.
6. Prentice AM. Intrauterine factors, adiposity and hyperinsulinaemia. BMJ 2003; 327:880–881.
7. Hiscock J, Legard R, Snape D. Listening to diabetes service users: qualitative findings for the Diabetes National Service Framework. London: Department of Health; 2000.
8. Roper NA, Bilous RW, Kelly WF, et al. Excess mortality in a population with diabetes and the impact of maternal deprivation: longitudinal population based study. BMJ 2001; 322:1389–1393.
9. Chaturvedi N, Jarett J, Shipley M, Fuller JH. Socio-economic gradient in morbidity and mortality in people with diabetes: cohort study findings from the Whitehall study and the WHO multi-national study of vascular disease in diabetes. BMJ 1998; 316:100–106.
10. Morgan C Ll, Currie CJ, Stott NCH, et al. The prevalence of multiple diabetes-related complications. Diabetic Medicine 2000; 17:146–151.
11. Audit Commission. Testing times – a review of diabetes services in England and Wales. London: Audit Commission; 2000.
12. HM Treasury. Securing our future health: taking a long term view (the Wanless Report). London: HM Treasury; 2002. Online. Available: http://www.hm-treasury.gov.uk/wanless
13. British Medical Association, Board of Science and Education. Diabetes mellitus: an update for healthcare professionals. London: BMA; 2004. Online. Available: http://www.bma.org.uk
14. Diabetes UK website www.diabetes.org.uk
15. Amos AF, McCarty DJ, Zimmet P. The rising gobal burden of diabetes and its complications: estimates and projections to the year 2010. Diabetic Medicine 1997; 14(suppl 5): S1–S85.
16. Riste L, Khan F, Cruickshank K. High prevalence of type 2 diabetes in all ethnic groups, including Europeans, in a British inner city. Relative poverty, history, inactivity, or 21st century Europe? Diabetes Care 2001; 24:1377–1383.
17. Department of Health. The NHS plan. London: The Stationery Office; 2000.
18. Nicolucci A, Carinci F, Ciampi A (on behalf of the SID–AMD Italian Study Group for the implementation of the St Vincent Declaration). Stratifying patients at risk of diabetic complications. Diabetes Care 1998; 21(9):1439–1444.
19. Pinkney J. Prevention and cure of type 2 diabetes. BMJ 2002; 325:232–233.

20. Mulvihill C, Quigley R. The management of obesity and overweight: an analysis of reviews of diet, physical activity and behavioural approaches. London: Health Development Agency; 2003. Online. Available: www.hda.nhs.uk/evidence

21. Royal College of Physicians. Storing up problems: the medical case for a slimmer nation. Report of a working party. London: RCGP; 2004. Online. Available: http://ww.rcplondon.ac.uk/pubs/brochures

22. Diabetes Prevention Program Research Group. Reductions in the incidence of type 2 diabetes with lifestyle intervention or metformin. New England Journal of Medicine 2002; 346:393–403.

23. Diabetes UK. Care recommendation physical activity and diabetes. London: Diabetes UK; 2003. Online. Available: http://www.diabetes.org.uk

24. Nutrition Subcommittee of the Diabetes Care Advisory Committee of Diabetes UK. The implementation of nutritional advice for people with diabetes. Diabetic Medicine 2003; 20:786–807. Online. Available: http://www.diabetes.org.uk

25. Rose G. The strategy of preventive medicine. Oxford: Oxford University Press; 1992.

26. National Institute for Clinical Excellence. Guidance on the use of patient-education models for diabetes.

Technology appraisal no. 60. London: NICE; 2003. Online. Available: http://www.nice.org.uk

27. BMJ Publishing Group. Clinical Evidence. Endocrinology. Issue 9, June 2003. Online. Available: http://www.nelh.nhs.uk

28. Griffin S, Kinmoth AL. Systems for routine surveillance for people with diabetes mellitus (Cochrane Review). In: The Cochrane Library, Issue 1. Chichester: John Wiley; 2004.

29. Diabetes UK. Recommendations for the management of diabetes in primary care. London: Diabetes UK; 2000. Online. Available: http://www.diabetes.org.uk

30. National Institute for Clinical Excellence. Management of type 2 diabetes. Renal disease – prevention and early management. Inherited clinical guideline F. London: NICE; 2002.

31. National Institute for Clinical Excellence. Management of type 2 diabetes. Retinopathy – screening and early management. Inherited clinical guideline E. London: NICE; 2002.

32. Diabetes UK. Position statement. Early identification of people with type 2 diabetes. London: Diabetes UK; 2002. Online. Available: http://www.diabetes.org.uk

Chapter 4

Smoking

Doreen McIntyre

SUMMARY OVERVIEW AND LINKS TO OTHER TOPICS

Smoking causes about one fifth of all deaths in the UK, most of them premature (on average, 21 years premature) and has hugely significant impacts on the wider environment and community through causing air pollution, fires and litter, and environmental damage in the countries where tobacco is grown.

Smoking is more common in people from poorer socio-economic groups, marginalized groups such as people with mental health problems and people in prison, and some ethnic groups. It is more prevalent in younger than older people. Steady falls in prevalence have slowed since the 1990s, levelling off at around 27% of the total adult population at the turn of the century.

National policy has addressed smoking since the publication of the White Paper *Smoking Kills*[1] in 1998, which heralded a range of measures including NHS help for people to stop smoking, bans on tobacco advertising and promotion, and rises in tobacco taxation (though not, as yet, a ban on smoking in workplaces and public places).

Effective ways to help individuals stop smoking include specialist services and nicotine replacement therapy. At a community level, we need to tackle changing social norms, influencing attitudes and supporting individual behaviour change with educational programmes, cessation treatment, bans on tobacco promotion, high prices for tobacco products and smoke-free environments, particularly workplaces.

There are many common myths about smoking, and many areas need further research, including measuring the impact of policies and programmes.

Cigarettes, alcohol and drugs are all 'drugs' so Chapter 10 'Alcohol use and misuse' and Chapter 11 'Drug use and misuse' may both be useful to read alongside this one. As health inequalities feature in smoking, and lifestyle changes are important for cessation, Chapter 13 'Tackling inequalities in health' and Chapter 14 'Helping individuals to change behaviour' are also relevant.

WHAT IS SMOKING?

It is helpful to answer this question in terms of three elements: the activity of smoking, the product smoked, and the market.

THE ACTIVITY

In developed countries like the UK smoking is largely the use of tobacco in manufactured and hand-rolled cigarettes. The cigarette has been the most common form of tobacco use since the early twentieth century, and the worldwide market for cigarettes continues to grow as the main manufacturing companies extend their marketing to less developed countries. Global production for cigarettes is now 5.5 trillion per year, of which 66 billion are smoked in the UK.[2] In the UK a very small percentage of smokers regularly use pipes or cigars. Cigarette smokers smoke an average of 15 cigarettes a day.[3]

THE PRODUCT

The manufactured cigarette consists of chopped tobacco rolled inside a paper tube with a filter at one end. The tobacco has been cured and mixed with a variety of additives to add flavour, increase nicotine availability from the smoke, and improve shelf life. The UK currently permits 600 of these additives,[4] most of which are relatively harmless individually but some of which are toxic in combination or when burnt.

The paper in manufactured cigarettes is treated with chemicals to prevent self-extinguishing after the cigarette is lit. The filter usually consists of cellulose acetate to trap some of the solid particles in smoke, and cool the smoke. The filters also have rings of small perforations whose purpose is to dilute the smoke with air as the smoker draws on the cigarette, although in normal smoking those holes are usually blocked by the smoker's lips or fingers.

The principal constituents of cigarette smoke are tar, carbon monoxide and nicotine:

- *Tar* is a complex mixture of substances produced when tobacco burns; over 60 known carcinogens have been identified among the estimated 4000 chemicals in tar.
- *Carbon monoxide* is one of the main gases given off during the combustion process; it is highly toxic, and is thought to be the main contributor to smoking-related heart disease.
- *Nicotine* is the active drug component; nicotine is toxic in its pure form.

THE MARKET

The UK is home to several of the world's major tobacco companies – British American Tobacco, Imperial Tobacco, Gallagher, and Rothmans UK, who together directly employ 9000 people in the UK and have over 90% of the UK cigarette market.[2] These companies are active in protecting their interests in matters of public policy related to tobacco.

The UK also has several non-governmental organizations that are active on tobacco issues – principally the registered charities ASH, No Smoking Day and Quit on the public health side, and the association FOREST on the pro-tobacco side. (See the 'Key sources of further information' section at the end of this chapter for details.)

The UK has for many years had one of the highest rates of cigarette tax in the world, but around 20% of the cigarettes consumed in the UK are supplied at cut price through the illegal black market.[5] The use of hand rolling tobacco to make home-made cigarettes has become more prevalent in recent years, principally because lower taxation of this tobacco makes it cheaper than manufactured cigarettes, prompting some smokers to switch. It is also widely available on the black market, which supplies over 70% of the hand-rolling tobacco consumed in the UK.[5]

WHY DO PEOPLE SMOKE?

Tobacco use in a community is primarily a socially determined phenomenon. In the UK, tobacco is a legal and socially acceptable consumer product, widely available and tolerated in public places. However, this consumer product contains the highly addictive drug nicotine, meaning that most people who start to use it go on to do so for many years – some for life.

Use of tobacco as a consumer product has also been greatly influenced by the promotional activities of its manufacturers. Until 2000, cigarettes could be widely advertised in the UK, and some forms of tobacco sponsorship (notably Formula 1 motor racing) will be permitted until 2005, ahead of the EU-wide ban due to come into force in 2006. As with any consumer product, advertising promotes not just individual brands but overall consumption – when it is banned, consumption tends to fall.[6]

Figure 4.1 Influences on an individual's decision to start or stop smoking.

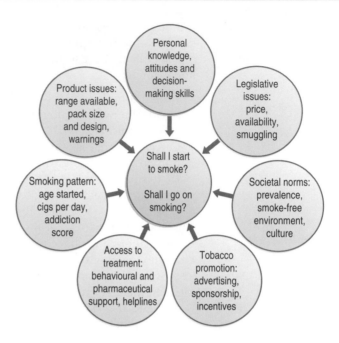

Most people who smoke start to do so in their teens. Experimentation quickly becomes a regular daily smoking pattern, sustained by nicotine addiction but reinforced by social norms. Groups of friends and families tend to adopt similar smoking patterns, and smoking becomes part of their social ritual. In working and social environments where smoking is freely permitted, smoking is perceived to be the norm and it becomes more difficult for individuals to opt out.

Figure 4.1 illustrates the complex set of influences that affect an individual's decision to start, continue or stop smoking. The societal influences are dominant, although the compelling influence of nicotine addiction on established smokers is a complicating factor.

WHY IS SMOKING AN IMPORTANT PUBLIC HEALTH ISSUE?

The impact of tobacco smoking on public health extends well beyond the direct effects on the individual smoker; it also extends beyond personal health effects, to economic, environmental and social effects.

The association between tobacco smoking and lung cancer was conclusively shown for the first time in the 1950s by Sir Richard Doll in his study of British doctors (updated in 1994).[7] Since then, thousands of researchers worldwide continue to document myriad health risks in tobacco smokers, from lip cancer to gangrene, from emphysema to early menopause, from childhood deafness to sight loss. Tobacco smoke is toxic to every human tissue it touches on its way into, through and out of the smoker's body.

Some key facts are:

- Smoking causes around a fifth of all deaths in the UK – approximately 114 000 each year,[8] most of them premature (on average, 21 years early).

- About half of all regular smokers will die from a smoking-related disease.[7]
- Most of the premature deaths are from one of the three main diseases:
  - lung and other cancers (42 800 per year);
  - coronary heart disease (30 600 per year);
  - chronic obstructive lung disease (29 100 per year).[8]
- Smoking also brings increased risk of many debilitating conditions, like asthma, angina, impotence, infertility, osteoporosis, gum disease and psoriasis.[9]

In the wider environment, smoking is the major cause of fatal fires, the major source of indoor air pollution in buildings where it is allowed, and a major cause of litter: 200 million cigarette ends are discarded in the UK every day, and each takes 18 months or more to biodegrade.[10] In countries where tobacco is grown for cigarette production, the environmental damage includes the consequences of intensive farming practices, and deforestation for the wood required in the curing process.[11]

HOW IS SMOKING ADDRESSED IN NATIONAL POLICY?

In the UK, smoking has been addressed systematically at government level since the publication of the White Paper *Smoking Kills* in 1998.[1] Specific measures to tackle smoking are outlined in the *National Service Framework for Coronary Heart Disease*,[12] and in *The NHS Cancer Plan*.[13] The main elements of the provisions are:

- government-funded mass media education campaigns;
- national telephone helplines and NHS specialist services for smokers who want to stop;
- pharmaceutical treatments on NHS prescription.

The White Paper and subsequent plans outline specific targets for smoking reduction, and emphasize that many strands of public policy will impact on their achievement. In some policy areas a legislative approach has been used, while in others progress has been sought through voluntary approaches.

POLICY MEASURES

Sales to under 16s

UK legislation prohibits the sale of tobacco products to people under 16 years old,[14] and since February 2003 all tobacco advertising has been banned[15] save for point-of-sale promotion – this too has been severely restricted from September 2004.

Taxation

Taxation has been used frequently to increase the price of smoking, with rises in duty imposed in each year's budget. Where such rises are meaningful, that is, significantly more than the rate of inflation, an immediate and lasting reduction in consumption is seen.

Oral tobacco

Certain types of oral tobacco (tobacco products that are not smoked, but held in the mouth for absorption through the cheek lining) have been banned in the UK since 1989, a ban that was subsequently extended to other countries under an EU Directive.[16]

Some other types of oral tobacco product, such as paan and gutkha, are widely used in minority ethnic populations. These are not currently regulated or comprehensively studied, but knowledge about their use is growing. It is apparent that smokeless products are more widely used by women in communities in which smoking is culturally unacceptable.

Smoking in public places and workplaces

There is currently no UK legislation on smoking in public places or workplaces save for the general obligations on employers under health and safety law.[17] However, an EU Directive requires employers to provide smoke-free rest areas for staff.[18]

International policy

The most recent major development at policy level has been the UK's signing of the international *WHO Framework Convention on Tobacco Control*[19] in 2003. This is the first global treaty for public health negotiated under the auspices of the World Health Organization and requires participating countries to implement a range of legislative and other measures to control smoking. These include action on passive smoking, banning tobacco promotion, providing services to smokers, monitoring smoking prevalence and international cooperation to control smuggling. The Convention comes into force in February 2005.

WHAT'S THE CURRENT PICTURE – WHO IS AT RISK?

SOCIAL CLASS

In the UK, smoking is strongly correlated with social class and deprivation. While there are few social class differences among young people taking up smoking, long term regular smoking is more likely to persist among more deprived groups. This produces the imbalance in smoking rates shown in Table 4.1: prevalence of smoking is more than doubled in low-paid groups compared with affluent groups.[3] Most of this social class difference in smoking rates is attributable to the greater difficulty people in less affluent groups experience in stopping smoking.

AGES

Across the age ranges, smoking is more prevalent in younger groups. Among 16–19 year olds, 25% of men and 31% of women are regular smokers, rising to 40% of men and 35% of women in the 20–24 age group. Smoking prevalence reduces with age, as smokers tend to give up in middle age or die of smoking-related illness, and the lowest smoking rates are seen in over 60s: 16% of men and 17% of women.[3] (See Table 4.2.)

The rate of uptake of smoking by children has barely changed in recent years: in 1982 11% of 11–15 year old boys and 11% of girls were regular

Table 4.1   Prevalence of cigarette smoking across social groups 2001, adults over 16[3]

	% Men who smoke	% Women who smoke
Overall prevalence of regular smoking	28	26
Prevalence in most affluent groups	16	15
Prevalence in low-paid groups	38	33

Table 4.2   Percentage who smoke cigarettes by sex and age, 1972–2001, Great Britain[3]

	Year															
	1972	1974	1976	1978	1980	1982	1984	1986	1988	1990	1992	1994	1996	1998	2000	2001
Men																
16–19	43	42	39	35	32	31	29	30	28	28	29	28	26	30	30	25
20–24	55	52	47	45	44	41	40	41	37	38	39	40	43	42	35	40
25–34	56	56	48	48	47	40	40	37	37	36	34	34	38	37	39	38
35–49	55	55	50	48	45	40	39	37	37	34	32	31	30	32	31	31
50–59	54	53	49	48	47	42	39	35	33	28	28	27	28	27	27	26
60+	47	44	40	38	36	33	30	29	26	24	21	18	18	16	16	16
All men	52	51	46	45	42	38	36	35	33	31	29	28	29	28	29	28
Women																
16–19	39	38	34	33	32	30	32	30	28	32	25	27	32	31	28	31
20–24	48	44	45	43	40	40	36	38	37	39	37	38	36	39	35	35
25–34	49	46	43	42	44	37	36	35	35	34	34	30	34	33	32	31
35–49	48	49	45	43	43	38	36	34	35	33	30	28	30	28	28	28
50–59	47	48	46	42	44	40	39	35	34	29	29	26	26	27	28	25
60+	25	26	24	24	24	23	23	22	21	20	19	17	19	16	15	17
All women	41	41	38	37	37	33	32	31	30	29	28	26	28	28	25	26
Total																
16–19	41	40	37	34	32	30	31	30	28	30	27	27	29	31	29	28
20–24	51	48	46	44	42	40	38	39	37	38	33	39	39	40	35	37
25–34	52	51	46	45	45	38	38	36	36	35	34	32	36	35	35	34
35–49	51	52	47	45	44	39	37	36	36	34	31	30	30	30	29	29
50–59	50	51	47	45	45	41	39	35	33	29	29	27	27	27	27	26
60+	34	34	31	30	29	27	26	25	23	21	20	17	18	16	16	17
All adults	46	45	42	40	39	35	34	33	32	30	28	27	28	27	27	27

smokers, and in 2002 the figures were 9% and 11% respectively.[20] (Data on children's smoking are not collected as consistently or widely as those on adult smoking. Adult smoking statistics are routinely collected throughout Great Britain in the annual General Household Survey. Children's smoking rates are collected separately, at different intervals and using different age groupings in England, Scotland, Wales and Northern Ireland.)

OTHER DIMENSIONS OF HIGHER RISK

In considering who is most at risk from smoking, many different dimensions of risk have to be acknowledged.

Current smokers

Most importantly, current smokers are at high risk of developing smoking-related disease: one in two smokers will die of such disease unless they stop. In that sense, all smokers should be considered at high risk.

Passive smokers

People who are exposed to passive smoking are also at risk: 85% of the smoke from a cigarette is emitted from the burning end, into the air breathed by people around the smoker.[21] That smoke contains the same toxins as the smoke inhaled directly by the smoker, and while it is more dilute, it is associated with a similar range of disease in exposed non-smokers.

Risk of starting to smoke

A further dimension of 'at risk' is the issue of uptake: which young people are most at risk of starting to smoke? The most reliable predictor of smoking in young people is smoking by other family members and peers, with children three times as likely to smoke if both their parents smoke.[22]

Risk to people in poor health

Lastly, the 'most at risk' groups must include those whose health is already compromised by other factors, such as existing medical conditions, extreme youth or old age, pregnancy, or use of certain medications. For example, tobacco smoke:

- aggravates conditions like asthma and diabetes;
- delays recovery from injury or surgery;
- can interfere with the action of some drugs;
- can damage the immature respiratory systems of babies;
- can hasten age-related deterioration in eyesight and other functions;
- restricts oxygen supply to the fetus in pregnant women;
- can make conception more difficult;
- increases the risk of coronary heart disease (20-fold) and stroke (7-fold) in users of oral contraception.[23]

IS THE PREVALENCE OF SMOKING INCREASING OR DECREASING?

Smoking has been in decline in the UK for many decades, although the steady falls in prevalence seen in the 1970s and 1980s have slowed considerably since the 1990s when overall smoking rates stabilized on or just below 30% of the adult population.[3] Figure 4.2 shows the trend in smoking prevalence for men and women since 1972. (Full details of age and gender-related changes in smoking over those years are shown in Table 4.2.)

Figure 4.2 Trends in smoking prevalence 1972–2001. (Source: Office for National Statistics. Living in Britain. Results from the 2001 General Household Survey. London: The Stationery Office; 2002 and previous editions.)

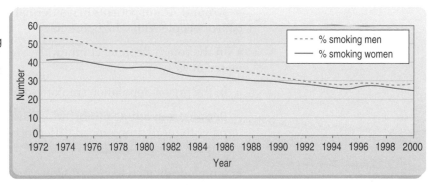

The picture in other countries varies according to their respective policy regimes. In other developed countries like Sweden, which has strong smoking prevention measures, smoking prevalence has continued to fall steadily, particularly among men: the overall adult smoking prevalence there was just 19% in 2001,[24] the lowest in Europe. In less developed countries, where tobacco control measures are relatively rare, smoking rates are rising as tobacco companies turn their attention there. Despite the overall decline of smoking in most of the developed world, it is estimated that the worldwide death toll from smoking-related disease will continue to rise from its current 4 million per year to 10 million per year by the year 2030,[25] with the majority of those deaths occurring in developing countries.

DO HEALTH INEQUALITIES FEATURE IN SMOKING?

LOW-INCOME GROUPS

Tobacco is widely recognized as a cause of health inequality in the UK. Not only is its use more common in deprived groups, but its use further compromises the already poorer health of deprived populations. A specific 'inequalities target' on smoking was set in *The NHS Cancer Plan*:[13] 'To reduce smoking rates among manual groups from 32% in 1998 to 26% by 2010, in order to narrow the health gap'.

The expense of smoking is a bigger drain on the budget of low-income families, particularly as people on low incomes, paradoxically, tend to be heavier smokers than those on higher incomes. The average household expenditure on cigarettes in smoking families is 2%, but the poorest tenth of the population spends around 15% of its weekly income on cigarettes, six times as much as those in the richest tenth.[26] Meaningful tax increases do prompt some smokers to stop: it is estimated that a 10% price increase prompts a 4% drop in consumption.[27] The impact of increases is harder on low-income groups; this is known as a 'regressive tax', and is discussed below in the 'Controversial issues' section of this chapter.

OTHER DIMENSIONS OF INEQUALITY

Marginalized groups, such as people with mental health problems, are more likely to smoke and less likely to access mainstream smoking cessation services.

● Around 70% of patients in residential psychiatric care smoke, and over 80% of people with schizophrenia.[28]

● In the rough sleeping community, smoking prevalence has been estimated at 90%.

● In the prison population smoking prevalence is around 80%.[29]

People from ethnic minorities show widely differing smoking patterns with more pronounced differences between men and women, for example:[30]

● Bangladeshi men have a smoking prevalence of around 42%, whereas smoking is rare among women in that community at only 4%.

● In the Chinese population, 17% of men smoke and 8% of women.

● In the black Caribbean population 34% of men smoke along with 23% of women.

(See Ch. 13 on 'Tackling inequalities in health'.)

WHAT CAN WE DO ABOUT PREVENTION AND HEALTH PROMOTION AT A COMMUNITY LEVEL?

Interventions have three sets of overlapping effects – changing social norms, influencing attitudes, and supporting individual behaviour change. Effectiveness reviews and national policy guidelines emphasize the importance of comprehensive approaches, which achieve greater impact through synergy, and the set of measures outlined in the international *WHO Framework Convention for Tobacco Control* reflects this need.[19] The US Surgeon General's Report *Reducing Tobacco Use*[31] explains:

> Approaches with the largest span of impact (economic, regulatory, and comprehensive) are likely to have the greatest long-term, population impact. Those with a smaller span of impact (educational and clinical) are of greater importance in helping individuals resist or abandon the use of tobacco.

The components of the comprehensive approach he and others outline[32] are educational programmes, cessation treatment programmes, bans on tobacco promotion, high prices for tobacco products (usually achieved through taxation), and smoke-free environments, particularly workplaces. The country that has best demonstrated the effectiveness of such a comprehensive approach is New Zealand, where consumption halved in 15 years and adult prevalence reduced by one quarter, from 32% in 1981 to 24% in 1996.[33]

This comprehensive approach is summarized in Figure 4.3.

At a local community level, strong smoke-free policies and enforcement of bans on tobacco promotion will help create an environment that encourages smokers to stop, in turn reinforcing a smoke-free norm that will discourage uptake by young people.

Figure 4.3   Public health measures for smoking prevention.

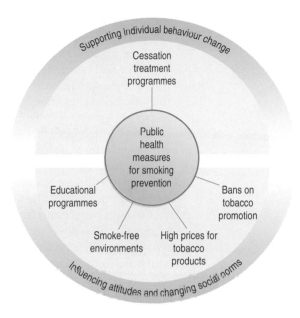

HOW CAN WE BEST HELP INDIVIDUALS?

There are two main categories of intervention with individuals: cessation and prevention.

CESSATION

This is the main intervention likely to be undertaken by healthcare professionals, principally in primary healthcare settings but also in others, including telephone enquiry centres, informal community settings, clinical care and rehabilitation settings.

Published guidelines outline the appropriate evidence-led intervention in each of these settings, and their cost effectiveness has been well demonstrated: the median cost of the 314 most common medical interventions was calculated in 1995 to be £17 000 per life year gained.[34] At 1998 costs, smoking cessation interventions were calculated to have a cost-effectiveness range of £212–£873 per life year gained.[35]

Smokers' feelings about smoking and stopping

Before considering the interventions, it is useful to understand what makes smokers want to stop, and what they experience in their attempts to do so.

Most smokers start to smoke in their teens, typically developing a regular daily smoking pattern and on average consuming 15 cigarettes a day. Many smokers report smoking rather more than their regular daily amount at weekends or on holiday, especially in situations where they consume more alcohol than usual.

Despite the early onset and prolonged regular use of tobacco (or perhaps because of it), smokers rapidly report regret about starting to smoke, often expressed as a wish to be able to stop: 70% of adult regular smokers say they would like to give up smoking[36] and 82% regret ever starting.[37] It is important to recognize this dissonance in smokers, and to understand the reasons behind it. For most, the regret stems from worries about current or future health. Other reasons include the cost of smoking, and dislike of feeling addicted. Many perceive social stigma about smoking, and some even feel repulsed by the smell and mess their own smoking creates. For women especially, this often translates into quite strong feelings of guilt about their smoking, particularly if they are pregnant or living with children. For men, it often translates into feelings of weakness.

Smokers often have these negative feelings about smoking from a very early stage in their smoking history, but most take refuge in the belief that they will be stopped 'within a couple of years'. Few start trying to stop before early middle age though, meaning that most will in fact smoke for 20 years or more. This phenomenon has been coined 'the delusion gap'[37] and needs to be recognized when approaching smokers, to create a sense of urgency about attempting to stop.

While stopping smoking at any age produces health gain, the greatest reductions in risk come from early attempts at stopping.[7] Men who stop smoking by age 35 attain similar longevity patterns to lifelong non-smokers, but stopping at older ages still increases life expectancy compared with continuing smoking. Cutting down does not achieve as big a risk reduction as stopping smoking completely.[38]

Intervention strategies

Several factors will influence the choice of intervention in given situations, principally:

- the level of expertise in the practitioner;
- the time available;
- opportunities for follow-up;
- access to pharmaceutical products.

The UK has a network of specialist NHS services for smokers who want to stop, providing intensive group or one-to-one support. Most health professionals will not be required to provide that level of support, but should rather view the aim of their intervention as triggering attempts to stop which more specialized professionals can then support.

Two main categories of pharmaceutical product are currently approved by the National Institute for Clinical Excellence (NICE), and are available on NHS prescription: nicotine replacement therapy (NRT) and bupropion (trade name Zyban).[39] Many NRT products are available over the counter in pharmacies or supermarkets.

Routine healthcare settings

Published national guidelines describe the evidence base and typical effectiveness outcomes of cessation interventions in routine healthcare settings, along with those of the more intensive interventions possible in specialist settings.[40] The recommendations for all healthcare professionals are that they should:

- routinely record patients' smoking status in case notes;
- raise the subject of smoking at least once a year;
- advise smoking patients to stop;
- offer information about sources of specialist help, referring where appropriate.

Many patients prefer to tackle their smoking without specialist help; if so they can be offered self-help information and referred to a pharmacist for NRT. Patients may simply be prescribed NRT, but its effectiveness in self-help situations is less well documented. Bupropion should not be prescribed unless the patient can be supervised in follow-up because of the higher risk of side effects with that drug.

Specialist cessation services

Specialist NHS cessation services provide the support of trained advisers and access to pharmaceutical products. Typically, smokers are offered structured group support over 6–8 weeks, and NRT or bupropion on prescription. A stop date is set during the course, and cessation rates at 4 weeks are monitored. Some services follow up clients and collect data for longer than the required 4 weeks. Quit rates at 4 weeks are typically around 50% (53% in 2002–2003[41]), and while there is some further relapse after 4 weeks, the quit rates remain considerably higher than those achieved by people attempting to stop without support. Much of the published literature compares cessation rates at 3, 6 or 12 months.

The specialist advisors in these services are often nurses, health visitors or counsellors, but all are required to undergo specialist training in smoking cessation. There is no formal registration process for such advisers, but guidelines exist on the recommended curriculum for establishments providing their training.[42] All healthcare professionals should find out about their local specialist services and refer interested patients there for support.

(See also Ch. 14 'Helping individuals to change behaviour'.)

PREVENTION

There is some scope for prevention work with individuals, although as previously described in this chapter, the most effective prevention measures are at the societal level.

In the healthcare setting, it is important that non-smoking status be recognized and valued as a self-care strategy. Healthcare settings should be smoke-free and provide information about smoking, and smoke-free lifestyles should be reinforced wherever possible, for example in health promotion clinic settings. In clinical settings with particularly vulnerable groups, such as family planning or diabetes clinics, the importance of remaining a non-smoker should be emphasized.

The most important target group for prevention messages are recent ex-smokers, who need sustained reassurance about the health gains they will attain by remaining smoke-free.

CONTROVERSIAL ISSUES

Tobacco has for many years been a relatively simple issue for healthcare practitioners: there is no safe level of exposure to tobacco smoke, whether active or passive, making abstinence the only message.

There are, however, some controversies in tobacco control. Most of them are deliberately created by tobacco company interests to try to dilute or delay tobacco control measures, as revealed in internal tobacco company documents. Others are debates among health professionals about the relative effectiveness of tobacco control measures and strategies, for example whether youth smoking prevention programmes are more important than cessation treatment programmes. Others are rooted in common myths and misunderstandings about smoking among the general public. The main controversy created by tobacco interests is on the appropriateness of measures to control passive smoking, and this is addressed in the 'Common myths' section below.

The three main genuine controversies are:

- the potential role of harm reduction strategies within a comprehensive tobacco control programme;
- the ethics of taxation strategies to discourage smoking;
- the effectiveness of youth smoking prevention programmes.

HARM REDUCTION

Traditional public health measures to tackle smoking have been aimed at promoting complete abstinence, as there is no safe way to smoke or safe level of consumption. Cutting down and so-called low tar cigarettes have been shown to have no value for harm reduction.

With the advent of new smokeless tobacco products, less hazardous ways to use nicotine are being made possible. While nicotine is not a benign substance, much of the harm of smoking is caused not by the nicotine but by the tar and carbon monoxide created in the tobacco combustion process, and by the fact that the major ingestion route is through the delicate tissues of the lung. Products that are not smoked do not carry this set of hazards, although they still involve the ingestion of nicotine.

The controversy for the UK is to decide whether to allow such products on to the market, in the hope that existing nicotine users (smokers) will switch to them, and that people who might otherwise have smoked will choose to use the smokeless options. For there to be a public health gain, any extra harm caused to people who would otherwise not have used any nicotine product must be outweighed by reduced harm to people who would otherwise have continued to smoke. The magnitude of risk reduction associated with different products allows for such assessments to be made in the course of policy development.

PRICE INCREASES AND THEIR EFFECT ON LOW-INCOME SMOKERS

High price helps deter young people from starting to smoke and prompts many smokers to stop, and the UK government frequently acts to keep tobacco prices high through taxation. However, as smoking is concentrated among the lowest paid sectors of society, and as it is likely to be the most addicted who will continue to smoke despite price rises, questions are often raised about the fairness of such tax: the poorest pay disproportionately more as a consequence of their acquired addiction.

Where significant amounts of the revenue obtained by government through this taxation are invested in programmes to help smokers stop, the policy is better accepted.

YOUTH SMOKING PREVENTION PROGRAMMES

It is a common misconception that the best way to tackle smoking is to undertake direct interventions with young people. These typically include school programmes, age-related sales restrictions and youth-oriented advertising. While these measures have a place in a comprehensive programme, they have very poor cost-effectiveness and will not succeed in isolation. At best, dedicated school-based programmes achieve a short delay in uptake of smoking among participants.

While smoking can and should be addressed through the normal curriculum, it is more important that schools should have strong policies prohibiting all smoking on school premises, for staff and visitors as well as pupils. The law prohibiting sales to under-16s adds to the allure of smoking as an adult activity, and can present an amusing challenge to young people's enterprising spirit in finding ways to get round it. Even where enforcement is strong, cigarettes are widely available to young people through black market routes, family bulk-buys of cigarettes and older siblings or friends. The usefulness of an age-related sales restriction is largely symbolic, as it marks some degree of undesirability of smoking.

Youth-oriented media campaigns have a notoriously poor record of credibility among young people, and it is often difficult to distinguish between those created by health organizations and those created by cigarette companies as part of their 'corporate social responsibility' programmes. Tobacco industry documents reveal the real strategy behind their youth programmes: to emphasize that smoking is for adults, and that smoking is an exercise of free choice, both of which make smoking more attractive to young people.[43] Media campaigns aimed at young people need to avoid these messages, as they reinforce rather than discourage smoking.

The evidence on effectiveness of interventions suggests that young people are most affected by adult-targeted campaigns: they smoke in an aspiration to be more adult, so discrediting smoking in the adult population will lessen its attraction for youth. Media campaigns aimed at adults have been shown to reach young people and have a high degree of credibility among them. Societal measures like smoke-free policies in the workplace and social settings have a denormalizing effect, dissociating smoking from the adult world.

The absence of cigarette advertising prevents the reinforcement of brand imagery, and the introduction of large stark warnings on packs makes the cigarette boxes themselves less attractive as fashion accessories. Some countries (Canada, Brazil and Thailand) have adopted pictorial warnings for cigarette packs, and they may in future be introduced in the EU.

COMMON MYTHS AND QUESTIONS

The jury's still out on passive smoking

This myth is widely promoted by tobacco industry interests, to disrupt attempts to have smoking banned in public places. Tobacco smoke has, however, already been recognized as a human carcinogen, and the British Medical Association's most conservative estimate of the annual death toll in the UK from passive smoking is at least 1000. Passive smoking is associated with heart disease, lung cancer, respiratory disease, aggravated asthma and pregnancy complications. The effects are compounded in babies and young children: an estimated 17 000 children are hospitalized each year because of parental smoking,[44] and many more suffer in other ways: respiratory infections, glue ear, impaired intellectual development.

People get addicted to cessation treatments

Some people who stop smoking by using nicotine replacement therapy continue to use the products beyond the recommended period. The level of nicotine in them is, however, very small compared with the levels in cigarettes, and long term use has not been shown to cause any harm to health. The nicotine delivery rate of these products is very slow compared to the hit of a cigarette, making their abuse potential low. When the alternative is relapse to smoking, long term use of NRT products is much preferable.

When you stop smoking you just get fat

Many people who stop smoking experience weight gain. This is invariably due to increased eating, unbalanced by any increased activity. Smoking does have a slight appetite suppressant effect, and smokers do tend to be slightly lighter than non-smokers. Weight gain on stopping smoking can be avoided by a sensible eating and exercise plan. A weight gain of 3 stones (19 kilograms) would be required to cancel out the heart health benefit of stopping smoking. (See Ch. 5 'Obesity' for more about tackling weight gain.)

Light cigarettes are healthier

So-called 'low-tar' or 'light' cigarettes were introduced to the market as a deliberate strategy by tobacco companies to address smokers' health concerns, as one document from British American Tobacco reveals:

> All work in this area should be directed towards providing consumer reassurance about cigarettes and the smoking habit. This can be provided in different ways, e.g. by claiming low deliveries, by the perception of low deliveries and by the perception of 'mildness'. Furthermore, advertising for low delivery or traditional brands should be constructed in ways so as not to provoke anxiety about health, but to alleviate it, and enable the smoker to feel assured about the habit and confident in maintaining it over time.[45]

There is, however, no reduced risk from these products: the 'low-tar' effect is created by a series of perforations in the cigarette filter, which quickly become blocked when a smoker draws on the cigarette. Smokers also self-regulate the amount of nicotine they absorb from each cigarette: they will draw harder on a 'light' cigarette in order to achieve the level of nicotine they desire, inhaling more smoke in the process. 'Light' cigarettes can in fact be even more harmful than regular cigarettes for this reason.

Cutting down reduces your risk

There is no safe level of smoking, and cutting down from a higher daily level to a lower level offers the smoker no reduction in risk – the smoker continues to accumulate risk, albeit at a slower rate. Risk reduction only occurs with complete cessation. It does appear, however, that smokers who do manage to sustain significant reductions in their daily cigarette consumption become more predisposed to make a complete quit attempt.

It's the only pleasure for poor people

Smoking rates are higher among people on low incomes, but they are just as likely to feel regret about their smoking and to want to stop. They traditionally need more support in achieving abstinence.

Cigars and pipes are safer than cigarettes

Puffing on cigars or pipes, even without inhaling, is associated with mouth, throat, head and neck cancers along with other oral disease. Some people believe that switching to pipes and cigars reduces their risk of tobacco-related disease, but such smokers tend to continue to inhale smoke, meaning that their risk of the full range of tobacco-related disease continues to rise.

The government needs people to smoke – the economy depends on it

Very few jobs in the UK are truly dependent on smoking: cigarette manufacturing is increasingly mechanized and moving overseas, and most tobacco-related jobs are now in sales, marketing and distribution. In the retail sector, most outlets sell cigarettes alongside other consumer products, and cigarette sales account for only a small part of their profit margin. The unique pricing structure of cigarettes in the UK, with such a large proportion of the cost being excise duty, means that expenditure on cigarettes does not stimulate the economy to the same extent as expenditure on other consumer products. The government obtains £8 billion per year from excise duty on tobacco products, approximately 2% of its annual revenue (£428 billion in 2003–2004[46]).

WHAT QUESTIONS ABOUT SMOKING STILL NEED ANSWERS?

The research agenda for tobacco control has been formally defined at global level by the World Health Organization,[47] which identifies eight main areas in which research is needed:

- country-level surveillance of trends in tobacco use, collecting standardized and comparable data;
- impact evaluation of policy interventions;
- methods and effectiveness of programme interventions;
- methods and effectiveness of treatment interventions;
- tobacco product design and regulation;
- tobacco industry analysis;
- tobacco farming issues;
- implementation and impact of the *WHO Framework Convention for Tobacco Control*.[19]

For public health practitioners in the UK, the research priorities are to monitor prevalence trends, measure policy and programme impact, and examine regulation issues.

Key sources of further information and help

Further reading

- **Tobacco Control:** A peer-reviewed professional journal published by BMJ Group. Online subscription available at www.tobaccocontrol.com.

Professional support and information networks

- **www.globalink.org:** an international online tobacco control network.
- **www.srnt.org:** Society for Research on Nicotine and Tobacco – for researchers, policy-makers and practitioners with an interest in scientific evidence.
- **www.tobacco-control.org:** British Medical Association's Tobacco Control Resource Centre for doctors.
- **www.treatobacco.net:** an online database of evidence-based interventions.

Organizations

- **Action on Smoking and Health: (ASH)** a registered charity at www.ash.org.uk, providing up-to-date, authoritative information and news on tobacco issues, as well as downloadable presentations and educational resources.

- **Department of Health:** dedicated tobacco web pages at www.dh.gov.uk/tobacco.
- **FOREST:** part-funded by tobacco industry interests, the Freedom Organization for the Right to Enjoy Smoking Tobacco challenges public health measures on smoking. Its website is at www.forestonline.org.uk.
- **No Smoking Day:** the registered charity that organizes the UK's annual event on smoking. Available at www.nosmokingday.org.uk, providing information for smokers, guidance, and downloadable materials for professionals running local campaigns.
- **Quit:** www.quit.org.uk, a registered charity that runs services for smokers who want to stop, and professional training courses in cessation.
- **World Health Organization Tobacco-Free Initiative:** www.who.int/tobacco.

Help for smokers

- **NHS Smoking Helpline:** 0800 690 169 or online at www.givingupsmoking.co.uk.

References

1. Department of Health. Smoking kills: a White Paper on tobacco. London: The Stationery Office; 1998.
2. UICC, WHO and ACS. Tobacco control country profiles 2003. Online. Available: http://www.globalink.org/tccp/United_Kingdom.pdf
3. Office for National Statistics. Living in Britain. Results from the 2001 General Household Survey. London: The Stationery Office; 2002 (and previous editions).
4. Department of Health. Permitted additives to tobacco products in the United Kingdom. London: DOH; 2000.
5. The Tobacco Manufacturers' Association. Online. Available: http://www.the-tma.org.uk February 2004.
6. Saffer H, Chaloupka F. The effect of tobacco advertising bans on tobacco consumption. Journal of Health Economics 2000; 19:1117–1137.
7. Doll R, Peto R, Wheatley K, et al. Mortality in relation to smoking: 40 years' observations on male British doctors. BMJ 1994; 309:901–911.

8. Peto R, Lopez A, Boreham J, et al. Mortality from smoking in developed countries 1950–2000. 2nd edn. Oxford: Oxford University Press; 2003.
9. American Council on Science and Health. Cigarettes: what the warning label doesn't tell you. 2nd edn. New York: American Council on Science and Health; 2003.
10. Novotny T, Zhao F. Consumption and production waste: another externality of tobacco use. Tobacco Control 1999; 8:75–80.
11. Geist HJ. Global assessment of deforestation related to tobacco farming. Tobacco Control 1999; 8:18–28.
12. Department of Health. National Service Framework for coronary heart disease. London: DOH; 2000.
13. Department of Health. The NHS cancer plan. London: DOH; 2000.
14. Children and Young Persons (Protection from Tobacco) Act 1991. London: HMSO. Online. Available: http://www.hmso.gov.uk/acts

15. Tobacco Advertising and Promotion Act 2002. London: HMSO. Online. Available: http://www.hmso.gov.uk/acts

16. European Parliament. Council Directive 2001/37/EC of the European Parliament and of the Council of 5 June 2001 on the approximation of the laws, regulations and administrative provisions of the member states concerning the manufacture, presentation and sale of tobacco products. Commission Statement. Official Journal L194, 18/07/2001: 0026–0035. Online. Available: http://www.hmso.gov.uk

17. Health and Safety at Work Act 1974. London: HMSO. Online. Available: http://www.healthandsafety.co.uk

18. European Parliament. Council Directive 89/654/EEC of 30 November 1989 concerning the minimum safety and health requirements for the workplace (First individual directive within the meaning of Article 16(1) of Directive 89/391/EEC). Official Journal L 393, 30/12/1989: 0001–0012. Online. Available: http://www.europa.eu.int

19. World Health Organization. WHO framework convention on tobacco control. Geneva: World Health Organization; 2003.

20. Office for National Statistics. Smoking, drinking and drug use among young people in England. London: The Stationery Office; 2002.

21. Fielding JE, Phenow KJ. Health effects of involuntary smoking. New England Journal of Medicine 1988; 319: 1452–1460.

22. Office for National Statistics. Teenage smoking attitudes in 1996. London: Office for National Statistics; 1997.

23. British Medical Association. Smoking and reproductive life. London: BMA; 2004.

24. World Health Organization. European Health for All statistical database. Geneva: WHO; 2003.

25. World Bank. Curbing the epidemic. Governments and the economics of tobacco control. Washington DC: World Bank; 1999.

26. Marsh A, Mackay S. Poor smokers. London: Policy Studies Institute; 1994.

27. Chaloupka F, Warner K. The economics of smoking: working paper 7047. Cambridge, Massachusetts: National Bureau of Economic Research, 1999.

28. McNeill A. Smoking and mental health – a review of the literature. London: ASH; 2001.

29. Singleton N, Farrell M, Meltzer H. Substance misuse among prisoners in England and Wales. London: Office for National Statistics; 1999.

30. Joint Health Surveys Unit. Health survey for England. The health of minority ethnic groups 1999. London: The Stationery Office; 2001.

31. US Department of Health and Human Services. Reducing tobacco use: a report of the Surgeon General. Atlanta, GA: US Department of Health and Human Services. Centers for Disease Control and Prevention,

National Center for Chronic Disease Prevention and Health Promotion, Office of Smoking and Health; 2000.

32. Laugesen M, Scollo M, Sweanor D, et al. World's best practice in tobacco control. Tobacco Control 2000; 9:228–236.

33. Laugesen M, Swinburn B. New Zealand's tobacco control programme 1985–1998. Tobacco Control 2000; 9:155–162.

34. Tengs TO, Adams ME, Pilskin JS, et al. Five hundred life saving interventions and their cost effectiveness. Risk Analysis 1995; 15:369–390.

35. Parrott S, Godfrey C, Raw M, et al. Guidance for commissioners on the cost effectiveness of smoking cessation interventions. Health Educational Authority. Thorax 1998; 53 (Suppl 5 Pt 2):S1–S38.

36. Office for National Statistics . Smoking related behaviour and attitudes, 2002. London: The Stationery Office; 2003.

37. Jarvis M, McIntyre D, Bates C. Efforts must take into account smokers' disillusionment with smoking and their delusions about stopping. BMJ 2002; 324:608.

38. Thun MJ, Myers DG, Day-Lally C, et al. Age and the exposure–response relationships between cigarette smoking and premature death in Cancer Prevention Study II. National Cancer Institute. Smoking and Tobacco Control Monograph 8, pp 383–475. National Institute of Health Publication no. 97–4213; 1997. Online. Available: http://www.cancer.gov

39. National Institute for Clinical Excellence. Technology appraisal guidance no. 39. Guidance on the use of nicotine replacement therapy (NRT) and bupropion for smoking cessation. London: NICE; 2002.

40. West R, McNeill A, Raw M. Smoking cessation guidelines for professionals: an update. Thorax 2000; 55:987–999.

41. Department of Health. Statistics on smoking cessation services in England, April 2002–March 2003. London: Department of Health; November 2003.

42. Health Development Agency. Standard for training in smoking cessation treatment. London: HDA: 2003.

43. Cancer Research UK and ASH. Danger! PR in the playground: tobacco industry initiatives on youth smoking. London: Cancer Research UK and ASH; 2002.

44. Royal College of Physicians. Smoking and the young. London: RCP; 1992.

45. Short PL, British American Tobacco Co. Smoking and health item 7: the effect on marketing. 14th April 1977. Minnesota Trial Exhibit 10 585.

46. HM Treasury. Budget 2003 summary: building a Britain of economic strength and social justice. London: The Stationery Office; 2003.

47. World Health Organization. Confronting the epidemic: a global agenda for tobacco control research. Geneva: WHO; 1999.

Chapter 5

Obesity

Dympna Pearson

SUMMARY OVERVIEW AND LINKS TO OTHER TOPICS

The increasing prevalence of overweight and obesity and its resulting health problems are now of major concern to governments, healthcare professionals and overweight individuals.

Obesity occurs when energy intake exceeds energy expenditure over a period of time. Our present environment is *obesogenic* – encouraging high consumption of calories coupled with low levels of activity – and this interacts with behavioural, genetic and other factors. Inequalities feature; some population groups are particularly at risk, including those who are socially deprived, on low income, with low levels of education, have learning difficulties or are from certain ethnic minorities.

Nationally, there are no effective strategies for tackling obesity yet, but a National Institute of Clinical Excellence (NICE) review is due in 2007. The Department of Health is developing a Food and Health

Action Plan, expected in 2005; a Commons Select Committee made a strong call for action on obesity in 2004.[1]

Action is clearly needed to prevent and tackle obesity at population level nationally and locally by creating a less obesogenic environment and promoting healthy eating; and to help obese individuals to access appropriate services and treatment regimes. There is much debate about how to meet the needs of obese people and how to engage the many stakeholders, especially those from the food industry, in preventing obesity, balancing freedom of individual choice with the responsibility to make our environment less obesogenic.

There is an urgent need for research on effective interventions for the prevention and treatment of obesity in children and adults.

Because activity is important in weight loss, weight maintenance and the prevention of obesity, this chapter should be read alongside Chapter 6 'Physical activity'. As obesity is a risk factor for cancer, heart disease and stroke, and type 2 diabetes, Chapters 1, 2 and 3 are also highly relevant. Chapter 13 'Tackling inequalities in health', and Chapter 14 'Helping individuals to change behaviour' cover pertinent issues in tackling obesity.

WHAT IS OBESITY?

Obesity is described by the World Health Organization (WHO) as: 'a disease in which excess body fat has accumulated to such an extent that health may be adversely affected'.[2] WHO also says: 'Obesity is a complex condition, one with serious social and psychological dimensions, that affects virtually all age and socioeconomic groups and threatens to overwhelm both developed and developing countries'.[3]

The rapid increase in obesity prevalence has crept up on this generation and awareness has only been highlighted in recent years.[1,2,4–6] As the Commons Health Select Committee report *Obesity* put it in 2004:

> Around two-thirds of the population of England are overweight or obese. Obesity has grown by almost 400% in the last 25 years and on present trends will soon surpass smoking as the greatest cause of premature loss of life. It will entail levels of sickness that will put enormous strains on the health service. On some predictions, today's generation of children will be the first for over a century for whom life-expectancy falls.[1] (p. 3)

DEFINING AND MEASURING OVERWEIGHT AND OBESITY

Body mass index

Overweight and obesity are most commonly defined using *body mass index* (BMI), a measure of relative weight for height. This is calculated by dividing weight in kilograms by height in metres squared (kg/m^2).

BMI provides the most useful population-level measure of obesity but it has some limitations, mainly:

- it does not take into account factors such as gender and age;
- it does not distinguish between weight associated with muscle and weight associated with fat; it is possible for people with well devel-

oped muscles (such as athletes) to have a high BMI and still be healthy.

The WHO classification of BMI is shown in Table 5.1.[2,7]

Waist measurement

People who are overweight and have central fat distribution are at greatest risk of developing heart disease and diabetes. This *central obesity* means that people are 'apple-shaped' with fat deposited around the abdomen, as opposed to 'pear-shaped' where there is more fat around the buttock area. Measurement of waist circumference is a convenient and simple method of identifying and recording central fat distribution. Table 5.2 indicates relative health risk in relation to waist measurement.[8]

Adults from the Indian subcontinent are particularly prone to central obesity and are very susceptible to diabetes and coronary heart disease. The cut-off points for BMI and waist measurements may need to be lower for the Asian population.

It is recommended that both waist and BMI measurements are used when working with overweight and obese individuals.[2,8,9]

Defining overweight and obesity in children

Obesity in children is defined as a BMI above the 98th centile and overweight as above the 91st centile of the UK reference charts for age and sex. (BMI centile charts, adjusted for growth, have been designed by the Child Growth Foundation. The charts are available to order from Harlow Printing Ltd via the website www.healthforallchildren.co.uk)

Measuring body fat

Bioelectrical impedance analysis (BIA) can be used to specifically measure body fat and lean tissue mass. It can distinguish between changes in fat and lean tissue during weight loss, which can be especially motivational in patients who become more active and improve body composition (increase muscle and decrease fat) in the absence of weight loss on the scales.

Table 5.1   WHO classification of obesity[2,7]

WHO classification	Terms more commonly used in UK	BMI (kg/m^2)
Underweight	Underweight	Below 18.5
Normal weight	Healthy weight	18.5–24.9
Pre-obese	Overweight	25–29.9
Obese class 1	Moderately obese	30–34.9
Obese class 2	Severely obese	35–39.9
Obese class 3	Morbidly obese	40 and above

Table 5.2   Health risk assessed by waist measurement[8]

	Increased risk	Substantial increased risk
Men	94 cm (= 37 inches) or more	102 cm (= 40 inches) or more
Women	80 cm (= 32 inches) or more	88 cm (= 35 inches) or more

Another indicator of body fat is skin fold thickness: the thickness of a pinch of skin and the fat layer beneath it, usually in the upper arm or below the shoulder blade. This is difficult to measure accurately and not recommended for general use. Research centres may also use other more sophisticated and accurate techniques to measure body composition.

CAUSES OF OBESITY

Obesity occurs when energy intake exceeds energy expenditure over a period of time. (Energy is usually measured in kilocalories – kcals – often just called calories.) The causes of obesity are multifactorial and often oversimplified; the reasons for the increasing trend in obesity are complex and varied.

Many factors, discussed below, interact to induce weight gain. In most cases it is not possible to identify a single factor as the cause of obesity.

AN OBESOGENIC ENVIRONMENT

Our present environment in the UK provides an abundance of energy dense foods and encourages an increase in sedentary behaviours, with a resulting decline in physical activity. This plays a major role in the development of obesity; it is often referred to as an obesogenic environment.

BEHAVIOURAL FACTORS

Behavioural causes of obesity are linked to an increased consumption of high calorie foods and a decrease in physical activity.

- **Physical activity:** the steady decline in physical activity levels of the population over the past 50 years is a key contributory factor in the rise in obesity. Occupational work has generally become more sedentary, and leisure time activities such as television viewing and computer games have replaced more active pastimes.[2]

- **Composition of diet:** there has been a marked shift in the composition of the diet, with an increase in the consumption of fat and a decrease in carbohydrate. As there is more than twice the number of calories in fat as in an equal weight of carbohydrate, this easily leads to over-consumption of calories without necessarily eating a greater total amount of food. High fat diets are associated with weight gain, especially in inactive people. Snacking and the loss of formalized meal patterns as well as frequent consumption of high calorie food and drinks are all linked to the increase in obesity.[2]

- **Eating patterns and portion sizes:** there has also been a major change in eating patterns over the past few decades. Eating outside the home and the use of 'convenience' foods has increased significantly. In many fast-food restaurants, high calorie foods are the predominant choices, and the price structure is often set to make bigger portion sizes more appealing. Studies have shown that if people are served larger portions, they are likely to eat them, encouraging them to develop larger appetites.[10]

PHYSIOLOGICAL
FACTORS

The metabolic control systems that govern regulation of body weight have been the focus of much research. Physiological controls include appetite, hunger, satiation and satiety, each of which has a different regulatory mechanism. (*Satiation* is the feeling of having had enough at the end of a meal; *satiety* is the feeling between meals of having eaten enough.) These controls involve highly complex interactions between neural and hormonal regulatory systems, which are often influenced by social and environmental factors.[11]

GENETIC FACTORS

Studies suggest that some people are genetically more susceptible to weight gain than others when exposed to our obesogenic environment.[2]

Estimates of the genetic contribution to weight gain in susceptible individuals range from 25–70%.[8] Obesity is regarded as a heterogeneous disorder rather than a single gene defect; single gene defects, for example Prader–Willi syndrome, are a rare cause of obesity. Over 200 genes have been identified as playing a role in the regulation of body weight, including those which influence appetite regulation, satiety signals and metabolic rate.[12]

MEDICAL FACTORS

● **Endocrine disorders:** certain rare endocrine disorders such as hypothyroidism, Cushing's disease and hypothalamic tumours result in hormone disturbances which can cause weight gain; these should be excluded as part of investigations into obesity in individuals.

● **Medication:** there are a number of drugs that can promote weight gain including corticosteroids, insulin, sulphonylureas (used in treatment of diabetes) and antidepressants.

LIFE CHANGES

● **Ageing:** most adults gradually increase their weight from early 20s up to their 50s. This is thought to be linked with a gradual decline in activity, without a compensating decrease in food intake.

● **Critical events:** dramatic changes in weight can occur at critical life stages such as after marriage, pregnancy or retirement. Those who stop playing sport are often vulnerable to weight gain in the same way as people who move from an active job to a less physically demanding job. People who become immobile through injury or illness can be liable to weight gain.

● **Smoking cessation:** Smoking cessation is often accompanied by some weight gain[2,8] and fear of putting on weight can be a barrier to giving up smoking. Smoking cessation advice needs to include help with weight management such as practical tips on choosing low calorie snacks and how to deal with cravings.

WHY IS OBESITY AN IMPORTANT PUBLIC HEALTH ISSUE?

Obesity is one of the greatest challenges facing modern society. The costs to the individual in terms of health and well-being, and to the NHS and the wider economy mean that it cannot be ignored.

ECONOMIC COSTS

The National Audit Office estimated that obesity cost the NHS at least £0.5 billion a year in 1998, with costs to the wider economy in England estimated at nearly £2 billion.[4] A further scrutiny in 2004 revised this, estimating that costs could be up to 42% higher.[1] Other estimates suggest that obesity-related disease costs the NHS in excess of £2 billion per year.[13]

PERSONAL IMPACT

Obesity has a major impact on individual health and well-being, both physically and emotionally. Social bias, prejudice and discrimination are not uncommon experiences for overweight and obese people; overweight children suffer name-calling and bullying, which is cited as one of the most distressing aspects of being overweight.[2]

HEALTH IMPACT

Thirty thousand premature deaths a year in England can be attributed to obesity, and it has been estimated that obesity shortens lives by 9 years.[4]

There are significant and wide-ranging health problems associated with obesity; the most common of these are:

- coronary heart disease
- type 2 diabetes
- hypertension
- certain types of cancer (postmenopausal breast, endometrial and ovarian cancer; cancer of the gallbladder and colon).

(See also Chs 1, 2 and 3 on 'Cancer', 'Diabetes' and 'Coronary heart disease and stroke' respectively.)

Other health consequences associated with obesity are:

- stroke
- hyperlipidaemia (raised levels of certain types of fat in the bloodstream)
- gallstones (but severe weight loss can also lead to an acute gallstone attack)
- breathlessness: respiratory disease, sleep apnoea (cessation of breathing during sleep)
- menstrual abnormalities
- pregnancy complications
- back and joint pain
- foot disorders
- stress incontinence
- psychological distress
- physical disability.

BENEFITS OF WEIGHT LOSS

Sustained weight loss is extremely difficult to achieve but it is worthwhile because intentional weight loss results in marked improvements in health. There is considerable evidence that even modest weight reduction produces important health benefits, including a reduction in overall mortality rates, type 2 diabetes and coronary heart disease.[8]

Table 5.3 shows the health benefits that can be gained from a 10% weight loss.[8] This is highly significant both from an individual and a

Table 5.3   The benefits of 10% weight loss[8]

Health parameter	Health benefits
Mortality rate	up to 20% fall in total mortality up to 30% fall in diabetes-related deaths up to 40% fall in obesity-related cancer deaths
Blood pressure	fall of 10 mmHg systolic fall of 20 mmHg diastolic
Diabetes	fall of 50% in fasting glucose
Lipids (levels of fats in the bloodstream)	fall of 10% total cholesterol fall of 15% LDL[a] fall of 30% triglycerides increase of 8% HDL[b]

[a]LDL – low density lipoprotein – undesirable fat
[b]HDL – high density lipoprotein – desirable because it signifies cholesterol being removed from the bloodstream to the liver

public health point of view. It means that, for example, a 20 stone woman losing 2 stone is significant in terms of health gain. It is no longer recommended that an 'ideal weight' (a BMI within the 18.5–25 'healthy' range) is a realistic target for most obese people. Aiming for unachievable weight loss can be demoralizing for both patient and practitioner.

WHO IS AT RISK? DO HEALTH INEQUALITIES FEATURE IN OBESITY?

It has already been mentioned that people are more at risk of becoming overweight or obese as they get older, when they experience life changes such as pregnancy or retirement, and if they stop smoking. In addition, specific population groups which are particularly at risk of becoming overweight or obese include:[2,8]

- children where one or both parents are overweight or obese;
- socially deprived groups or those on low income;
- those with low levels of education;
- some ethnic minority groups;
- people with learning difficulties.

Some of these are considered below in more detail. (See also Ch. 14 'Tackling inequalities in health'.)

LOW INCOME GROUPS

Those on low incomes often live in socially deprived circumstances, with poor access to shops and lack of transport to out-of-town supermarkets, relying on local shops where food is often more expensive. They also have less disposable income to bulk-buy or take advantage of special offers. For those on very low incomes, eating healthily is often not their top priority and feeding families with the cheapest foods available may be the only option.[5]

LOW LEVELS OF
EDUCATION

Obesity has been linked with low levels of education, though not exclusively.[2,8] Effective weight management requires a level of knowledge and understanding of the problem, along with the skills relating to menu planning, shopping and cooking.

ETHNIC MINORITY
GROUPS

Obesity rates are higher in certain ethnic groups such as people of South Asian origin and black Caribbean women.[2,8] Ethnic groups need special consideration for weight management advice, often best achieved through a combination of community activities and individual interventions. Special consideration needs to be given to suitable food choices and methods of cooking as well as culturally acceptable methods for increasing physical activity.

LEARNING
DIFFICULTIES

Interventions need to be targeted towards families and carers as well as individuals.[2,8] Support may need to include help with shopping and cooking choices as well as emphasizing the importance of physical activity.

TRENDS IN PREVALENCE OF OBESITY

As previously stressed, the prevalence of obesity has reached epidemic proportions. The majority of European countries have seen obesity increase by about 10–50% over the past 10 years and similar trends have been observed in other developed and less developed countries across the world.[14] Figure 5.1 shows obesity levels in selected European countries, with England particularly high in the 'league table'.[15]

The rise in obesity prevalence in the United Kingdom has been dramatic: it has trebled since 1980. In 2002 one in five adults (22% of men and 23% of women) were classified as obese, with nearly half of the population (48% of men and 40% of women) classified as overweight or obese.[16] These figures equate to 24 million adults in England[4] and figures are similar for Scotland and Wales.

Figure 5.1   Male and female obesity levels in selected European countries. Collated by the International Obesity Task Force from recent surveys. (Reproduced with permission from International Obesity Task Force.[15])

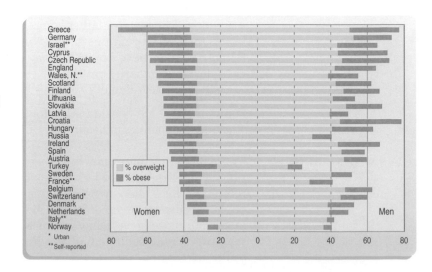

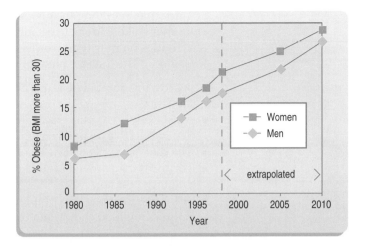

Figure 5.2   Trends in the prevalence of obesity in England. Adapted from the National Audit Office analysis of data from the Health Survey of England. (Reproduced with permission from National Audit Office 2001.[4])

If the current trend continues, it is estimated that over a quarter of the population in England will be obese (BMI above 30) by 2010 (see Fig. 5.2.)[4]

Childhood obesity

The increasing proportion of overweight and obese children is of particular concern. In 2001 in England 8.5% of 6 year olds and 15% of 15 year olds were obese and in the period between 1996 and 2001 the proportion of overweight children (aged 6–15 years) had increased by 7% and obese children by 3.5%.[5]

NATIONAL POLICY

NHS POLICY

Within the NHS the prevention and treatment of obesity is currently addressed through the National Service Frameworks for coronary heart disease, diabetes and mental health[17,18,19] and national strategies for cancer.[20] However, this has not led to effective strategies for tackling obesity. Many experts believe that obesity treatment and prevention should have a higher priority, bearing in mind its role in the development of diabetes, coronary heart disease and many other serious medical conditions.[1,6]

Current NICE guidance exists for drug use and surgery in obesity management.[21,22,23] A fully comprehensive NICE review on obesity and overweight, covering prevention and treatment, and produced in collaboration with the Health Development Agency, is due in 2007.[24] This needs to be backed by a comprehensive and coordinated approach at national and local level to meet the needs of individuals and local populations, making the best use of available resources.

WIDER GOVERNMENT POLICY

At a wider national level, the Department of Health has taken the government lead in addressing food and health issues. It published a *Food and Health Action Plan: Food and Health Problem Analysis* for comment in 2003.[25] (The Department of Health's website (www.dh.gov.uk) also publishes a summary of responses from a wide range of agencies with interests in health, food policy and food industry.) This was the first phase of an initiative involving the government working with the food industry and other stakeholders 'to establish a coherent and effective programme of activities on nutrition in order to achieve a healthier diet for people in England.'[25] The issues it highlighted included the following:

- A growing number of adults and children are affected by cardiovascular diseases, obesity, cancers and diabetes linked to poor diet.
- Most people eat more saturated fat, salt and sugar and less fruit and vegetables than experts recommend.
- The diet of people on low income is an area of particular concern.
- For most consumers, food choices are driven by value, convenience and lack of time.
- Attitudes to eating are complex and there are many non-health factors influencing food choice, such as price.

The next phase is the publication of the *Food and Health Action Plan*, planned for 2005.

Other government initiatives which have a bearing on healthy eating include Sure Start (www.surestart.gov.uk) and work in schools such as the Health Promoting Schools programme (www.euro.who.int) and the 5 a day National School Fruit Scheme (www.dh.gov.uk) to increase consumption of fruit and vegetables.

The next section discusses what more needs to be done at national and local level.

WHAT CAN WE DO ABOUT PREVENTION AND HEALTH PROMOTION?

This question is tackled looking at:

- promoting healthy eating (including breast feeding);
- preventing and tackling obesity at population level: what sort of approaches are needed; what national initiatives and calls to action have been initiated; what can be done at local level, including addressing overweight in children;
- helping obese and overweight individuals with appropriate services and treatments.

PROMOTING HEALTHY EATING

Healthy eating and adequate levels of physical activity are the basis for:

- primary prevention of obesity;
- secondary prevention of related heath problems (such as type 2 diabetes) by helping overweight or obese people to attain a healthier weight.

Physical activity is discussed in Chapter 6; here the focus is on what is meant by healthy eating.

What is 'healthy eating'?

The Food Standards Agency (website www.foodstandards.gov.uk) is an independent UK food safety watchdog set up by an Act of Parliament in 2000 to protect the public's health and consumer interests in relation to food. In 2001 it published guidelines on the recommended balance of

Box 5.1   Healthy eating: Food Standards Agency *Balance of Good Health* **(2001)[26]**

The Balance of Good Health aims to give people a practical message about healthy eating which applies to adults and children over 5.

Recommendations about what to eat and how much are based on five commonly accepted food groups:

- *Bread, cereals and potatoes* (including breakfast cereals, pasta, rice, noodles, maize, millet and cornmeal)
- *Fruit and vegetables* (5 portions a day are recommended including fresh, frozen, canned and dried; a glass of fruit juice also counts)
- *Milk and dairy* (milk, cheese, yoghurt and fromage frais; this group *excludes* butter, eggs and cream)
- *Meat, fish and alternatives* such as nuts, beans and pulses; one portion per week of oily fish such as salmon or sardines is recommended

- Foods containing *fat* (margarine, butter, spreading fats, cooking oils, cream, high fat foods such as chocolate, crisps and pastries); foods and drinks containing **sugar** (soft drinks, sweets, jam, sugar, cakes, puddings and biscuits).

Encouraging people to choose a variety of foods from the first four groups every day will help ensure that they obtain the wide range of nutrients their bodies need to remain healthy and function properly. Foods in the fifth group – foods principally containing fat and sugar – add extra variety, choice and palatability to meals. This group of foods should form the smallest part of the diet.

The key message is the *balance* of foods that should be consumed to achieve a healthy diet. This is shown by the different area occupied by each of the food groups in a 'plate' model (Fig. 5.3). However much food people need, the proportion of food from the different groups should remain the same.

Figure 5.3   Balance of good health: the plate model of food groups.

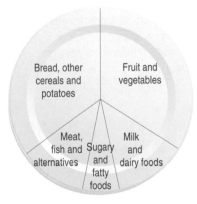

food in the diet (see Food Standards Agency website above, and British Nutrition Foundation website www.nutrition.org.uk). The main points are summarized in Box 5.1.

Breast feeding

There is growing interest in whether breast feeding has a role in preventing obesity in later life. The balance of evidence and expert opinion now seems to be that breast feeding does confer a protective effect for childhood obesity.[27] Also, of course, it brings many other benefits for mother and child, so there is nothing to be lost and much to be gained from promoting breast feeding. No discussion of 'what is healthy eating' should omit breast feeding, so key information from a Health Development Agency evidence briefing *The effectiveness of public health interventions to promote the initiation of breast feeding*[27] is summarized in Box 5.2.

Box 5.2   Breast feeding

Breast feeding provides complete nutrition for the development of healthy infants and is important for protection against gastroenteritis and respiratory infection in babies. There are strong indications that breast feeding also plays an important role preventing:

- otitis media (inflammation of the middle ear)
- urinary tract infection
- atopic disease (hypersensitivity reactions, e.g. hay fever, allergic asthma, atopic eczema) if a family history of atopy is present
- type 1 diabetes
- obesity.

Breast feeding is also beneficial to the mother's health:

- Women who do not breast feed are more likely to develop epithelial ovarian cancer.
- Women who breast feed are more likely to use up the body fat deposited in pregnancy and therefore less likely to be overweight following the pregnancy.

The World Health Organization recommends that wherever possible infants should be fed exclusively on breast milk from birth to 6 months, a position which is endorsed in the UK.

Rates of breast feeding are low: in 2002, the percentage of mothers who initially breast fed their babies was 71% in England and Wales, 63% in Scotland, and 54% in Northern Ireland, with mothers more likely to breast feed if they are from higher socio-economic groups, had reached higher educational levels, were aged over 30, and were feeding the first baby. Qualitative research on why some women on low incomes do not want to breast feed concluded that breast feeding is a practical skill; the confidence and commitment to breast feed successfully are best achieved by exposure to breast feeding rather than talking or reading about it.

Evidence on the most effective ways to increase breast feeding in the UK is scanty, but antenatal and postnatal intensive group and one-to-one education and counselling by trained healthcare professionals and peer counsellors show some evidence of effectiveness. Media campaigns can be effective in improving attitudes towards breast feeding. Multifaceted programmes have been shown to increase rates of mothers initiating breast feeding; this includes elements of media campaigning, health education, training of professionals, peer support for mothers, and structural changes in healthcare provision to encourage breast feeding.

PREVENTING AND TACKLING OBESITY AT POPULATION LEVEL

Prevention and management of obesity needs a public health approach[2] focusing on:

- elements of the social, cultural, political, physical and structural environment that affect the weight status of the population; in other words, creating a less obesogenic environment;
- processes and programmes to deal with those individuals and groups who are particularly at risk of developing obesity and related health problems;
- services for those individuals with existing obesity, focusing on weight reduction and maintenance, and secondary prevention of obesity-related conditions.

There are lessons to be learnt from successful public health approaches in other areas such as smoking.[2] The main features are:

- adequate duration and persistency
- a slow and staged approach
- legislative action

- education
- advocacy
- shared responsibility by consumers, communities, food industry and governments.

It is clear that prevention of obesity needs to be tackled at many different levels, involving many different agencies, as discussed below.

National initiatives and calls for action

A Leaner, Fitter Future is an initiative by the Medical Research Council Human Nutrition Research with the Association for the Study of Obesity and the London School of Hygiene and Tropical Medicine, launched in 2003.[28,29] It has brought together a wide range of stakeholders to discuss what is needed and identify opportunities for action, calling for a clear lead from government.

Secondly, in 2004 a working party of the Royal College of Physicians, the Royal College of Paediatrics and Child Health, and the Faculty of Public Health Medicine published *Storing up Problems: the Medical Case for a Slimmer Nation*, which discussed the impact and consequences of the 'obesity time bomb' and strategies to prevent obesity.[6] It recommended a comprehensive range of public health measures to address the obesity 'epidemic', and these are summarized in Box 5.3. It is to be hoped that a comprehensive approach such as this will be developed.

Finally, also in 2004, the House of Commons Health Select Committee published a report *Obesity*[1] which examined the prevalence, impact and causes of obesity, set out solutions in terms of both nutrition and physical activity, and made recommendations. It advocated a wide-ranging approach, similar to that in *Storing up Problems* (Box 5.3).[6] The Select Committee's report generated much media coverage, especially because it emphasized the scale and urgency of the problem, and strongly criticized the food industry, government departments and the NHS for failing to tackle the issues. It concluded thus:

> ... we note that it is difficult to establish the impact of any individual measure to combat so complex and challenging an issue as obesity; this is not, in our view, an excuse to delay and measures must be taken to tackle the nation's diet and its levels of activity. We acknowledge the responsibility of the individual in respect of his or her own health but believe that the Government must resist inaction caused by political anxiety over accusations of 'nanny statism'.[1] (p. 5)

Local community level

Meantime, what can be done at local level? There is scope for local action in a variety of ways, including:

- individual interventions as part of healthcare consultations
- public health messages through the media
- school-based programmes
- community development programmes
- workplace interventions.

An example of a community initiative was a US pilot campaign 'Colorado on the Move' (see www.uchsc.edu/nutrition/Coloradoonthemove) which

---

Box 5.3   Recommendations from Storing up Problems[6]

● **A cross-governmental task force** to develop and implement national strategies, which would include health, education, fiscal policies, transport, food and agriculture, sport and culture. It would engage the public, public services, local government, schools, the voluntary sector, industry and business. Specific priorities would be the promotion of healthy lifestyles for children and young people.

● **A government-led public education campaign** to improve people's understanding of the benefits of healthy eating and active living, to motivate people to eat a healthier diet and adopt a more active lifestyle. This should particularly aim to engage children, young people, disadvantaged people and those from ethnic groups at increased risk of increased fatness.

● **New standards in nutritional content, food labelling, and food marketing and promotion,** and incentives to encourage the production, promotion and sale of healthier foods.

● **Population-wide initiatives at local level to tackle obesity.** Public services should take the lead by promoting healthy eating and increased physical activity in public places and institutions, such as schools and hospitals. This should include reducing dependency on cars and increasing opportunities for walking, cycling, using stairs and other active forms of recreation and transport. All planning applications and public policies should require an assessment/prediction of health impact and encourage the incorporation of features to support healthy eating and physical activity.

● **NHS services:** the prevention and management of overweight and obesity should be included in all NHS plans, policies and clinical care strategies, with appropriate training for healthcare professionals.

● **Research** to improve understanding of the societal and cultural factors behind the epidemic of overweight and obesity, and the development and implementation of effective prevention and treatment.

Guiding principles for the implementation of such a strategy include:

● being long term and sustainable, recognizing that behaviour change is complex, difficult and takes time;
● helping those in most need and closing the health gap between different population groups resulting from geography, ethnicity and socio-economic status;
● promoting the positive benefits of healthy eating, active living and healthy weight;
● avoiding 'victim-blaming' which creates its own problems of guilt, stigma and alienation and bullying.

---

demonstrated that weight gain can be prevented by two small daily changes:

● take 2000 more steps (an extra mile)
● eat 100 calories less.

This was so successful that it has now been extended to a much larger campaign, 'America on the Move' (website: www.americaonthemove.org).

Prevention and treatment of obesity needs a coordinated and comprehensive response from NHS organizations and local authorities, along with the cooperation of food, sports and leisure industries.[5] Local healthcare services need to work closely with education and leisure services, public transport and food provision outlets to ensure that being more active and eating healthily are realistic options for all members of the community. Initiatives which encourage physical activity need to be promoted at every opportunity and the appointment of local physical activity and/or healthy eating coordinators by primary care trusts is a welcome move to support this.

The move away from traditional diet has led to a loss of cooking, menu planning and shopping skills which needs to be addressed, both through the school curriculum and through community-based programmes such as those aiming to help people gain skills and knowledge about shopping and preparing food. The availability of healthy food choices in shops, restaurants and take-away outlets is essential if the rising tide of obesity is to be combated.

In its evidence review on the management of obesity and overweight,[30] the Health Development Agency drew the following conclusions:

- The evidence base for treating obesity and overweight is sound, but this learning is not always translated into changes in practice.

- There is a lack of evidence on strategies to prevent excessive weight gain, and strategies for maintenance of weight loss.

- For treatment of obesity, targeted programmes can be effective. There is evidence to support the use of workplace interventions for the treatment of obesity.

Prevention and treatment of obesity and overweight in children

A focus on children is clearly desirable in an attempt to prevent the development of obesity in adult life. Children from families where one or both parents are overweight are most at risk of developing obesity.[8] Basic issues are that:

- obesity in children may be prevented by increasing activity and decreasing inactive occupations (such as watching TV) and eating a well balanced healthy diet;
- family support is necessary for children to achieve a healthy lifestyle;
- healthy schools initiatives can also contribute to the prevention of obesity in children.[2]

Evidence supports the use of multifaceted school-based interventions to reduce obesity and overweight in schoolchildren, particularly girls.[30] These interventions include:

- nutrition education
- physical activity promotion
- reduction in sedentary behaviour
- behavioural therapy
- teacher training
- curricular material
- modification of school meals and tuck shops.

More narrowly focused school and family interventions had limited or no evidence to support them as a means of preventing obesity.[30]

Approaches to treatment of individual children should generally aim to help children to maintain their weight so they can 'grow into it'.[31] Family-based behaviour modification programmes have also been shown to be effective.[30]

HELPING OBESE AND OVERWEIGHT INDIVIDUALS

Successfully helping an obese individual to lose weight is important to achieve physical, emotional and psychological benefits for the patient, and because it can help to prevent associated problems such as heart disease, strokes and type 2 diabetes.

Service provision

Although obesity is classified as a chronic disease by the WHO,[2] there are limited NHS services in place which offer effective treatment.

Obesity needs to be managed mainly at primary care level by primary care trusts with support from specialist services for more severe and complicated cases. Well structured obesity and overweight management services are needed to provide effective care for individuals with a condition which now affects about half of the population. The NHS cannot cope with this burden alone and therefore close links need to be established with non-NHS obesity services to provide a structured, coordinated service. Quality controls need to be in place to ensure that high quality, evidence-based services are developed.

With the increasing demand for effective services for obesity management, there is an urgent need to develop training for all those involved in their provision. Because obesity has traditionally not been viewed as a serious medical condition, training has not been in place to equip healthcare professionals and others with the knowledge and skills to manage this complex condition.

Attitudes towards obesity

An appreciation of the difficulties that some people experience in managing their weight is essential for an effective helping relationship. Healthcare professionals and others such as people who work in leisure industries are not immune to being influenced by the attitudes of society, and sometimes retain attitudes linking negative stereotypes with people who are overweight or obese. A sensitive manner that demonstrates empathy and understanding is required.

Many healthcare professionals express concerns about how to deal with weight management issues, as talking about lifestyle changes is very different from treating medical conditions such as an infection or acute pain. Most people are already aware that they are overweight and do not welcome comments like 'you need to do something about your weight'. Few patients see weight as their primary problem and so it is helpful to link it with a presenting medical condition.

Screening

Screening for overweight and obesity can be done by GP practices recording BMIs for all patients and targeting those most at risk from obesity and its associated problems. Also, concerned individuals often approach their doctor or nurse for help.

Assessment

Simply telling patients to exercise more and eat less is not effective and research shows that a more skilled approach is required.[29]

For patients who would benefit from medical supervision, assessment forms the basis of any intervention. A full medical history is essential, along with listening empathically to the patient's experience of previous weight loss attempts, understanding their social background, and having a clear picture of current eating and activity patterns. This will indicate where beneficial changes can be made. Difficulties in making proposed changes need to be discussed along with exploring ways to overcome potential barriers.

Behaviour modification

There is evidence to support the use of behaviour modification in conjunction with changes to diet and levels of activity.[30] Changing eating and physical activity behaviour is complex; it is often the most challenging aspect of obesity management, both for the person and the practitioner. An understanding of what influences health behaviour and how to facilitate change is essential for effective weight management. Practitioners need to be equipped with high level skills to treat this complex condition.

Approaches taken from the world of psychology, such as motivational interviewing and cognitive behaviour therapy, are discussed in Chapter 14 'Helping individuals to change behaviour'. Specific strategies include assessing readiness to change, exploring ambivalence to change, self-monitoring, goal setting, problem solving, self-rewards, relapse prevention, stress management, social support, stimulus control (identifying and modifying environmental barriers) and cognitive restructuring.[32,33]

It is best to make changes to lifestyle in small steps and to focus on those that can be maintained long term. Support is a key factor in achieving change and it is therefore important to establish where support will come from and what type of support is required.

Dietary changes

First line treatment for obesity should always commence with appropriate changes to diet and levels of activity. Physical activity is particularly important for helping to prevent weight regain; ways to increase activity are discussed in detail in Chapter 6 'Physical activity'.

Energy balance

The basic undisputed fact about weight loss is that in order to lose weight, the body needs to be in a state of negative energy balance. A deficit of 500 kcals per day, achieved through a combination of diet and physical activity, will result in weight loss at the desirable rate in most people.

The desirable rate of weight loss is 1–2 pounds (0.5–1 kg) per week and a realistic goal is 5–10% weight loss over 3–6 months, after which progress and goals should be reviewed.[34]

In practice, most men will lose 0.5 kg a week on 1800 to 2000 kcals per day, and most women on 1400 to 1500 kcals per day. People with a high BMI have higher energy requirements than people of 'normal' weight, so will lose weight on higher calorie intakes.

Changes to diet

These should focus on the following:[35]

● Establish regular meal patterns. Many overweight people have erratic eating habits, going without food for long periods of time, only to overcompensate when they do eat. In the obese population, the prevalence of binge eating has been estimated to be 20–40%, so helping people to establish regular eating patterns is key to weight management programmes.[36]

● Ensure the nutritional adequacy of the diet; dietary advice should be based on the model in Box 5.1.

● Reduce calorie intake. This can often be achieved with surprising ease for some people by focusing on a few key calorie-dense foods and/or portion sizes of foods such cheese, butter and oil. But for others, it is considerably more challenging.

Other dietary options include:

● Meal replacements (milk shakes, soups, bars or portion controlled ready-meals providing 1200–1400 calories per day): these can be a valuable method for some people to achieve a reduced calorie intake. There is good evidence to support their efficacy for use with people who struggle to lose weight using more traditional dietary approaches.[37]

● Very low calorie diets: these can be used for patients requiring rapid weight loss for medical reasons; they consist of liquid meal replacements which provide 800 kcals or less per day and are nutritionally complete. Patients require close medical and dietetic supervision.[9,38]

● Commercial slimming clubs: many people find that attending a group programme is an excellent way of helping them to manage their weight. It is important that healthcare professionals have good knowledge about local options and continue to provide ongoing support to patients, and that the programme directly meets their needs.[38] Evaluation of commercial slimming clubs is a major research priority; little is known about attendance rates, short and long term weight loss, the effects on clients' health, and psychosocial factors.[39]

Weight maintenance

One of the biggest challenges in weight management is *sustaining* weight loss; many people have a history of repeated cycles of weight gain and loss. Practitioners have an important role in emphasizing the chronic nature of obesity and the importance of lifelong weight management. Therefore it is more helpful to talk about weight management programmes, which have a *weight loss* and a *weight maintenance* phase.

Patients should be encouraged to make changes to diet and physical activity which they can sustain, and to continue monitoring their weight and waist measurement, so that any weight regain can be tracked and appropriate action taken.

Maintaining weight lost – what works?

Over the past decade an increasing number of studies have been directed towards the achievement of weight maintenance. Whilst no simple solution has been highlighted, a number of different strategies have been evaluated. Those emerging as most significant are extended support along with continued changes to diet and physical activity.[40]

The Health Development Agency's review of strategies for weight treatment and maintenance[30] also found evidence to support:

● continued therapist contact when combined with behavioural therapy and relapse prevention training;
● continued therapist contact by mail and telephone.

A theme which emerges clearly is the need to emphasize permanent 'lifestyle changes', as opposed to 'quick fixes', and continue to offer lifelong support to patients. There are implications for practitioners about how best to provide long term contact and support. It may be offered by different members of the multidisciplinary team at different times throughout the patient's life. It is also important to recognize the supportive role that family, friends, peers and other agencies such as leisure services, commercial slimming clubs and home-based programmes can play.

A US study gives further pointers about what may help weight maintenance. Data from the National Weight Control Registry in the USA provide information on 3000 subjects who lost 30 pounds or more and successfully maintained the weight lost for a year or more.[41] The common factors highlighted are listed below:

● The majority were eating a high carbohydrate, low fat diet, which is consistent with current healthy eating guidelines. Less than 1% reported following a high protein, low carbohydrate (Atkins type) diet. Most meals were eaten in the home.

● The majority monitor their weight and food intake and levels of activity. This highlights the benefits of self-monitoring as a behavioural strategy which helps with weight management.

● The majority ate regular meals and only 4% never ate breakfast. It appears that skipping meals leads to over consumption at another time.

● The majority engage in high levels of physical activity. Walking was the most popular activity. This was measured by using a pedometer; subjects averaged 11 000 steps per day, which is equivalent to about 4 miles or one hour of walking daily.

Drug treatment and surgery

The use of medication is appropriate for obese patients who also have other related medical conditions and for whom lifestyle changes have not been successful. Currently there are two drugs which are licensed for use on the NHS (orlistat, which works by reducing fat absorption, and sibutramine, which acts to produce feelings of satiety) with strict criteria governing their use.[21,22] Further guidance is given by the Royal College of Physicians[42] and the National Obesity Forum.[43]

Surgery to treat obesity (bariatric surgery) can be used for patients with clinically severe obesity, following NICE guidelines, but in reality currently there is limited availability on the NHS.[23] The surgery modifies the size of the stomach and/or bypasses some of the gut, so that less food is eaten and/or less is absorbed. Patients who have had bariatric surgery need lifelong monitoring and support. (For further information on bariatric surgery visit the NICE website www.nice.org.uk. For patients, the website www.wlsinfo.com provides useful information.)

CURRENT DEBATES AND DILEMMAS

In summary, at local and national level, there is debate about addressing the needs of obese people: what services to provide, how to provide them, and how to resource them given competing demands for limited NHS funds.

Nationally, the debate is wider: how to engage the many interests, including those of the food and advertising industry, in tackling obesity; and how to balance the freedom of individuals to eat what they choose and be as active (or not) as they like, with the responsibility to make our environment less obesogenic.

COMMON MYTHS AND QUESTIONS

Obese individuals have a slower metabolism than lean individuals

This is *false*. Resting metabolic rate (RMR) accounts for approximately 70% of total energy expenditure. RMR is related to lean body mass, which is usually greater in overweight people.

Overweight people are less active than lean individuals

This is *false*. Studies show that on average, overweight people are not particularly inactive compared with lean individuals, although high levels of obesity can result in lower levels of exercise.

Some people are genetically predisposed to obesity

This is *true*. There is increasing evidence that genetic factors relating to metabolism, appetite, and satiety signals contribute to the development of obesity. Estimates of a genetic component range from 25–70% in susceptible individuals.[8]

Do special 'slimming diets' work?

There is no 'magic cure' for overweight. So-called 'slimming diets' may help people to lose weight in the short term, but they are usually 'fad' diets, best avoided because they:

- may not ensure adequate nutritional intake;
- may result in abnormalities of metabolism and body chemistry;
- may cause health damage in the long term;
- do not encourage the establishment of lifelong, sustainable healthy eating and activity patterns which will maintain weight loss.

The British Dietetic Association stresses the importance of making sustainable changes to achieve long term success, cautioning against a 'quick-fix' diet.[44] It's a quick-fix diet if it:

- recommends 'magic' or 'miracle' foods to burn fat – foods can't burn fat;
- promotes bizarre quantities of only one food or type of food, e.g. eating only grapefruit, meat or cabbage soup;
- suggests rigid menus, limiting food choice and the times you can eat;
- suggests a rapid weight loss of more than 2 pounds (1 kg) a week;
- allows foods to be eaten only in specific combinations;
- fails to warn people with diabetes, high blood pressure or a kidney disorder to seek medical advice before commencing the diet;
- focuses on appearance rather than the health benefits of being a healthier weight.

WHAT DON'T WE KNOW ENOUGH ABOUT YET?

There is an urgent need for research on effective interventions for the prevention and treatment of obesity in children and in adults. The Health Development Agency calls for research which assesses the effectiveness of interventions and particularly highlights the need to include lower socio-economic, ethnic minority and vulnerable population groups in intervention studies to help address known inequalities.[30]

The Royal College of Physicians 2004 report[6] recommends research:

- to improve understanding of the social and cultural factors behind the epidemic of overweight and obesity – expanding the evidence base on the causes of obesity;
- on the development and implementation of effective prevention and treatment – expanding the evidence base on the health benefits and cost-effectiveness of prevention and treatments.

Finally, studies show that many people who successfully lose weight put it on again within 5 years.[40] Future research also needs to focus on effective weight maintenance.

Key sources of further information and help

Organizations and websites

- **Association for the Study for Obesity:** www.aso.org.uk. Promotes research into the causes, prevention and treatment of obesity, encourages action to reduce the prevalence of obesity, and facilitates contact between individuals and organizations interested in obesity and weight management.
- **British Dietetic Association:** www.bda.uk.com. The professional association for dietitians in the UK. Publishes strategy and policy documents, briefings and position papers on dietetics and nutritional issues.
- **British Nutrition Foundation:** www.nutrition.org.uk. A charitable organization which promotes the nutritional well-being of society through the impartial interpretation and effective dissemination of scientifically based nutritional knowledge and advice. Provides information on food, nutrition and healthy eating.
- **Dietitians Working in Obesity Management (UK):** www.domuk.org. An interest group for dietitians, aiming to improve prevention and management of obesity in the UK. Provides training, update and resources.
- **Food Standards Agency:** www.food.gov.uk/healthiereating/. The Food Standards Agency is an independent food safety watchdog set up in 2000 to protect the public's health and consumer interests in relation to food. Provides information on healthy eating, and food and weight.

- **National Institute of Clinical Excellence:** www.nice.org.uk. Provides guidance on medical and surgical treatment of obesity.
- **National Obesity Forum:** www.nationalobesityforum.org.uk. An independent medical organization established in 2000 to raise awareness of the growing impact of obesity and overweight on patients and the NHS. For healthcare professionals, aiming to use all available resources in the media, politically, educationally and professionally to enable all practitioners to confidently treat overweight patients.
- **Weightwise:** www.bdaweightwise.com. A consumer website of the British Dietetic Association.

Reports

- **Commons Select Committee** report.[1] Can be downloaded from: www.parliament.the-stationery-office.co.uk/pa/cm/cmhealth.htm.
- **Department of Health:** *Food and Health Action Plan.*[25]
- **Health Development Agency** www.hda-online.org.uk. The national authority on what works to improve people's health and reduce health inequalities. It gathers evidence and produces advice for policy makers, professionals and practitioners, working alongside them to get evidence into practice. See HDA evidence briefings.[27,30]
- **Royal College of Physicians**, the Royal College of Paediatrics and Child Health, and the Faculty of Public Health Medicine report.[6]

References

1. House of Commons Select Committee. Obesity. London: The Stationery Office; 2004. Online. Available: http://www.parliament.the-stationery-office.co.uk/pa/cm/cmhealth.htm
2. World Health Organization. Obesity: preventing and managing the global epidemic. Geneva: WHO; 2000.
3. World Health Organization. Controlling the global obesity epidemic. Online. Available: http://www.who.int/nut 9 March 2003.
4. National Audit Office. Tackling obesity in England. Report by the Comptroller and Auditor General. Norwich: The Stationery Office; 2001.
5. Department of Health. Annual report of the Chief Medical Officer. London: DOH; 2002.
6. Royal College of Physicians, the Royal College of Paediatrics and Child Health and the Faculty of Public Health Medicine. Storing up problems: the medical case for a slimmer nation. London: Royal College of Physicians; 2004. Online. Available: http://www.rcplondon.ac.uk
7. Thomas B, ed. In conjunction with the British Dietetic Association. Manual of dietetic practice. 3rd edn. Oxford: Blackwell; 2001.
8. Scottish Intercollegiate Guidelines Network. Obesity in Scotland: a national clinical guideline for use in Scotland (SIGN 8). Edinburgh: SIGN; 1996.
9. National Obesity Forum (NOF). Guidelines on management of adult obesity and overweight in primary care. 2003. Online. Available: http://www.nationalobesityforum.org.uk
10. Nielsen SM, Popkin BM. Patterns and trends in food portion sizes, 1977–1998. JAMA 2003; 289:450–453.
11. Prentice A, Stubbs J. Aetiology of obesity. In: British Nutrition Foundation. Obesity: report of the British Nutrition Foundation's task force. London: BNF; 1999.
12. Price AR. Genetics and common obesities. In: Wadden T A, Stunkard A J. Handbook of obesity treatment. New York: Guilford; 2002; 73–94
13. Medical Research Council. Online. Available: http://www.mrc-hnr.cam.ac.uk/NutHlth/Obesity May 2004.
14. World Health Organization. Diet, nutrition and the prevention of chronic diseases. Geneva: World Health Organization; 2003.
15. International Obesity Task Force. www.iotf.org. Personal communication.
16. Joint Health Surveys Unit (on behalf of the Department of Health). Health survey for England, 2002. Norwich: The Stationery Office; 2003.
17. Department of Health. National Service Framework for coronary heart disease. London: DOH; 2000. Online. Available: http://www.doh.gov.uk/nsf/chd
18. Department of Health. National Service Framework for diabetes: standards. London: DOH; 2001. Online. Available: http://www.doh.gov.uk/nsf/diabetes
19. Department of Health. National Service Framework for mental health. London: HMSO; 1999. Online. Available: http://www.doh.gov.uk/nsf/mentalhealth
20. Department of Health. The NHS cancer plan. London: DOH; 2000.
21. National Institute of Clinical Excellence. NICE Technology Appraisal No. 22. The use of orlistat for the treatment of obesity in adults. London: NICE; 2004. Online. Available: http://www.nice.org.uk
22. National Institute of Clinical Excellence. NICE Technology Appraisal No. 31. The use of sibutramine for the treatment of obesity in adults. London: NICE; 2004. Online. Available: http://www.nice.org.uk
23. National Institute of Clinical Excellence. NICE Technology Appraisal No. 46. The use of surgery to aid weight reduction for people with morbid obesity. London: NICE; 2002. Online. Available: http://www.nice.org.uk
24. National Institute of Clinical Excellence. Obesity: the prevention, identification, evaluation, treatment and weight maintenance of overweight and obesity in adults. London: NICE; expected 2007. (See www.nice.org.uk)
25. Department of Health. Food and health action plan: food and health problem analysis for comment. London: DOH; 2003. Online. Available: http://www.dh.gov.uk
26. Food Standards Agency (www.foodstandards.gov.uk) and British Nutrition Foundation (www.nutrition.org.uk). The balance of good health; 2001.
27. Health Development Agency. The effectiveness of public health interventions to promote the initiation of breast feeding. London: HDA; 2003.
28. Medical Research Council Association for the Study of Obesity. A leaner, fitter future: options for action. A multi-sectoral perspective on overweight in children. London: London School of Hygiene and Tropical Medicine; November 2003. Online. Available: http://www.mrc-hnr.cam.ac.uk May 2004.
29. Jebb S. Obesity tsar: dealing with population obesity in the UK. Dietetic Adviser (British Dietetic Association) April 2004; p. 20.
30. Health Development Agency. The management of obesity and overweight: an analysis of reviews of diet, physical activity and behavioural approaches. London: HDA; 2003.
31. Scottish Intercollegiate Guidelines Network. Management of Obesity in Children and Young People (SIGN 69). Edinburgh: SIGN; 2003.
32. Rollnick S, Mason P, Butler C. Health behaviour change: a guide for practitioners. London: Churchill Livingstone; 1999.
33. Foreyt JP, Paschali AA. Behaviour therapy. In: Kopleman P. The management of obesity and related disorders. London: Martin Dunitz; 2001;165–178.
34. Lean M. Clinical handbook of weight management. 2nd edn. London: Martin Dunitz; 2002;53–63.
35. British Dietetic Association. Position paper. Obesity treatment: future directions and the contributions of dietitians. J Hum Nutr Dietetics 1997; 10:95–101.

36. Marcus DM. Binge eating and obesity. In: Brownell KD, Fairburn CG. Eating disorders and obesity. London: Guilford Press; 1995;441–444.

37. Heymsfield SB, Mierlo CAJ, Knaap HCM, et al. Weight management using a meal replacement strategy: meta and pooling analysis from six studies. IJO 2003; 27(5): 537–549.

38. Jackson D, Kushner R. Commercial programmes. In: Bessesen DH, Kushner R. Evaluation and management of obesity. Philadelphia: Hanley and Belfus; 2002;47–51.

39. Cormillot A. Commercial and self-help approaches to weight management. In: Brownell KD, Fairburn CG. Eating disorders and obesity. London: Guilford; 1995;498–503.

40. Perri MG, Corsica JA. Improving the maintenance of weight lost in behavioural treatment of obesity. In: Wadden TA, Stunkard AJ. Handbook of obesity treatment. New York: Guilford Press; 2002;357–379.

41. Klem ML, Wing RR, McGuire MT, et al. A descriptive study of individuals successful at longterm maintenance of substantial weight loss. Am J Clin Nutr 1997; 66:239–246.

42. Royal College of Physicians. Clinical management of overweight and obese patients with particular reference to the use of drugs. London: RCP; 1998.

43. National Obesity Forum. Pharmacotherapy guidelines for obesity management in adults. 2002. Online. Available: http://www.nationalobesityforum.org.uk

44. The British Dietetic Association. Food facts. Want to lose weight and keep it off. Birmingham: BDA; 2003. Online. Available: http://www.bda.uk.com

Chapter 6

Physical activity

Chris Riddoch

SUMMARY OVERVIEW AND LINKS TO OTHER TOPICS

Low levels of physical activity are now a major public health problem, affecting children as well as adults. The public health impact of inactivity is as great as that of smoking cigarettes or unhealthy eating, and the health benefits of increased activity are substantial.

Inactivity results from changed patterns of transport and work, and sedentary occupations and entertainment, over the last decades. Most adults do not meet current activity recommendations, and only around two thirds of 2–11 year olds report activity levels that meet recommendations for children. The trend of decreasing activity seems to be getting worse for adults, whereas children's activity levels seem to be stable over recent years.

People of higher socio-economic status are more physically active in their leisure time, and walk more. Men in the lowest social class (which includes manual workers) are more physically active at work than those in higher social classes, but there is little difference by social class among women.

The importance of physical activity is now recognized in national policy, with recommendations for healthy levels of physical activity set since 1996.

In general, changes to the physical environment which make activity easier and more pleasant can result in greater improvements in population health than attempts to change people's individual lifestyle. However, interventions targeting individuals, including those in healthcare settings, can also be effective in helping people to become more active. From a public health perspective, assisting all people to improve their activity levels will produce the greatest population health benefit, with the least active people having the most to gain.

We need to know more about the barriers which stop adults and children from being active in order to plan more effective interventions.

Other chapters particularly linked with physical activity are Chapter 5 'Obesity', Chapter 13 'Tackling inequalities in health' and Chapter 14 'Helping individuals to change behaviour'. Physical activity is also a factor in cancer, coronary heart disease and strokes, diabetes and mental health, so the chapters dealing with those issues – Chapters 1, 2, 3 and 12 respectively – are also relevant.

WHAT IS PHYSICAL ACTIVITY?

Physical activity can be defined as 'any force exerted by skeletal muscle that results in energy expenditure above resting level'.[1] The term therefore includes the full range of human movement, from competitive sport and exercise to active hobbies, walking, cycling, or the physical activities of daily living.

The term is often used interchangeably with the similar term *exercise*, but technically, exercise is different: 'planned bouts of physical activity usually pursued for personal health and fitness goals. A subset of physical activity, which is volitional, planned, structured, repetitive and aimed at improvement or maintenance of any aspect of fitness or health.'[1]

Physical activity has several dimensions (see Box 6.1).

Aerobic activity

One important type of physical activity – for health – is *aerobic activity*. This is activity that predominantly uses aerobic energy metabolism: the production of energy by the oxidation of the various fuels used for exercise – carbohydrate, fat and (to a lesser extent) protein. Light and moderate intensity exercise is predominantly aerobic. More vigorous exercise uses more anaerobic energy metabolism – the production of energy in the absence of oxygen. Most activities involve a mixture of both energy pathways.

Aerobic activity is intended to increase oxygen consumption and benefit the lungs and cardiovascular (heart and circulation) systems.

Box 6.1   Dimensions of physical activity

All physical activity can be described in terms of its principal dimensions:

- *Frequency*: how often you are active
- *Time*: the length of a single bout of activity
- *Intensity*: how hard the activity is
- *Mode*: the type of activity, e.g. walking, swimming
- *Volume*: the total amount of activity – the total energy you expended.

Intensity is the most complicated to understand. It is the rate of energy expenditure during the activity – in other words, how hard a person is working. A fitter individual will perceive the intensity of a specific activity to be lower compared with an unfit individual because the fitter individual uses a smaller proportion of their fitness reserve (or capacity). The fitter body copes with the physical task more comfortably.

Lifestyle activity

Activities that are performed as part of everyday life, such as climbing stairs, commuting on foot or bicycle can be termed *lifestyle activities*. They are normally contrasted with *programmed activities* such as attending a dance class or fitness training session.

Fitness

It is common to see physical activity used synonymously with fitness. However, the two are very different. Whereas physical activity is a behaviour – as described above – fitness is 'a set of attributes that people have or achieve that relates to the ability to perform physical activity'.[1] Specifically, it refers to the ability to perform a given physical task in a specified physical, social and psychological environment.[2]

The main elements of fitness are:

- aerobic capacity (your maximal ability to exercise aerobically)
- strength
- flexibility
- speed
- power.

Optimum levels of body fat are also considered an element of fitness. Fitness components can be sports-related or health-related, or both.

An important dimension of fitness in terms of health is aerobic fitness, often referred to as cardiorespiratory (heart and lung) fitness. The technically correct term is *aerobic power*: the body's maximal capacity to perform aerobic physical activity. It comprises two elements:

- the ability of the heart and circulatory system to deliver blood (containing fuel and oxygen) to the working muscles, and
- the ability of the cells of the working muscles to extract and utilize the fuel and oxygen and perform aerobic work (via aerobic metabolism).

Health-related fitness

Health-related fitness is a dimension of fitness that goes beyond pure physical function.[2] It encompasses the following:

- Sufficient functional capacity to perform activities of daily living without undue discomfort. The main determinants are the physical condition of the cardiorespiratory and musculoskeletal (muscle and bone) systems.
- Optimal weight control. The main determinants are regular physical activity and healthy diet.
- Low levels of risk factors for major diseases, for example, normal levels of body fat, blood pressure, lipids (fats in the bloodstream) and insulin sensitivity.
- Optimal psychological and social well-being, for example, good mental health and membership of social networks.

Sport

Finally, the term 'sport' is often used when speaking about physical activity. But this is different again: 'a subset of physical activity, which involves structured competitive situations governed by rules. In Europe, sport is often used in a wider context to include all exercise and leisure physical activity'.[3]

WHY IS PHYSICAL ACTIVITY AN IMPORTANT PUBLIC HEALTH ISSUE?

Low levels of physical activity are now a major public health problem, affecting children as well as adults.

Health impact of inactivity

The overall health impact of inactivity is as great as that of smoking cigarettes or unhealthy eating.[4] The disease and disability caused by inactivity bring about serious and unnecessary human suffering and reductions in quality of life for individuals, families and the wider community.

The World Health Organization has reported that physical inactivity is one of the ten leading causes of death in developed countries, producing 1.9 million deaths worldwide per year.[5] It estimates that physical inactivity is responsible for the following proportions of some of the most common diseases in developed countries:

- 23% of ischaemic heart disease for men and 22% for women
- 16% of colon cancer for men and 17% for women
- 15% of diabetes mellitus
- 12% of strokes for men and 13% for women
- 11% of breast cancer.

The 2004 Chief Medical Officer's report *At Least 5 a Week: Evidence on the Impact of Physical Activity and its Relationship to Health* contains a detailed review of the role of physical activity with respect to prevention and treatment of the major chronic diseases.[6] In this report the full impact of sedentary lifestyles is described, together with the potential health gain from becoming more active:

> This report must be the wake-up call that changes attitudes to active lifestyles in every household. Being active is no longer simply an option – it is essential if we are to live healthy and fulfilling lives into old age.[6] (p. iii)

Low levels of physical activity in England are a significant factor in the dramatic increase in prevalence of obesity. Maintaining activity throughout life is important in avoiding weight gain. Physical activity by itself can result in modest weight loss of around 0.5 kg–1 kg per month, but the most effective way to lose weight is by a combination of activity and dietary restriction. Only a small proportion of people following weight loss programmes maintain their weight loss in the long term, but those people who achieve and maintain regular physical activity are the most likely to be successful. (See also Ch. 5 'Obesity' for further reading on overweight and obesity.)

Financial costs of inactivity

Estimated costs which take into account the direct expense of treatment and the indirect effects through increased sickness absence are £8.2 billion annually.[7] This does not include the contribution of inactivity to obesity which in itself has been estimated to cost £2.5 billion annually.[8] If the proportion of insufficiently active people were reduced by just 5%, theoretically a £300 million saving in costs per year would be achieved.

The benefits of activity

There is no doubt that the human body thrives on regular physical activity and reacts adversely to inactivity. Humans have inherited a genome within which important genes may only express themselves appropriately within an environment of regular physical activity. When activity levels fall below critical thresholds, gene expression changes and overt clinical disorders such as heart disease and some cancers manifest themselves.[9] With the industrial revolution and more recently the emergence of computerization, food availability and the energy required to access food have become seriously mismatched, leading to a new pandemic of metabolic diseases such as obesity and diabetes.

The benefits of physical activity are summarized in Box 6.2.

Becoming more active can bring substantial benefit. With regard to all-cause mortality and some aspects of disease, such as coronary heart disease and diabetes, a clear dose–response relationship with physical

---

Box 6.2   The benefits of physical activity

Regular physical activity can:

- help to control weight and reduce body fat
- lower blood cholesterol levels
- improve circulation and lower blood pressure
- strengthen the heart
- tone muscles
- strengthen bones
- keep joints mobile
- help to regulate blood glucose and prevent diabetes
- improve sleep patterns
- promote mental health and well-being.

Figure 6.1   Relationship between health risk and physical activity or fitness level.[6] (Reproduced with permission from the Department of Health.)

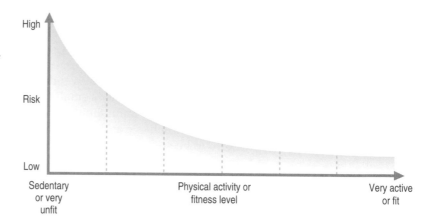

activity exists: greater benefits occur with greater activity participation (see Fig. 6.1).[6]

A physical activity energy expenditure of 500–1000 kcals per week (about 6–12 miles of walking for an average-weight individual, compatible with current recommended physical activity guidelines for adults) reduces the risk of dying from all causes by 20–30%. These considerable health benefits hold for both women and men and are evident even up to the age of 80 years.[10]

From a public health perspective, promoting activity to all people will produce the greatest health gain, with the least active having the most to gain.

WHAT CAUSES THE PROBLEM OF SEDENTARY LIVING?

The fitness boom of the latter part of the twentieth century has essentially failed to compensate for the loss of more traditional physical activities, especially the physical activity of work.[11]

Changing patterns of transport and work, electronic communication, internet shopping, energy-saving devices such as escalators, motorized lawn mowers, washing machines and remote controls, as well as sedentary entertainment such as television and computer games, have made it possible for us to be virtually inactive the whole time – but with our minds occupied. While the loss of any one of these activities will have only a marginal impact on energy expenditure, the combined effect of all these lifestyle changes together is substantial.

The most visible sign of these changes is the increasing prevalence of obesity, as people find it impossible to eat only a small amount of food to compensate for their very low energy expenditure.

HOW IS PHYSICAL ACTIVITY ADDRESSED IN NATIONAL POLICY?

National health policies

Physical activity has not been at the forefront of national policy until relatively recently. However, physical activity is mentioned in most of the

National Service Frameworks[12,13,14,15] and there are many local initiatives such as exercise referral schemes[16,17] and community-based activity promotion schemes.

Recommendations for healthy levels of physical activity have been set for the nation[18] and have been refined to be more specific for individual diseases[6] (see Box 6.3).

In 2004, the Chief Medical Officer's report *At Least 5 a Week*[6] firmly established physical activity as a major public health issue. This followed a similar major policy document in the United States.[19]

Sport England

A further major policy shift has been the radical change in emphasis of the role of Sport England. Sport England is now as much concerned with the role of sport and physical activity as health promoting behaviours as it is in fostering high levels of achievement in sport. Policies, initiatives and strategies such as these culminate in an Action Plan for England – a

---

Box 6.3   Guidelines for physical activity[6]

Children and young people

- Children and young people should achieve a total of at least 60 minutes of at least moderate intensity physical activity each day.

- At least twice a week this should include activities to improve bone health (activities that produce high physical stresses on the bones), muscle strength and flexibility.

Adults

- Adults should achieve a total of at least 30 minutes of at least moderate intensity physical activity a day, on 5 or more days a week.

- The 30 minutes can be achieved in bouts of at least 10 minutes.

- More specific activity recommendations are made for beneficial effects within individual diseases and conditions.

- *All* movement contributes to energy expenditure and is important for weight management.

- For bone health, activities that produce high physical stresses on the bones are necessary.

Older adults

- The recommendations for adults are also appropriate for older adults.

- Older people should take particular care to keep moving and retain their mobility through daily activity.

- Additionally, specific activities that promote improved strength, coordination and balance are particularly beneficial for older people.

national strategy for the nation to improve levels of activity. Initiatives such as this in England and other UK countries aim to get at least half the population active at healthy levels over the next two decades.

WHAT'S THE CURRENT PICTURE – WHO IS AT RISK?

ADULTS

Only a minority of people in England take enough physical activity to be healthy. About two thirds of men and three quarters of women do not meet current health-related activity recommendations (see Box 6.3[6]) of at least 30 minutes of moderate intensity physical activity on 5 or more days of the week. In addition, about a third of men and between a third and a half of women can be classed as 'inactive' (defined as participating in less than 30 minutes of moderate intensity activity per week). The prevalence of inactivity is even higher in women than men and increases with age in both men and women. Just over 7 out of 10 men and 8 out of 10 women aged 75 years and above are inactive.

CHILDREN

Children are more likely to be driven to school, spend more time in front of the television, and experience less school sport and physical education than in the past.

Boys spend a mean of 14.2 hours and girls 12.2 hours per week participating in physical activities that are considered to be beneficial for health.[20] This means that most children achieve healthy levels of activity when measured against the current recommendation of 1 hour a day. (This is contrary to what most people believe, but it is what the evidence tells us.) For boys this figure holds steady to age 15, whereas for girls there is a steady decline. Large proportions of children report very high levels of activity, with 42% of boys and 33% of girls being active for at least 2 hours per day on at least 5 of the previous 7 days. At all ages, over one third of boys are active at this high level.[20]

IS THE PROBLEM OF INACTIVITY GETTING BETTER OR WORSE?

The problem seems to be getting worse, although as more and more people become sedentary there is likely to be a 'floor' effect where the trend flattens out because more and more people become totally sedentary.

Between 1994 and 1998 there was a distinct increase in the proportion of people who are inactive.[21,22] Both walking, which is the most common form of physical activity, and cycling on the public highway declined steadily between 1975–1976 and 1999–2001. Total miles travelled per year on foot fell by 26% and miles travelled by bicycle also fell by 26%.[23] This produced a difference of 66 fewer miles per person walked per year between 1976 and 2001. For a 65 kg person this represents an annual reduction in energy expenditure equivalent of almost 1 kg of fat.

In contrast, adults are now *more* likely to undertake walks for leisure over 2 miles, go swimming and participate in cycling for leisure.[24]

Taken together these data suggest an increase in the proportion of people taking physical activity for leisure, but a decrease in physical activity as part of daily routines.

CHILDREN

Children's activity levels seem to be stable – at least over recent years. It is possible to compare the 2002 activity data on children with similar data collected in the 1997 *Health Survey for England*.[25] Using variables that were consistent in both surveys, no increase or decrease in activity levels is detectable between 1997 and 2002. Prior to 1997, no nationally representative activity data were collected in England. However, from indirect evidence it appears that this generation of children may be less active than past generations.[26]

There are many perceived threats to children's activity levels:

- They are transported more often in cars even on short journeys.

- Parents are more reluctant to allow children to play outdoors because of perceived dangers within the physical environment (for example, heavy traffic and 'stranger danger').

- Children are now given less 'licence' to act independently away from the home at later ages than they were a generation ago.[27]

- There is more access to television and computers and other sedentary alternatives that attract children.[28]

Modes of travelling to school are a significant factor in children's activity levels.[23]

- In 1985–1986, 67% of children aged 5–10 years walked to school, whereas in 1999–2000 the figure had fallen to 54%.

- Primary school age children transported to school by car over the same period increased from 22% to 39%.

- For primary school children, cycling to school had become almost non-existent in 1999–2000.

- In secondary school children, the figure has fallen from 6% in 1985–1986 to just 2% in 1999–2000.

In comparison, in the Netherlands and Denmark, over 60% of children cycle to school.

DO HEALTH INEQUALITIES FEATURE IN PHYSICAL ACTIVITY?

People of higher socio-economic status take part in more physical activity in their leisure time. In men, rates of walking are 38% higher in social class I compared with social class V. In women, rates are 67% higher in social class I compared with social class V. Similar trends are observed for sports participation.[21] In all age and gender groups, low educational attainment predicts higher levels of inactivity.[29]

Where surveys have included work-related physical activity, men in the lowest social class (which includes manual workers) are more physically active than those in higher social classes, with little difference by social class among women.[21,29]

See also Chapter 13 'Tackling inequalities in health'.

WHAT CAN WE DO TO PROMOTE PHYSICAL ACTIVITY?

The Health Development Agency reviewed current evidence from selected good quality systematic reviews and meta-analyses published between 1996 and November 2001 on effectiveness of public health interventions for increasing physical activity among adults.[30]

LIFESTYLE CHANGE APPROACHES

To date, most efforts to increase physical activity levels that have focused on educational and motivational strategies have been unsuccessful.[31,32] It may be unreasonable to expect individuals to become more active when inactivity is so strongly reinforced by their environment and prevailing social norms.[33] Individual, behavioural approaches may not only be unrealistic, it may also be counter-productive in contemporary social and physical infrastructures.[31,33] For example, trying to persuade drivers to adopt more active commuting options is unlikely to succeed in the absence of an integrated and reliable public transport system.

Behavioural and educational interventions have focused principally on leisure time activity. However, people in modern societies spend the great majority of their time at work, in transit, and performing household chores.[32] Encouraging either programmed or lifestyle activity at these times and within these settings may be more effective. Lifestyle activities may be more likely to respond to intervention[34] and are more susceptible to environmental change.[32] Walking and stair-climbing, for example, could be undertaken easily by most people every day, and may be particularly amenable to environmental reinforcement.[32]

ENVIRONMENTAL CHANGE APPROACHES

In general terms, it has been argued that the modification of social, economic, and environmental factors can yield greater population-health dividends than individual lifestyle approaches.[35] Environmental interventions can reach larger and broader constituencies,[36] including low-income groups where environmental barriers may be particularly constraining.[31] Modification of the social, cultural and physical environment(s) may be necessary to initiate population level changes in activity patterns. To date, modification of the physical environment has received most attention. It has been suggested that environmental approaches may result in longer lasting effects as environmental change is assimilated into structures, systems, policies, and sociocultural norms.[37]

Environmental change is likely to be the most successful intervention to increase activity levels, but it is expensive. The greatest barrier to environmental change may be its sheer complexity.

Ultimately, the aim of environmental change should be to facilitate increased activity in all sections of society.[38] The potential benefits of environmental change in this context are clear. Unlike behavioural and

Box 6.4   Case study: an intervention in the physical environment to promote increased physical activity levels at the community level

Aim

Evaluation of a (physical) environmental intervention to promote increased physical activity levels at the community level.

Setting

Bristol inner city.

Research partnership

Bristol University, Bristol City Council, Sustrans.

The community

A well defined community geographically, housing a distinctive, relatively deprived community. The community is a priority for urban regeneration.

The capacity for change

The community has particular features thought to restrict opportunities for active lifestyles. These features include major physical barriers to active transport in and out of the area and high levels of motorized commuter traffic.

There is considerable perceived scope for improvements in active recreation and informal play opportunities for children.

Scope also exists for increased everyday journeys to school, work and shops.

Evaluation methods

- Mixed methods – quantitative and qualitative – will be used.

- Both children and adults will be measured.
- Comparisons will be made with a 'control' community who are unaffected by the intervention.
- Methods include interviews, focus groups, surveys, document searches, participant observation, Geographical Information Systems (GIS), cycle counters.

The intervention

1. A new section of traffic-free route will be constructed to connect the area to a major recreation and commuting route for cycling and walking.
2. A 'home zone' will be created, affording a more pleasant urban living environment and traffic calming strategies. A 'home zone' is a group of streets designed primarily to meet the interests of pedestrians and cyclists rather than motorists, opening up the street for social use. Features include traffic calming, shared surfaces, trees and planters, benches and play areas.
3. There are further plans for investment in the area via the VIVALDI (*VI*sionary and *VI*brant *A*ctions through *L*ocal transport *D*emonstration *I*nitiatives) project.

Timescale

September 2003–August 2005
(For further information, see: www.vivaldiproject.org/pdf/fact_sheet_home_zone.pdf)

educational approaches, environmental initiatives do not hold individuals responsible for change.

Box 6.4 describes an environmental approach to promoting increased physical activity levels at the community level.

INTERVENTIONS IN COMMUNITY SETTINGS

Community-based interventions targeting individuals are effective in producing short term, and mid to long term changes in physical activity.[30] In particular:

● Interventions based on theories of behaviour change, which teach behavioural skills and that are tailored to individual needs, are also associated with longer term changes in behaviour.

● Interventions that promote moderate intensity physical activity, particularly walking, and are not dependent on special exercise facilities, are also associated with longer term changes in behaviour.

● Interventions that incorporate regular contact with an exercise specialist tend to elicit more sustained changes in physical activity.

Older people

The effectiveness of interventions in older adults has been reported:[11]

● Interventions designed specifically for adults aged 50 and above are generally effective in producing short term and mid to long term changes in physical activity.

● Interventions that use behavioural or cognitive approaches with a combination of group and home-based exercise sessions rather than a class or group-only format are associated with longer term changes in behaviour.

● Interventions that promote moderate and non-endurance physical activities (for example, flexibility exercises) are associated with long term changes in behaviour.

● Interventions that use telephone support and follow-up are also associated with long term behaviour change.

Disadvantaged groups

Interventions that are specifically effective in disadvantaged groups have not been examined. However, population surveys have reported that the prevalence of physical inactivity is higher in some ethnic minority groups, people in low-income households, in the lower social classes and people with low levels of education. Ethnicity, income, social class and education are interrelated and we need to examine the independent association between these factors and physical activity to inform appropriate interventions.

INTERVENTIONS IN HEALTHCARE SETTINGS

Both brief advice from a doctor, and referral to an exercise specialist based in the community, have been shown to have modest effect on activity levels.

These exercise referral schemes identify patients whose clinical condition can be improved by physical activity. GPs identify the initial need for increased activity and the patients are then referred to an accredited activity specialist for an individually tailored exercise prescription that will ameliorate their specific condition.[39] For individuals who have specific motivational problems individual counselling sessions can be employed. Motivational interviewing has been shown to be particularly effective for physical activity. (Motivational interviewing is discussed in Ch. 14 'Helping individuals to change behaviour'.)

But as described above, individuals operate within a cultural, social and physical environment. Each of these can inhibit activity. One of the most powerful of ways of helping individuals may therefore be to modify the environments in which they live.

CONTROVERSIAL ISSUES

WHICH ACTIVITY PATTERNS ARE BEST?

It is generally accepted that physical activity, in its broadest sense, is beneficial for health. However, we are not clear which modes, intensities, durations, volumes and frequencies of people's activity – their activity 'patterns' – are most conducive to improved health. It is generally accepted that the most critical factor is the overall *volume* of activity and for general benefit across a broad spectrum of clinical conditions 30 minutes of moderate intensity activity performed 5 days per week confers substantial benefit. However, for improving bone health, for example, weight-bearing, high-impact activities are necessary, whereas activities such as swimming have minimal benefit. For weight management, 45–60 minutes of activity daily may be necessary. More precise prescriptions of activity types and amounts that are most beneficial in other diseases, such as reducing risk of cancer, are beyond the scope of this chapter, but can be found in the 2004 Chief Medical Officer report *At Least 5 a Week.*[6]

HOW TO MEASURE PHYSICAL ACTIVITY?

Measurement of physical activity remains exceptionally difficult. Because physical activity is a complex, multidimensional and infinitely variable human behaviour, it is difficult to quantify it, that is, to describe it in terms of a number. The accurate assessment of individual activity levels remains a controversial and difficult area.[40] Advances in measurement technology – notably the use of accelerometers (movement sensors) – offers a way forward for more precise quantification of activity levels and patterns.[41]

COMMON MYTHS AND QUESTIONS

Physical activity abounds with myths. Many of these myths involve heavily marketed machines and products which promise, for example, fitness without effort, or weight loss without activity. A typical example is exercises that are advertised to reduce the size of a specific part of the body – spot reduction – but this is physiologically impossible.

WHAT QUESTIONS STILL NEED ANSWERS?

There are two major areas where further research is necessary.

First, as mentioned above, we need a more accurate assessment of activity levels. Motion sensors are being increasingly used, but there is a need for a more accurate research instrument that can characterize the full complexity of a person's behaviour with high precision.

Secondly, we do not know what the real barriers to increased activity are.

Furthermore, we have limited knowledge of how the barriers vary between individuals of different age, gender, ethnicity, and socio-economic position. Without a detailed knowledge of barriers, we cannot design effective interventions – which must focus on removing the barriers.

All of these problems are heightened when children are the focus of study. This is critical, as there are strong indications that promotion of activity during childhood may be one of the most effective ways to improve the health of future generations.

Key sources of further information and help

Further reading

- Department of Health. At least 5 a week: evidence on the impact of physical activity and its relationship to health. A report from the Chief Medical Officer. London: Department of Health; 2004. Online. Available: http://www.dh.gov.uk.
- Hardman A, Stensel D. Physical activity and health. London: Routledge; 2003.
- Hillsdon MC, Foster C, et al. A review of the evidence on the effectiveness of public health interventions for increasing physical activity amongst adults: a review of reviews. London:

Health Development Agency; 2003. Online. Available: http://www.hda.nhs.uk/evidence.
- McKenna J, Riddoch CJ. Perspectives on health and exercise. Basingstoke: Palgrave Macmillan; 2003.
- US Department of Health and Human Services. Physical activity and health: a report of the Surgeon General. Atlanta, GA: US Department of Health and Human Services, Centers for Disease Control and Prevention, National Center for Chronic Disease Prevention and Health Promotion; 1996. Online. Available: http://www.cdc.gov/nccdphp/sgr/sgr.htm.

References

1. Caspersen CJ, Powell KE, et al. Physical activity, exercise and physical fitness: definitions and distinctions of health-related research. Public Health Reports 1985; 100:126–131.
2. Bouchard C, Shephard RJ, et al. Physical activity, fitness, and health: international proceedings and consensus document. Champaign, Ill. Human Kinetics; 1994.
3. Fox KR, Riddoch C. Charting the physical activity patterns of contemporary children and adolescents. Proc Nutr Soc 2000; 59(4):497–504.
4. McPherson K, Britton A, et al. Coronary heart disease. Estimating the impact of changes in risk factors. London: The Stationery Office; 2002.
5. World Health Organization. World health report. Geneva: World Health Organization; 2002.
6. Department of Health. At least 5 a week: evidence on the impact of physical activity and its relationship to health. A report from the Chief Medical Officer. London:

Department of Health; 2004. Online. Available: http://www.dh.gov.uk
7. Department for Culture, Media and Sport/Strategy Unit. Game plan: a strategy for delivering the government's sport and physical activity objectives. London: Strategy Unit; 2002.
8. National Audit Office. Tackling obesity in England. London: The Stationery Office; 2001.
9. Booth FW, Gordon SE, et al. Waging war on modern chronic diseases: primary prevention through exercise biology. Journal of Applied Physiology 2000; 88:774–787.
10. Lee IM, Skerrett PJ. Physical activity and all-cause mortality: what is the dose–response relation? Med Sci Sports Exerc 2001; 33(6 Suppl):S459–471; discussion S493–494.
11. King AC, Rejeski WJ, et al. Physical activity interventions targeting older adults. A critical review and recommendations. American Journal of Preventative Medicine 1998; 15:316–333.

12. Department of Health. National Service Framework for mental health. London: Department of Health; 1999.

13. Department of Health. National Service Framework for coronary heart disease. London: Department of Health; 2000.

14. Department of Health. National Service Framework for diabetes: standards. London: Department of Health; 2001.

15. Department of Health. National Service Framework for older people. London: Department of Health; 2001.

16. Fox K, Biddle S, et al. Physical activity promotion through primary health care in England. British Journal of General Practice 1997; 47:367–369.

17. Riddoch C, Puig-Ribera A, et al. Effectiveness of physical activity promotion schemes in primary care: a review. London: Health Education Authority; 1998.

18. Department of Health and Social Services. Strategy statement on physical activity. London: Department of Health; 1996.

19. US Department of Health and Human Services. Physical activity and health: a report of the Surgeon General. Atlanta, GA: US Department of Health and Human Services, Centers for Disease Control and Prevention, National Center for Chronic Disease Prevention and Health Promotion; 1996.

20. Department of Health. Health survey for England 2002. London: The Stationery Office; 2003.

21. Department of Health. Health survey for England 1998. London: The Stationery Office; 2000.

22. Office for National Statistics. The UK 2000 time use survey. Office for National Statistics; 2003. Online. Available: http://www.statistics.gov.uk/timeuse/default.asp

23. Department for Transport. National travel survey; 1999–2001 update. London: DfT; 2001.

24. Office of National Statistics. Living in Britain: Results from the 1996 General Household Survey. London: The Stationery Office; 1998.

25. Department of Health. Health survey for England: the health of young people 1995–1997. London: The Stationery Office; 1998.

26. Durnin JVGA. Physical activity levels – past and present. In: Norgan NG. Physical activity and health: symposium of the Society for the Study of Human Biology. Cambridge: Cambridge University Press; 1992: 20–27.

27. Hillman M. One false move: an overview of the findings and issues they raise. Children, transport and the quality of life. London: Policy Studies Institute; 1993: 7–18.

28. Epstein LH, Paluch RA, et al. Decreasing sedentary behaviours in treating paediatric obesity. Archives of Paediatrics and Adolescent Medicine 2000; 154:220–226.

29. Health Education Authority and Sports Council. Allied Dunbar National Fitness Survey: main findings. London: Sports Council and Health Education Authority; 1992.

30. Hillsdon M, Foster C, et al. A review of the evidence on the effectiveness of public health interventions for increasing physical activity amongst adults: a review of reviews. London: Health Development Agency; 2003. Online. Available: http://www.hda.nhs.uk/evidence

31. Sallis JF, Bauman A, et al. Environmental and policy interventions to promote physical activity. Am J Prev Med 1998; 15(4):379–397.

32. King AC. Environmental and policy approaches to the promotion of physical activity. In: Rippe JM. Lifestyle medicine. Norwalk, CT: Blackwell Science; 1999.

33. Schmid TL, Pratt M, et al. Policy as intervention: environmental and policy approaches to the prevention of cardiovascular diseases. American Journal of Public Health 1995; 85:1207–1211.

34. Hillsdon M, Thorogood M, et al. Randomised controlled trials of physical activity promotion in free living populations: a review. Journal of Epidemiology and Community Health 49; 1995:448–453.

35. Nutbeam D. Creating health-promoting environments: overcoming barriers to action. Australian and New Zealand Journal of Public Health 1997; 21:355–359.

36. Bauman A, Smith B, et al. Geographical influences upon physical activity participation, evidence of a 'coastal effect'. Australian and New Zealand Journal of Public Health 1999; 23:322–324.

37. Swinburn B, Egger G, et al. Dissecting obesogenic environments: the development and application of a framework for identifying and prioritizing environmental interventions for obesity. Preventive Medicine 1999; 29:563–570.

38. Richter K, Harris KJ, et al. Measuring the health environment for physical activity and nutrition among youth: a review of the literature and applications for community initiatives. Preventive Medicine 2000; 31:S98–S111.

39. Department of Health. NHS national quality assurance framework: exercise referral systems. London: Department of Health; 2001.

40. Harro M, Riddoch CJ. Physical activity. In: Armstrong N, Van Mechelen W, eds. Paediatric exercise science and medicine. Oxford: Oxford University Press; 2000:77–84.

41. Cooper AR. Objective measurement of physical activity. In: McKenna J, Riddoch CJ, eds. Critical perspectives in physical activity and health. London: Palgrave; 2002.

Chapter 7

Injury prevention

Gail Errington and Elizabeth Towner

SUMMARY OVERVIEW AND LINKS TO OTHER TOPICS

Unintentional injuries (the term we use in preference to 'accidents' which implies something that cannot be prevented) represent the greatest single threat to life for children and young people and are a major cause of death and disability in older people in the UK. Those most at risk are the most vulnerable: children and young people, older people, and those living in poorer socio-economic circumstances.

Injury prevention is addressed across national policies by a range of agencies concerned with health, transport, fire, health and safety at work, consumer affairs and education.

Many factors work together to cause injuries: to do with the person who is injured, the physical hazard which caused the injury, and the set of circumstances. Analysing these, and knowing who is most at risk, helps us to understand what can be done about prevention. At a community level, education, legislation and environmental modification are particularly relevant, and require many agencies working together to coordinate multifaceted injury prevention programmes. The approaches most likely to be successful in helping individuals to avoid injury are education and improving access to safety equipment.

Since injury is more common among people living in poorer circumstances, Chapter 13 'Tackling inequalities in health' is especially relevant to injury prevention.

WHAT IS INJURY PREVENTION?

Injury is currently responsible for 7% of world mortality and poses a considerable threat to the health of the population in every country. The burden of injury falls disproportionately on the most vulnerable in society – those living in poverty. In the UK children, young adults and older people are particularly at risk.

Injury has been defined by the US National Committee for Prevention and Control as: 'any unintentional or intentional damage to the body resulting from acute exposure to thermal, mechanical, electrical or chemical energy or the absence of such essentials as heat or oxygen'.[1]

Such damage can result in physical and psychological harm, disability and, in the worst cases, death.

Injury prevention is based on an understanding of the epidemiology of injury, that such events are not random occurrences but are predictable and therefore amenable to intervention. Within this chapter we have chosen not to use the word 'accident' since this implies a chance happening, the outcome of which cannot be avoided.

In the UK context, the focus has been on the prevention of unintentional injury, excluding events resulting from violence and suicide. Prevention strategies fall into three broad categories – primary, secondary and tertiary prevention.

● *Primary prevention* looks to prevent the event leading to injury – for example, the installation of a fireguard creating a physical barrier which denies access to the hazard (the fire).

● *Secondary prevention*, whilst not preventing the actual event, aims to prevent or reduce the severity of injury – for example, the wearing of seatbelts or cycle helmets.

● *Tertiary prevention* focuses on the development of optimal treatment and rehabilitation to minimize the impact of injury on the individual – administration of appropriate emergency aid and referral for medical care after a burn, for example.

WHAT CAUSES INJURIES?

The causes of injury are multifaceted and interrelated, necessitating a wide range of potential solutions. Responsibility for the prevention of injury does not fall neatly into the remit of one agency, a fact which may contribute to the relatively low priority given to the area in terms of both research funding and the national health agenda. The complex nature of injury does, however, make it an ideal challenge for partnership working and many of the more successful approaches to injury prevention have, as their core, a strong ethos of collaborative working.

Any given injury event results from the dynamic interaction of three key elements:

- *host* (the individual person suffering the injury);
- *agent* (the physical hazard which causes the injury);
- *environment* (the set of circumstances which results in the host and agent coming into contact with each other).

Each of these elements can be explored further to reveal some of the underlying causes of injury.

Characteristics of the host may predispose certain groups or individuals to a greater risk of injury, for example young children often display unpredictable behaviour which puts them at danger in the road environment. Some people are by nature 'risk-takers' or choose to indulge in risky activities – extreme sports for example. In older people, factors such as balance, confidence and the effects of medication may have a bearing on the individual's risk of injury.

Exposure of the host to a specific agent at a given time is largely an issue of access. In some cases this can be restricted to reduce the risk of injury, for example removing potential hazards such as medicines or small objects from a child's reach to prevent poisoning or choking. In other cases, say where an older person chooses not to go out on an icy day for fear of falling on a slippery pavement, the hazard remains and the host avoids contact and thereby prevents the risk of injury.

The concept of the environment embraces both the physical surroundings and the structure of society. It is, in part, the social inequalities in the distribution of wealth and power which result in some groups being more vulnerable to the risk of injury than others. Children, for example, live and play in an environment designed by adults mainly for adults and which takes little account of their natural inquisitiveness and need to explore. People living in poor housing may be placed at greater risk of injury by the material structure of their homes – factors such as older properties in need of repair, faulty electrics and so on are compounded by the stresses resulting from having a low income, overcrowding and lack of social support.

WHY IS INJURY PREVENTION AN IMPORTANT PUBLIC HEALTH ISSUE?

Injuries are a leading cause of the global burden of disease. They represent the greatest single threat to life for children and young people and in the UK are a major cause of death and disability in older people. Every year 10 000 people die from unintentional injury in England and Wales. It is the leading cause of death among children aged 0–14 years. In the

Figure 7.1 Pyramid of injury. (Reproduced with permission from British Medical Association.)[3]

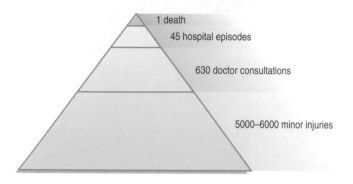

period 1998–2000 in England, 1003 children aged 0–14 years died as a result of an unintentional injury.[2] In addition there are many millions of non-fatal injury events each year. Deaths are thus just the tip of the iceberg – for each person who dies, many more are admitted to hospital, attend Accident and Emergency departments or visit their GP (see Fig. 7.1).[3]

The treatment of injuries to people of all ages costs the NHS around £1.2 billion annually.[4] The Department for Transport estimates the average cost of a road traffic accident resulting in injury as £72 560. This is based on the loss of earnings, medical costs, police and administration costs, damage to property and allowance for pain, suffering and grief as calculated in 2000. Similar studies estimate the value for preventing a serious home injury to be £28 830.[5]

In 2001, the British Medical Association published a report recommending that injury prevention be recognized as one of the major public health priorities in the UK.[3] Injury disproportionately affects the most vulnerable groups in society. For children this burden includes the cost to society of life years lost, treatment and ongoing care costs. Amongst older people, around one in five falls requires medical care contributing greatly to NHS costs including the cost of rehabilitation. In addition to these, each event leading to serious injury, disability or death can bring with it terrible emotional and psychological consequences for both victim and family.

HOW IS INJURY PREVENTION ADDRESSED IN NATIONAL POLICY?

The major policies addressing injury prevention are outlined in Box 7.1 together with specific targets where these are set out in policies.

WHAT IS THE CURRENT PICTURE – WHO IS AT RISK?

Those most at risk of injury are the vulnerable in society – the young, older people and those living in deprived or disadvantaged circumstances. We discuss the key factors in childhood and older people below, and say more about deprivation when we discuss health inequalities.

Box 7.1   Injury prevention in major national policies

Department of Health (1999): *Saving Lives: Our Healthier Nation*[4][*]

Target: ● to reduce the death rate from accidents by at least one fifth and to reduce the rate of serious injury from accidents by at least one tenth by 2010 – saving up to 12 000 lives in total.

Department of Transport, Environment and the Regions (2000): *Tomorrow's Roads – Safer for Everyone*[6]

Targets (by 2010, compared with 1994–1998):
  ● 40% reduction in number of people killed or seriously injured in road accidents
  ● 50% reduction in number of children (under 16 years of age) killed or seriously injured
  ● 10% reduction in slight casualty rate, expressed as number of people slightly injured.

Community Fire Safety Task Force (1997): *Safe as Houses*[7]

Target: ● to reduce number of accidental fire-related deaths in the home by 20% over a 5 year period from 1994–1998 average by March 2004 and to reduce the number of fires overall.

Injury prevention is also an integral part of the following:

Health and Safety Executive (1999/2002): *Health and Safety Commission Strategic Plan*[8]

HSE's mission is to ensure that risks to people's health and safety from work activities are properly controlled. The plan sets out intention to work in partnership with others, to reduce the unacceptable suffering and costs caused by work-related ill health and injury.

Department of Trade and Industry (DTI) Consumer Affairs Directorate: *Consumer Safety Division*

Aims to help consumers make well-informed purchases and protect them from unsafe products and practice. Responsible for establishment of Home and Leisure Accident Surveillance Systems using hospital-based injury data. Data collection ceased May 2003, databases 1978–2002 can be interrogated by contacting the Royal Society for the Prevention of Accidents (RoSPA).

Department for Education and Employment, and Department of Health (1997): *Excellence in Schools*[9]

The White Paper set out the government's intention to help all schools to become 'healthy schools'. The National Healthy Schools Standard, introduced as part of the Healthy Schools Programme, encourages schools to work towards achieving progressive levels of award through implementing a healthy schools charter in which the whole school and wider community work together. Safety is a key theme within this, encompassing the development of a healthy and safe school environment, encouragement for training pupils in first aid skills and promotion of opportunities for pupils and staff to cycle or walk to school.

Department for Education and Skills, and Department of Health (2003/4–2005/6): *Sure Start Service Delivery Agreement Targets*[10]

Sure Start is part of the government's drive to tackle poverty and social exclusion and is concentrated in neighbourhoods with the highest levels of poverty. This joint initiative aims to improve the health and well-being of families and children before starting school in an attempt to break the cycle of disadvantage.

Within the aim of improving health, a specific target is set:

  ● 10% reduction in children aged 0–4 years admitted to hospital with severe injury.

[*] Similar strategies including targets related to death and injury rates have been developed for Scotland,[11] Wales[12] and Northern Ireland.[13]

INFLUENCING FACTORS IN CHILDHOOD

Age

Age, or more accurately the stage of maturation and development reached, can predict the type of injury from which children are most at risk. Pre-school children spend most of their time in the home and accordingly the majority of injuries to this age group occur in the home as slips, trips and falls. As independence increases with age, so the risk of injury outside the home increases, particularly in the road environment.

Gender

Boys are at greater risk of most types of injury than girls. The mechanisms behind this are not fully understood. They may relate to increased exposure for boys in certain activities (e.g. cycling), or to the more adventurous nature of boys, whose tendency towards competitiveness may encourage them to indulge in more risk-taking behaviours.

Social class

The risk of death from injury in childhood rises steeply with poverty. The social gradient is particularly apparent for certain types of injury, for example road traffic accidents, where there are four times as many pedestrian deaths for children from social class V as for those in social class I. For domestic house fires, the difference is even more marked, with children from social class V being 16 times more likely to die in a house fire than their counterparts in social class I.[14] This will be discussed in greater detail when we consider health inequalities.

Culture/ethnicity

There is some evidence that children from minority groups in Britain have different injury experiences, but findings related to the scale and type of injuries suffered by children in different cultural groups are mixed, and as with other aspects of inequality may be complicated by factors such as age, gender and social circumstances.[15]

INFLUENCING FACTORS IN OLDER PEOPLE (65 YEARS AND OLDER)

Older people are amongst those at greatest risk of falling, a risk which increases with age. Although older people drive cars less than their younger counterparts, the risk of an older driver being killed from motor vehicle related injuries is well out of proportion to the level of exposure.[16] For all age groups, the injury death rate for men is greater than for women. However, more women than men die or are admitted to hospital following injury beyond the age of 75, reflecting the increased life expectancy of women. There is currently very little research available relating to inequalities in unintentional injury amongst older people.[17]

Factors affecting risk of injury to older people can be broadly divided into:

- intrinsic factors – characteristics relating to the process of ageing, for example muscle strength, flexibility, balance as well as the effects caused by medication;
- extrinsic factors – relating to the environment, such as uneven pavements, slippery surfaces, inadequate lighting.

IS THE PROBLEM GETTING BETTER OR WORSE?

In the 40 year period from 1950 to 1990, deaths of young people (aged 1–19 years) in England and Wales from causes other than injury fell by nearly three quarters. By contrast over the same time, injury-related deaths fell by only one quarter.[18] As the death rate from injury gradually declines, there is debate as to whether this can be attributed to an increase in injury prevention activity, or whether other factors such as reduced exposure to risk or improved emergency medical care come into play.

In developing countries, as deaths from infectious diseases have fallen, so injury has become responsible for a growing proportion of lives lost in childhood and young adolescence. The World Health Organization (WHO) suggests that by 2020 injury will account for the greatest single reason for loss of healthy human life-years.[19]

Despite a reduction in falls-related mortality amongst older people, as a result of having an ageing population the rates of fractures to bones already weakened by osteoporosis are predicted to double over the next 50 years.[20]

DO HEALTH INEQUALITIES FEATURE IN THIS TOPIC?

We discussed the major risk factors for unintentional injury earlier in this chapter. Social deprivation is an underlying cause closely associated with unintentional injury in childhood. In the UK, a steep gradient exists between injury rates amongst socially deprived populations and those of more affluent groups, with children from poorer families having higher mortality rates than their richer counterparts. This association has also been found in other developed countries.[14] Roberts and Power report a widening of the gap between rich and poor children's deaths from injury over the ten years 1981–1991.[21]

There are a number of ways in which children living in socially deprived circumstances may be placed at greater risk of injury, including the following:

- Poverty, poor housing, overcrowding and lack of social support may result in lower levels of child supervision.

- High stress levels and poor mental health are risk factors for injury for both the sufferers and their dependants.

- Poor families have less money with which to purchase safety equipment such as stair gates and fireguards as a form of protection against injury.

- The area in which they live may comprise older housing stock with its associated problems of maintenance.

- There may be a lack of suitable play facilities so that children are exposed to risks from traffic when playing outside.

No direct evidence of social class associations has been identified in relation to older people, although the relative effect of affluence and deprivation is difficult to define amongst a population no longer in paid employment.

(See also Ch. 13 'Tackling inequalities in health'.)

WHAT CAN WE DO ABOUT PREVENTING INJURIES AT A COMMUNITY LEVEL?

Whitehead[22] sets out four different approaches to reducing inequalities in health generally under the headings:

- strengthening individuals;
- strengthening communities;
- improving access to services;
- broad economic and cultural change.

Table 7.1 illustrates how each of these can contribute to preventing injuries, in this case for child pedestrians.[23]

This combination of approaches involving components of education, legislation and environmental modification is particularly relevant in the field of injury prevention. Such complex programmes requiring multi-agency collaboration and coordination are well suited to delivery at a community level. This effectively shifts the focus of responsibility from the individual to society as a whole and combines passive measures with active behavioural solutions affording an opportunity to change the culture of safety within a community.

Intervention programmes have the potential to be effective in more deprived communities through their ability to strengthen neighbourhoods and increase social capital using both top-down and bottom-up approaches.

The WHO Safe Communities initiative launched in Stockholm in 1989[24] encourages a broad-based approach to injury prevention, successful elements of which include:

- good local data;
- interagency collaboration;

Table 7.1   Prevention of child pedestrian injuries[23]

Approach	Methods
Strengthening individuals	• Parent and child education, e.g. traffic clubs, pedestrian skills training, driver education
Strengthening communities	• Supervising child pedestrian journeys to school • Developing safer play areas • Developing safer road environments • Safer routes to school programmes
Improving access to services	• Developing professional knowledge/skills • Targeting those most at risk • Information in different languages
Broad economic and cultural change	• Slower speeds • Car design • Driver legislation • Land-use policies (e.g. school location) • Transport policies – recognize needs of all road users • Encouraging walking

- leadership;
- time needed to establish and develop networks and local programmes.

The case study described in Box 7.2 illustrates these principles being put into practice. A systematic review of ten community-based intervention programmes targeting children found increasing evidence of the effectiveness of such approaches.[25]

HOW CAN WE BEST HELP INDIVIDUALS?

EDUCATIONAL PROGRAMMES AND CAMPAIGNS

Educational programmes and campaigns aimed at improving safety have been subject to considerable criticism owing to their reliance on the need for individuals to make changes to their own behaviour. Some examples of education/skills development which have been shown to be effective are given below.[19]

- **Pedestrian education aimed at the child/parent** – Children's Traffic Clubs providing educational, age appropriate material relating to road safety knowledge, skills training and adult supervision. An evaluation of the UK-based schemes has shown good evidence of positive behaviour change.

- **Pedestrian skills training** – programmes aimed at developing child pedestrian skills (children aged between 4 and 10 years) using a variety of methods including simulated road layouts, table-top models in the classroom and training in the road environment. Programmes have been

---

Box 7.2   Case study: community approach to injury prevention

OUCH Safety Equipment Scheme – Gateshead

In 2000, outreach sessions by a worker from a local child safety project identified the need for provision of a low-cost home safety equipment scheme within a community in Gateshead.

Following consultation with parents, local authority and health workers and a local housing association, the scheme was established in February 2002. A management committee of enthusiastic and determined parents run the scheme with the part-time support of a Sure Start worker. To assist committee members in their role, an extensive training programme has been developed, covering areas such as use of computers, confidence building, accounting and book-keeping, and health and safety.

Just after the scheme was launched, the premises were subject to an arson attack in which all the equipment was lost. Despite this huge setback, the scheme has continued in temporary accommodation and has expanded to include additional areas of Gateshead. The role of the worker initially involved in setting up the scheme is acknowledged as invaluable.

In addition to providing a much needed resource, the scheme has afforded the opportunity for members of the local community to gain skills and confidence through their involvement in its management. One of the original members is now paid as a part-time worker for the group, and two further members have gone on to train as community and youth workers. (Based on personal communication with S. Warlock.)

shown to improve children's skills where these have been specifically targeted.

- **Bicycle skills training** – programmes aimed at developing skills amongst children aged 8–10 years produce general evidence that bicycle training schemes can have a positive effect in improving children's cycling behaviour.

- **Promoting exercise and physical activity for older people** – a review of randomized controlled trials involving exercise as a means of preventing falls and fall-related injuries concluded that exercise is effective in lowering the risk in selected groups of people and should form part of falls prevention programmes.[26]

- **Assessment of individual circumstances for older people** – taking into account the individual and combined effects of medication, dietary supplements (in particular vitamin D and/or calcium) and vision assessment, which have all been shown to have an association with the risk of falls.

IMPROVING ACCESS TO SAFETY EQUIPMENT

Improving access to safety equipment, for example through the provision of low-cost purchase or loan schemes, can remove some of the economic barriers encountered by lower-income groups. The success of such schemes has been shown to increase where equipment is made available alongside an educational campaign to raise awareness of injury risk and encourage appropriate use, such as those designed to promote the use of smoke detectors.[27]

Compliance in using safety equipment by those most at risk of injury is a huge issue. The reluctance of young people to wear cycle helmets and of older people to wear hip protectors has considerably limited the potential of helmets and hip protectors to reduce injury rates.

PRODUCT MODIFICATION AND LEGISLATION

Whilst the provision of education and skills training can go some way towards changing individual behaviour and reducing risk, by far the most dramatic reductions in injury rates have been brought about by product modification and legislation. Two illustrative case studies are given in Box 7.3.

CONTROVERSIAL ISSUES

SHOULD WE TACKLE INTENTIONAL INJURY ALONGSIDE UNINTENTIONAL INJURY?

In the UK injury prevention encompasses those circumstances and events leading to an unintentional injury. Injuries occurring as a result of violent actions or attempts at self-harm are not currently included in the field. This is at odds with the approach taken in the USA, from where much of the international research literature arises. Recent government initiatives in the UK focus on community safety. Given the similar issues involved with collaborative working, using a combination of approaches and models of community participation, a move towards the inclusion of intentional injury may merit consideration. Tackling the problem of injuries from this broader base may help to shed light on those areas which are sometimes overlooked, such as bullying.

Box 7.3   Case study: product modification and legislation approach to injury prevention

Product modification: child resistant packaging

The introduction of child resistant packaging for medications resulted in a reduction of 85% in episodes of fatal poisonings in Britain and the USA.[28]

The limitations of such measures relate to the number of substances using child resistant closures and reliance on the individual remembering to replace them correctly after use.

Legislation: bicycle helmets

Wearing bicycle helmets is not mandatory in the UK. Evidence presented here is drawn from experience in the USA and Australia where several federal states have introduced legislation covering compulsory helmet wearing.

Towner et al identified 13 studies on helmet legislation, many of which cited a period of health promotion prior to the introduction of the law in order to increase helmet wearing rates.[29] For example, in New Zealand, voluntary wearing rates of 84% in the 5–12 year age group were achieved before legislation was introduced. The evidence shows legislation to be effective in increasing the rates of helmet wearing, and associated with reductions in head injuries.

However, one Australian study estimated cycling exposure for teenagers to have decreased by 44%, suggesting that compulsory wearing of helmets may discourage some from cycling and lead to an undesirable reduction in physical activity.

BALANCING SAFETY WITH INDEPENDENCE AND PHYSICAL ACTIVITY

Preventing injuries to children can create conflict between a desire to keep them safe and to allow them to experience the risks necessary to encourage and develop their independence.

Parental concern over their children's perceived safety can lead to restrictions on their activities, sometimes completely out of proportion to the actual risk itself. Worries about the dangers of heavy traffic and congested roads result in fewer children walking or cycling to school, in favour of being driven from home to the school gates. This leads to a reduced risk of injury for children as car passengers but an increased risk for those children who remain as pedestrians. A reduction in levels of physical activity brings concerns about increasing levels of obesity in children. (See Chs 5 and 6 on 'Obesity' and 'Physical activity' respectively.)

For older people, anxieties about uneven pavements, increased traffic flow, busy public places and the threat of violence and crime outdoors may also reduce their levels of walking. Ironically, this can lead to a loss of confidence and/or a reduction in physical flexibility and mobility, which in themselves can contribute to the risk of injury.

COMMON MYTHS AND QUESTIONS

Accidents are unavoidable, they just happen

Perhaps this is the biggest myth relating to unintentional injury. There is now a considerable body of research evidence which confirms exactly the opposite, that when viewed as a public health issue, unintentional injuries display clear patterns. At population level they are both predictable and preventable.

Aren't some people just 'accident–prone'?

Anecdotally it may seem that certain individuals have more than their fair share of accidents. Evidence from the literature on childhood injury has focused mainly on children with hyperactive and attentiveness disorders, such as attention deficit hyperactivity disorder (ADHD). A review of 11 general child injury studies and 6 child pedestrian studies reported that aggressive behaviour was a constant risk factor for general injuries, though not for pedestrian injuries, and that an inconsistent link existed between hyperactivity and all types of injury.[30] It is important to note that the overall contribution to risk from such conditions is small compared to the effect of environmental and social class risk factors.

Safety equipment, rules and laws make you safe

Using safety equipment – cycle helmets, seatbelts etc – does not in itself prevent the occurrence of injury, although it can dramatically reduce the severity of any injuries which may occur. Similarly, rules and legislation encourage certain models of behaviour, but do not ensure complete avoidance of injury.

The idea of risk compensation suggests that when using safety equipment or when faced with the limitations imposed by law, we may alter our behaviour and take more risks in order to maintain a balance in our personal 'risk-level'.[31] This may go some way to explaining why some people – the 'thrill-seekers' – are drawn to more risky activities, whilst others are by nature more cautious. On a practical level this has implications, for example by installing less challenging play equipment and impact-absorbing surfaces, we may inadvertently encourage some children to indulge in more adventurous behaviour. Whilst the idea of risk compensation has gathered some support, it does not lend itself to rigorous testing and remains an area of debate.[32, 33]

You can't teach young children about safety

Incomplete development of cognitive and reasoning skills in young children has led to a view, illustrated by the work of Sandels[34] looking at children in the road environment, that 'they are biologically incapable of managing its many demands'.

This view is disputed by Thomson et al who consider that properly targeted, practical training programmes have considerable potential in training children in road crossing skills.[35] Whilst it is not disputed that safety education must take into account the learning capabilities of the child, it may be the case that it is never too early to teach children about safety.

WHAT QUESTIONS STILL NEED ANSWERS?

GENERAL RESEARCH NEEDS

The field of injury prevention is relatively new and whilst the evidence base is growing rapidly, there remain a number of substantial questions yet to be addressed. When we consider research in injury prevention, the following issues are especially significant:

- Access to comprehensive, accurate and timely injury event data, coded for severity, continues to present problems at international, national and local level. This complicates attempts to evaluate intervention programmes and is of particular frustration to practitioners who are constantly called upon to justify their efforts.

● Further evidence on the cost-effectiveness of injury prevention measures would add weight to the battle to secure funding (which is ever-decreasing) and commitment for intervention programmes.

● Comparative UK-based research using the same research methodology in different settings would help to assess the transferability of successful interventions and provide an opportunity to learn from the vast amount of work which has been undertaken worldwide, particularly in the USA, Australia and Sweden.

● The importance of evaluating both new and existing injury prevention programmes cannot be overemphasized. This is particularly true in the area of community-based interventions which by their very nature are complex, and where the detailed process of implementation is an essential component in interpreting the outcomes.

● As our knowledge and understanding of the science of injury prevention continues to increase, it is vital that practitioners are kept up-to-date with current thinking. The literature is vast and covers a diverse range of disciplines, making it difficult to keep abreast of the latest developments. Systematic reviews and best practice guides, produced and presented in an accessible and meaningful format, are good ways of helping practitioners to make sense of it all.

RESEARCH ON SPECIFIC TARGET GROUPS

There are also some issues specific to certain target groups, notably children and young people, and older people.[36]

Children and young people

We still need to know:

● what the current picture of unintentional injury and prevention is amongst 12–14 and 15–24 year olds;
● more about injuries and what works to prevent them for children living or playing in rural areas;
● more about disability and its effect on quality of life for children and their families.

Older people

We still need further information on:

● the description of the causes of falls and falls-related injury using the evidence in a systematic way;
● developing a validated risk factor assessment tool to identify people at high risk of falling;
● what the components of a falls prevention programme should be – which risk factors can be modified and would these lead to a reduction in falls;
● which sub-groups of older people should be targeted for falls prevention – and who would benefit most;

- what might be the most effective strategies for increasing the participation of older people in multifaceted prevention and physical activity programmes;
- what association (if any) exists between accidents and social deprivation and ethnicity among older people.

Key sources of further information and help

Further reading

- Accidental Injury Task Force. Preventing accidental injury – priorities for action. London: The Stationery Office; 2000. Online. Available: http://www.doh.gov.uk/accidents/accinjuryreport.htm.
- British Medical Association. Injury prevention. London: British Medical Association Board of Education and Science; 2001.
- Cryer C. Priorities for prevention. Accidental Injury Task Force's Working Group on Older People. December 2001. Online. Available: http://www.doh.gov.uk/accidents/accinjuryreport.htm.
- Hayes M. Preventing childhood accidents: guidance on effective action. London: Child Accident Prevention Trust; 2003.
- Millward LM, Morgan A, Kelly MP. Prevention and reduction of accidental injury in children and older people. Evidence briefing. London: Health Development Agency; 2003. Online. Available: http://www.hda.nhs.uk/evidence.
- Pless B, Towner E, eds. Action on injury. Injury prevention 1998; 4(S1). Online. Available: http://www.injuryprevention.com.
- Towner E. The prevention of childhood injury. Background paper prepared for the Accidental Injury Task Force. September 2003. Online. Available: http://www.doh.gov.uk/accidents/accinjuryreport.htm.
- UNICEF. A league table of child deaths by injury in rich nations. Florence, Italy: UNICEF Innocenti Research Centre; 2001.

Useful websites

- Child Accident Prevention Trust – national charity concerned with reducing death, disability and serious injury to children and young people. Variety of resources available.

  www.capt.org.uk

- Information and resources on safety in education.

  www.dfes.gov.uk www.teachernet.gov.uk

- Injury Control and Safety Promotion is an international journal, an initiative of ECOSA (European Community Safety Association) that promotes safety through injury epidemiology, research and practice.

  www.szp.swets.nl

- Injury Prevention is a multidisciplinary peer reviewed journal, published since 1995. It is the official journal of the International Society for Child and Adolescent Injury Prevention.

  www.injuryprevention.com

- Royal Society for the Prevention of Accidents – provides information, advice, resources and training in all aspects of safety.

  www.rospa.org.uk

- Whoops! Child Safety Project – an arts-based initiative working creatively to reduce childhood injuries in Gateshead.

  www.whoopschildsafety.co.uk

References

1. National Committee for Injury Prevention and Control. Injury prevention: meeting the challenge. New York: Oxford University Press; 1989.
2. Accidental Injury Task Force. Preventing accidental injury – priorities for action. London: The Stationery Office; 2000. Online. Available: http://www.doh.gov.uk/accidents/accinjuryreport.htm
3. British Medical Association. Injury prevention. London: British Medical Association Board of Education and Science; 2001.
4. Department of Health, Secretary of State for Health. Saving lives: our healthier nation. London: The Stationery Office; 1999.
5. Hopkin JM, Simpson HF. Valuation of home accidents: a comparative review of home and road accidents. TRL Report 225. Crowthorne: Transport Research Laboratory; 1996.
6. Department of Transport, Environment and the Regions. Tomorrow's roads: safer for everyone. The Government's road safety strategy and casualty reduction targets for 2010. London: DTER; 2000.
7. Community Fire Safety Task Force. Safe as houses. London: Home Office; 1999.
8. Health and Safety Executive. Health and Safety Commission strategic plan for 1999/2002. London: HSE Books; 1999.
9. Department of Education and Employment. Excellence in schools. London: The Stationery Office; 1997.
10. Department for Education and Skills, Department of Health. Sure Start service delivery agreement targets 2003/4–2004/5. Online. Available: http://www.surestart.gov.uk/-doc/152-BBC938.doc
11. Scottish Office Department of Health. Working together for a healthier Scotland: a consultation document. Edinburgh: The Stationery Office; 1998.
12. Health Promotion Authority for Wales. Health for all Wales: plans for action. Cardiff: HPAW; 1992.
13. DHSS Northern Ireland. Health and wellbeing into the next millennium. Original strategy for health and social wellbeing 1997–2000. Belfast: Strategic Planning Branch, DHSS Northern Ireland; 1997.
14. Office of Population Censuses and Surveys. Occupational mortality: childhood supplement. Registrar General's decennial supplement for England and Wales, 1970–1972. DS No. 1. London: HMSO; 1988.
15. Towner E, Dowswell T, Errington G, et al. Injuries in children aged 0–14 years and inequalities. London Health Development Agency, 2004.
16. Binder S. Injuries amongst older adults: the challenge of optimizing safety and minimizing unintended consequences. Inj Prev 2002; 8 (suppl IV):iv2–iv4.
17. Millward LM, Morgan A, Kelly MP. Prevention and reduction of accidental injury in children and older people: evidence briefing. London: Health Development Agency; 2003.
18. Woodroffe C, Glickman M, Barker M, et al. Children, teenagers and health. The key data. Buckingham: Open University Press; 1993.
19. Towner E, Dowswell T, Mackereth C, et al. What works in preventing unintentional injuries in children and young adolescents? An updated systematic review. London: Health Development Agency; 2001.
20. Cryer C. What works to prevent accidental injury amongst older people. Report to the Health Development Agency. London. Centre for Health Services Studies, University of Kent; 2001.
21. Roberts I, Power C. Does the decline in child injury mortality vary by social class? A comparison of class specific mortality in 1981 and 1991. BMJ 1996; 313:784–786.
22. Whitehead M. Tackling inequalities: a review of policy initiatives. In: Benzeval M, Judge K, Whitehead M, eds. Tackling inequalities in health. An agenda for action. London: King's Fund; 1995.
23. Towner E. The prevention of childhood injury. Background paper prepared for the Accidental Injury Task Force. September 2003. Online. Available: http://www.doh.gov.uk/accidents/accinjuryreport.htm
24. World Health Organization. Manifesto for safe communities. Proceedings of the first World Conference on Accident and Injury Prevention, Stockholm. Geneva: WHO; 1989.
25. Towner E, Dowswell T. Community-based childhood injury prevention: what works? Hlth Prom Int 2002; 17(3):273–284.
26. Gardner M, Robertson M, Campbell A. Exercise in preventing falls and fall-related injuries in older people: a review of randomized controlled trials. Brit J Sports Med 2000; 34:7–17.
27. DiGuiseppi C, Roberts I. Individual-level injury prevention strategies in the clinical setting. In: The future of children. Unintentional injuries in childhood. Los Altos, CA: The David and Lucile Packard Foundation; 2000:53–82.
28. Health Evidence Bulletins for Wales. Injury prevention 1998. Online. Available: http://hebw.uwcm.ac.uk/injury/chapter1.html
29. Towner E, Dowswell T, Burkes M, et al. Bicycle helmets – a review of their effectiveness. A critical review of the literature. Road Safety Research Report No.30. London: Department for Transport; 2002.
30. Wazana A. Are there injury prone children? A critical review of the literature. Canadian J Psychiatry 1997; 42(6):600–610.
31. Hedlund J. Risky business, safety regulations, risk compensation and individual behaviour. Inj Prev 2000; 6:82–89.
32. Adams J, Hillman M. The risk compensation theory and bicycle helmets. Inj Prev 2001; 7:89–91.
33. Thompson D, Thompson R, Rivara F. Risk compensation theory should be subject to systematic reviews of the scientific evidence. Inj Prev 2001; 7:86–88.

34. Sandels S. Children in traffic. Revised edn. Surrey: Elek Books; 1975.

35. Thomson J, Ampofo-Boateng K, Pitcairn T, et al. Behavioural group training of children to find safe routes to cross the road. Brit J of Educ Psych 1992; 62:173.

36. Cryer C. Developing the future of public health research relating to accidents and unintentional injury. Paper to the Health Development Agency, London. Canterbury: Centre for Health Services Studies, University of Kent; 2001.

Chapter 8

Teenage pregnancy

Catherine Dennison and Alison Hadley

SUMMARY OVERVIEW AND LINKS TO OTHER TOPICS

In England, data for 2002 indicate that about 43 in every 1000 15–17 year old girls (1 in 23) became pregnant; about half these pregnancies ended in abortion.[1]

Teenage pregnancy is an important public health issue: teenage parenthood is far more common in disadvantaged groups, including those who have disengaged from education, and spent time in the care system and/or in prison. Levels of sexually transmitted infections are unacceptably high in teenagers and teenage parents experience more poverty, unemployment and health problems than other parents, as do their children. Addressing teenage pregnancy needs to be central to tackling social exclusion, child poverty and cycles of deprivation.

UK rates of teenage pregnancy have not fallen in recent decades as they have in other European countries, largely because of teenagers' low expectations of their futures, ignorance about sexual matters, mixed media messages, and poor communication and education about sexual relationships.

A national strategy was launched in England in 1999[2] to tackle teenage pregnancy on four fronts: coordinated action across all agencies from government level to local communities; a national media campaign to reach young people and their parents; improved sex and relationships education and access to contraception; and better support for teenage parents. Early indicators of falling conception rates and higher proportions of young mothers in education, training and employment are encouraging.

Other UK countries have also begun to address this issue in systematic ways. Northern Ireland, Scotland and Wales each have national strategies which share the aim of reducing teenage conceptions and employ similar measures, such as enhancing sexual health service provision for young people and supporting local implementation and coordination.

Teenage pregnancy often provokes sensationalized media coverage and polarized debate, where myths flourish and research evidence is ignored: this chapter addresses common topical controversial questions.

This chapter needs to be read alongside Chapter 9 'Sexually transmitted infections', since both are key aspects of sexual health. Chapters 10 and 11 on alcohol and drugs respectively are also linked: many teenagers become pregnant after drinking or using drugs. As health inequalities feature strongly in the incidence of teenage pregnancy, Chapter 13 'Tackling inequalities in health' is also highly relevant.

WHAT DO WE MEAN BY 'TEENAGE PREGNANCY'?

Teenage pregnancy is a term which is often loosely used in the media to refer to under 16s, unmarried teenage mothers or teenage abortions. However, for those working in the field and in the compilation of statistics, teenage pregnancy refers to conceptions in young women under 20 which end in live birth or abortion. (An unknown number of conceptions may also end in miscarriages.)

Within the under 20s, specific age brackets may be identified in relation to a strategy target, such as in England which has set a goal to halve the conception rate in under 18s. Data on teenage pregnancy are usually described in rates rather than numbers, i.e. the number of 15–17 year old conceptions per 1000 15–17 year old female population. This describes the proportion of young women conceiving within the population and is a more accurate indicator of the size of the issue.

WHAT IS THE CURRENT PICTURE?

In 2002, the most recent year for which figures are available, data for England indicate that around 39 000 young women under 18 became pregnant – a rate of 42.6 per 1000 15–17 year olds.[1]

● In England, 91 200 young women under 20 conceived, a rate of 60.2 per 1000 15–19 year olds; the majority of these pregnancies were amongst women aged 18 and over.

● Of those who conceived, 46% of under 18s chose to have an abortion. The percentage increases the younger the teenager, with 56% of under 16s deciding to terminate their pregnancies.

● In England and Wales, less than 400 girls under 14 conceived – undoubtedly a major event for each individual but a reminder that despite what the headlines imply, pregnancy in very young teenagers always was and continues to be very unusual.

Across the UK rates vary between the different countries. Scotland and Northern Ireland have similar levels of conceptions and births to those in England; Wales is slightly higher.[1] In contrast, birth rates across Western Europe are significantly lower.[3] Rates of teenage (under 20s) births in the UK are five times those in the Netherlands, three times those in France, and twice those in Germany. These comparisons are for 1998, the most recent year for which comparable data are available. In contrast to these other countries, where rates fell during the 1970s, 1980s and 1990s, UK rates have remained at similar levels since the 1980s.

WHO BECOMES PREGNANT AS A TEENAGER?

Fig. 8.1 summarizes factors affecting the likelihood of teenage pregnancy.

Figure 8.1   Factors affecting the likelihood of teenage pregnancy.

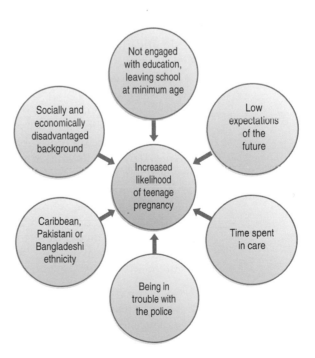

In the UK, as elsewhere in the developed world, teenage pregnancy occurs in all social classes, ethnic groups and religions. However, conceiving as a teenager and deciding to continue the pregnancy are both considerably more common among young people who:[4]

- are from disadvantaged backgrounds;
- have become disengaged from education;
- have low expectations for their futures.

Young women from the lowest social class are around ten times more likely to become teenage mothers compared with the highest social class. Young men who become fathers are also more likely to come from lower socio-economic families and to leave school at the minimum age.

Those who have spent time in the care system and those who have been in trouble with the police are also at higher risk. Estimates suggest that around 39% of young women and 25% of young men under the age of 21 in prison are already a parent.[5]

Although national conception rate statistics are not compiled according to ethnicity, survey data suggest that teenage birth rates show ethnic differences.[6] Caribbean, Pakistani and Bangladeshi women have higher teenage birth rates than white young women. In contrast, Indian young women have lower rates than white young women.

(See also Ch. 14 'Tackling inequalities in health'.)

WHY IS TEENAGE PREGNANCY A 'PROBLEM' AND AN IMPORTANT PUBLIC HEALTH ISSUE?

The high proportion of pregnancies that end in abortion indicates that significant proportions of teenage conceptions are unplanned and unwanted.

Levels of sexually transmitted infections (STIs) in young people are also unacceptably high, with STIs highest in 16–19 year old women and an estimated one in ten sexually active teenagers infected. These high levels of abortion and infections represent a significant public health issue and indicate that substantial numbers of young people lack the knowledge, skills and confidence to use contraception and condoms effectively, or to say 'no' to sexual activity before they are ready. (See also Ch. 9 'Sexually transmitted infections'.)

Amongst those who go on to parenthood, we know that a large proportion become good and committed parents and their children do well. However, we also know that they frequently face a whole range of disadvantages. Compared with older mothers, teenage mothers:

- are three times more likely to experience postnatal depression;
- are half as likely to breast feed;
- have a higher incidence of smoking during pregnancy.

Research has shown that even when they are in their thirties, those who became parents as teenagers are more likely than their peers to:[7]

- live in poverty;
- experience unemployment;
- not have qualifications;
- be receiving welfare payments.

The children of teenage parents:

- are 60% more likely to die in the first year of life;
- are 25% more likely to be of low birth weight;
- are at considerably greater risk of growing up in poverty, living in poor housing and having poor nutrition;
- in the longer term, have a higher chance of becoming teenage mothers themselves.

Research suggests that this greater risk of negative outcomes arises partly from the fact that already disadvantaged teenagers are more likely to become young mothers.[8] However, becoming a young parent does seem to confer additional difficulties. Notably, young mothers are at a considerably greater risk of poor mental health for 3 years postnatally. In addition, young mothers appear to fare significantly worse in the 'marriage market', tending to find partners who are also experiencing poverty and lack of opportunity. This reinforces the disadvantages of both and increases the likelihood of the child growing up in poverty. Therefore, tackling teenage pregnancy and its consequences needs to be central to attempts to tackle social exclusion, child poverty and cycles of deprivation.

WHY ARE RATES IN THE UK SO HIGH?

In the early 1970s, the UK had similar teenage birth rates to other European countries. But while Europe achieved dramatic falls in the 1980s and 1990s, rates in the UK remained static.[2] There is no single explanation for the UK's failure to tackle its relatively high rates, but the four factors described below stand out.

LOW EXPECTATIONS   The higher rates of teenage conceptions and births in lower socio-economic groups make clear the link between teenage pregnancy, disadvantage and low educational attainment. Currently too many young people are outside of education, employment and training. As a result there are substantial numbers of young people who feel they have few prospects for their future and see little reason to delay becoming a parent. Indeed, without employment to confer the status of adulthood, pregnancy and parenthood may well appear to be the only passport out of adolescence.

IGNORANCE   Research shows that many young people lack accurate knowledge about mutually agreed and safe sexual relationships. One study[9] found over a quarter of 14–15 year olds thought the pill protected them from STIs, while seasoned myths still circulate the grapevine, such as not being able to get pregnant the first time they have sex.

To many adults who see the world of teenagers saturated with images of sex, this ignorance seems unbelievable. But ice cream advertisements with sexualized images are not sex education, and many young people are only picking up pieces of the sex education jigsaw without being shown the whole picture. Young parents also often say how little they knew of the reality of bringing up a child, often alone and usually on a low income.

In short, far too many young people do not know how easy it is to get pregnant and how hard it is to be a parent.

MIXED MESSAGES

Every day the UK media bombards teenagers with messages that sexual activity is the norm, enjoyable and an essential part of romantic relationships. For many young people, girls and boys, this will add to the weight of pressure to have sex young, to conform to the apparent norm of the peer group and avoid the stigma of being the odd one out. Indeed, 46% of 13–17 year olds believe that over half of under 16s are sexually active, whereas less than a third have actually had sex.[10]

In contrast to the plethora of sexual images and storylines, there are virtually no references in TV soaps or films to the consequences of unprotected sex or how to discuss and obtain contraception and condoms. As one teenager put it, 'It sometimes seems as if sex is compulsory but contraception is illegal.'[2]

POOR COMMUNICATION

Aside from the 'media noise', there is very little communication in UK society about sex, relationships or contraception. Most public institutions and many parents remain too embarrassed to talk about sex or believe, mistakenly, that by doing so they will hasten the onset of sexual activity. And young people themselves seldom discuss contraception before having sex, in stark contrast to their Dutch peers who are much more likely to talk about protection before first sex. The net result of pressure and poor communication is not less sex, but less protected sex.

A NATIONAL STRATEGY FOR TACKLING TEENAGE PREGNANCY

Reflecting on our high rates of teenage pregnancy and woeful comparison with our European neighbours, the Prime Minister stated:

> Britain has the worst record on teenage pregnancies in Europe. It is not a record in which we can take any pride . . . As a country, we can't afford to continue to ignore this shameful record. Few societies find it easy to talk honestly about teenagers, sex and parenthood. It can seem easier to sweep such uncomfortable issues under the carpet. But the consequences of doing this can be seen all round us in shattered lives and blighted futures.[11]

In response to these concerns, Tony Blair charged the Social Exclusion Unit (SEU) with developing a teenage pregnancy strategy, known as the

National Teenage Pregnancy Strategy. It is important to point out that the SEU's remit related to England only. However, it was made explicit that recognition of the need to tackle the issue was shared by the recently devolved administrations of Scotland, Wales and Northern Ireland and that they would look to instigate their own locally appropriate responses. Subsequently each administration has developed, or is in the process of developing, its own national strategy.[12,13,14] This has been either as part of a wider sexual health strategy (Scotland and Wales) or by a specific teenage pregnancy and parenthood strategy (Northern Ireland).

These strategies share many elements in common with the English one, for example:

- the evidence base on which they draw;
- targets to reduce teenage conceptions;
- an action plan for implementation;
- multidisciplinary working;
- a focus on improving the quality of and access to sexual health services and the education young people receive about sex and relationships.

Consequently, although this chapter concentrates on the English strategy developed by the SEU, much of what follows, for example evidence cited and practice examples, will be of interest to those working across the UK.

The SEU's report was based on a review of international research evidence, exploration of existing good practice, and consultation with a wide group of people including young people and young parents. The report laid the foundations of a 10 year government strategy for England, launched in 1999.[2]

THE EVIDENCE BASE FOR THE STRATEGY

In order to inform the direction the Strategy should take, the SEU drew on the available evidence for what works in preventing teenage conceptions and supporting teenage parents. Staying on top of the developing evidence base has remained a priority. It is important to highlight that the majority of systematic evaluation is still carried out in the North American context, therefore the extent to which findings are transferable to the UK context needs to be considered.

Prevention

Regarding prevention, reviews of the best available research conclude that there is good evidence for:[15]

- the effectiveness of school-based sex and relationships education (SRE), especially when linked to contraceptive services;
- including teenagers' parents in information and prevention;
- programmes that combine a long term, multidimensional approach, e.g. bringing together self-esteem building, voluntary work, educational support and SRE.

Provision of sexual health services

There has been little evaluation of the impact of contraceptive provision, but there is good evidence that services should adopt the following characteristics:

- long term provision;
- clear, unambiguous information and messages;

- tailoring services and interventions to meet local needs;
- focusing on local high risk groups;
- taking key opportunities to deliver information and advice, e.g. on receipt of a negative pregnancy test;
- checking that interventions and services are accessible to young people;
- selecting and training staff who are committed to programme and service goals;
- respecting the confidentiality of young people;
- joining up services and interventions aimed at preventing pregnancy with other services for young people.

Abstinence approaches

In contrast there is no strong evidence for the effectiveness of abstinence only ('just say no') approaches. Proponents of abstinence approaches have argued that such methods have been responsible for substantial decreases in teenage birth rates in the USA. However, the decline in birth rates began several years before abstinence education came to prominence. Instead, it is thought that the decrease is due as much to the increased use of effective methods of contraception, particularly to prevent second pregnancies. Reviewing international evidence, UNICEF concluded that developed countries with low rates of teenage births have good access to contraception, provide quality sex education and build incentives to avoid early parenthood.[3]

Support for teenage parents

Regarding support for young parents, the available evidence is more sparse. There is strong evidence, though, that pregnancy outcomes for mothers and their children are improved by:[15]

- good antenatal care;
- home visiting and emotional support interventions;
- individual and group-based parenting programmes.

As poor housing has a strong adverse impact on health, improving the quality of housing available to young parents and their children is also likely to be of real benefit.

WHAT ARE THE OBJECTIVES OF THE NATIONAL TEENAGE PREGNANCY STRATEGY?

The current National Teenage Pregnancy Strategy[2] contrasts dramatically with previous government responses to tackling teenage pregnancy. Drawing on the evidence base and wide consultation with those working in the area, it was recognized that there will be no 'quick fix'. Instead, a concerted effort is needed over several years, to achieve the necessary cultural shift in attitudes and behaviours amongst professionals, parents and young people. The 10 year span of the Strategy is vital. Change will not happen overnight.

In addition, it was realized that change cannot be achieved by action on just a small number of fronts: activity must be multifaceted and must tackle the causes of teenage conceptions and disadvantage among young parents wherever they occur.

As a consequence, it was clear that no single body could be charged with implementing this strategy. Whereas previous attempts to reduce teenage pregnancy had rested solely with health services, the National

Teenage Pregnancy Strategy recognized that there must be a 'joined-up' approach:

- between government departments;
- between national, regional and local government;
- between government and non-government organizations.

In short, every initiative, policy and individual playing a part in young people's lives has a role to play in effective implementation of the Strategy.

The Strategy is also the first to recognize the importance not only of preventing unplanned and unwanted teenage pregnancies but also of supporting those who choose to become young parents to improve their own and their children's life chances. As a result, the Strategy has two main goals:

- first, to halve the under 18 conception rate by 2010 and set a firmly established downward trend in under 16 conceptions;
- second, to increase to 60% the proportion of teenage parents in education, training or employment in order to reduce their risk of long term social exclusion.

AN AGENDA FOR ACTION

The Strategy has a 30 point action plan organized under four main themes, depicted in Figure 8.2:

- Joined-up action;
- National media campaign to reach young people and parents;
- Better prevention: improved sex and relationships education and access to contraception and sexual health advice services;
- Better support for teenage parents.

The following sections detail how the Strategy has progressed and include examples of innovative practice at local level.

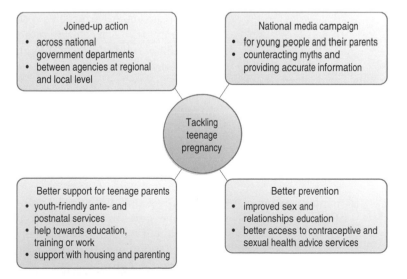

Figure 8.2   Themes of the National Teenage Pregnancy Strategy (England) 1999.[2]

'JOINED–UP' ACTION

A comprehensive structure has been put in place to ensure the Strategy is implemented across all areas of England. The emphasis is being placed upon all these groups working together so that action is coordinated and strengthened and clear messages about sex and pregnancy are sent to young people.

At national level

At national level the Teenage Pregnancy Unit was established to coordinate and drive forward the Strategy's implementation. Funded by all government departments but initially based in the Department of Health, in 2003 the Unit moved into the Children, Young People and Families Directorate in the Department for Education and Skills. This move signalled the government's aim, set out in the Green Paper *Every Child Matters*,[16] to bring together all programmes and strategies relating to children and young people to improve their health and well-being. The Unit continues to work across government departments to drive forward the elements of the action plan.

The importance of the Strategy in tackling inequalities and social exclusion is underlined by the inclusion of the target to halve the under 18 conception rate by 2010 as a government priority for the Department for Education and Skills, the Department of Health, local NHS services and local authorities. The importance of reducing teenage pregnancy and supporting teenage parents will also be highlighted in the forthcoming *National Service Framework for Children and Young People*,[17] and is highlighted in the Green Paper *Every Child Matters*.[16]

At local level

Every top tier local authority in England has a 10 year teenage pregnancy strategy in place, reflecting the themes of the national strategy, to reach agreed local 2010 reduction targets of between 40 and 60%.

Each strategy is led by a Teenage Pregnancy Coordinator working with a Teenage Pregnancy Partnership Board. Representation on the Board comprises the local authority (including education, housing and social services), local primary care trusts, Connexions (a support and information service for teenagers), Sure Start and relevant voluntary sector organizations. All strategies receive a grant to fund the coordinator and to pump prime, accelerate or add value to Strategy-related activity. The amount of funding is weighted to areas of high rates and numbers of under 18 conceptions.

At regional level

Local Teenage Pregnancy Coordinators are supported by nine Regional Teenage Pregnancy Coordinators, one in each Government Office of the Regions. The Regional Coordinators work closely with Government Office and regional colleagues from relevant programmes, to support and strengthen local implementation and provide assessment of each strategy's annual report on progress.

An independent advisory group

An advisory group, with an independent chair and a wide-ranging membership of experts from outside of government, advises government on the direction of the Strategy and the work of the Teenage Pregnancy Unit. Individual members also act as advocates for the Strategy among their own professional groups.

NATIONAL MEDIA CAMPAIGN FOR YOUNG PEOPLE

In 2000, a national media campaign was launched aimed at counteracting myths and providing young people – boys as well as girls – with accurate information to help them make safe and well informed choices. The campaign was developed after an extensive literature review of youth campaigns across the world, which made clear that effective messages need to be non-authoritarian, non-patronizing and unambiguous. They also have to be sustained over a long period of time, both to reinforce the message and to ensure they are heard by every new wave of teenagers.

As a result, under the campaign slogan 'Sex, are you thinking about it enough?' the advertisements use humour and straight talking to convey the key messages:

- resisting pressure to have sex before you're ready;
- awareness of STIs;
- the importance of using condoms and contraception if you're sexually active.

Advertisements feature in teenage magazines, on commercial radio stations and on washroom doors in some shopping centres. Recent research shows that around 80% of young people in the target group of 13–17 year olds recognize the campaign materials, an awareness level usually only achieved by television advertising.[10] The radio advertisements are particularly effective at reaching boys.

The campaign is supported by the national Sexwise helpline, which provides young people under 18 with advice and signposting to confidential services in their local area. Sexwise answers nearly 1.5 million calls a year, over 50% of which are from boys. An accompanying website – www.ruthinking.co.uk – provides extensive information as well as the database of local services, and receives over 40 000 visits a month.

At a local level, teenage pregnancy strategies can use the advertisements in poster and postcard form to distribute to community and leisure venues popular with young people. In addition, the strategies are charged with publicizing their local services to young people with specially designed credit card style materials, as well as ensuring all professionals have a referral checklist of services to which they can speedily refer young people in need of advice.

... AND THEIR PARENTS

Research shows that young people growing up in families where sex is talked about openly and without embarrassment have sex later and are more likely to use contraception.[18] Surveys show that parents want to talk to their children about sex and relationships and 86% believe there would be fewer teenage pregnancies if parents did discuss these issues with their children. Young people too cite parents as their preferred source of advice, yet nearly half (46%) say they receive little or no information, with boys receiving the least.

To address this, a 'Time to Talk' media initiative is run by the parenting support organization Parentline Plus (www.parentlineplus.org.uk) to help parents develop confidence and skills in talking to their children about sex and relationships. 'Time to Talk' prompts discussion in local, regional and national media and provides support to parents through a freephone helpline and website. Posters and leaflets highlighting the importance of discussing sex and relationships are available for display in general practice and other community settings. This work is complemented by a range of local parenting support projects and initiatives incorporating sex and relationships issues, in schools and other community venues.

BETTER PREVENTION

Alongside the campaign messages promoting accurate information and open discussion, the Strategy aims to improve sex and relationships education and enable better access to confidential contraceptive and sexual health services.

Sex and relationships education

Contrary to the expectations of older generations, the content, amount and quality of sex and relationships education (SRE) that young people receive in schools is very variable. Although some schools have well thought out SRE programmes that are delivered by confident, skilled staff, this is still not the norm. Young people still commonly report that SRE is given too late, often by embarrassed teachers, and focuses only on facts and biology. What they would like is more discussion about relationships and the realities of negotiating real life situations.

A range of initiatives has been developed to encourage improved provision of SRE, within the framework of Personal Social and Health Education (PSHE). In 2000 the Department for Education and Skills issued guidance to schools on how SRE should be delivered, to boys as well as girls, against which all schools are expected to review and develop their individual policies.[19]

Subsequently, OFSTED published a review of current SRE provision, making recommendations for improvement and setting clear learning outcomes for each Key Stage.[20] OFSTED now also include PSHE within their full inspections of schools.

To develop the skills and confidence of teachers to deliver PSHE and SRE effectively, a programme of professional development in PSHE was introduced in 2002 to award teachers specialist PSHE certification status. Recognizing the important contribution nurses can make to PSHE both in and out of school settings, a complementary specialist PSHE certification programme has been developed for community nurses. By 2006 the aim is for all secondary schools to have a specialist PSHE teacher and the 1000 schools in the most deprived communities also to have access to a specialist PSHE community nurse, providing a 'package' of expertise to lead and develop high quality PSHE and SRE for young people.

The SRE needs of more vulnerable young people are also being addressed; these include looked after children and young offenders. Specific training packages have been developed for social care professionals and all young offenders institutions have to offer inmates an SRE and parenting module.

Contraception and sexual health advice

Providing pupils with precise details of local sources of confidential contraceptive advice services is a requirement of the SRE guidance. However, it is clear from research with young people that services will not be used unless they are easily accessible and trusted. Concerns about lack of confidentiality, judgemental or disapproving staff, and formal clinical environments, combined with practical difficulties of transport and opening hours clashing with school commitments, often deter teenagers from seeking early advice.

The Teenage Pregnancy Unit's *Best Practice Guidance on the Provision of Effective Contraception and Advice Services* sets out the criteria by which services are expected to be commissioned and provided in all areas.[21] These highlight the importance of services:

- being focused on young people – with an upper age limit of 25;
- ensuring confidentiality with visible posters and clear statements to clients;
- being in the right locations – accessible by public transport;
- being open at the right times – after school and preferably at weekends;
- creating a youth friendly atmosphere – culturally appropriate to the young people in the community and welcoming to boys and young men;
- having staff with a smile – to welcome and reassure young people at reception and during consultations;
- posting publicity in places where young people meet – linked to local strategies' service publicity plans;
- providing as full a range of contraception, pregnancy testing and sexual health advice and treatment as possible, but helping young people to access other services when necessary.

Recognizing the significant role general practice plays in supporting young people on a range of issues, including teenage pregnancy and sexual health, an initiative has been developed with the Royal College of General Practitioners. *Getting it Right for Teenagers in Your Practice*[22] and the 'Confidentiality Toolkit'[23] both aim to help practices review and improve teenagers' trust in and uptake of advice from general practice. A resource to help services develop young people-friendly standards, and examples of 'Getting it Right' initiatives in general practice are being published in 2005. Box 8.1 shows an example of a 'badged' young people-friendly service.

Box 8.1   4YP contraception and sexual health advice services[24]

In Enfield and Harringay a 4YP 'brand' has been developed for all local contraception and sexual health services for young people. This includes clinics, a sexual health bus and 4YP pharmacies which provide emergency contraception under NHS arrangements.

The consistent use of the 4YP brand gives young people a recognizable image, indicating that the services are confidential and welcoming. The logo is clearly displayed on all publicity materials. Advertisements written and performed by young people have also been broadcast on Choice FM and community radio stations, promoting 4YP services.

To take advice closer to those young people who do not easily access mainstream services, local strategies are also integrating contraception and sexual health services into non-traditional youth-based settings. Mobile units, youth projects, Connexions Centres and schools have all been successful in involving sexual health professionals, to make advice hard to miss, not difficult to find. This new approach to service delivery is largely led by nurses, providing contraception under a 'patient group direction' (an arrangement whereby medicines can be provided by nurses to specified groups of patients without the direct involvement of a doctor). To increase the numbers of nurses skilled to work in the growing number of integrated services, the Teenage Pregnancy Unit has supported the Royal College of Nursing (RCN) to develop an RCN accredited sexual health distance learning programme.

Since 2002, the number of school-based health services which include the provision of contraception has increased significantly. Some provide pupils with school nurse liaison direct to the local general practice. Others have combinations of youth workers with nurses from relevant services such as family planning and Child and Adolescent Mental Health Services, providing weekly or sometimes daily drop-in sessions during school lunch hours. Some have developed innovative ways of improving access through a mobile phone helpline, staffed by a rota of school nurses. Pupils can text or talk to the nurse and, if necessary, arrange to meet at a suitable location, on or off the school site, if speedy treatment is needed, such as emergency contraception. Interestingly the mobile phone service is particularly well used by boys who did not previously use the school drop-in.

Any school-based service is developed at the discretion of the individual governing body, in consultation with parents, pupils and staff. However, schools with drop-in services consistently report benefits to pupils and staff, and support from parents. The provision of health services on site is one of the options in the government's Extended Schools Programme which aims to increase the potential of schools to be a wide resource for the local community. All local authorities are expected to have a full Extended School by 2006. (See www.teachernet.gov.uk/wholeschool/extendedschool for more information on extended schools.)

BETTER SUPPORT FOR TEENAGE PARENTS

An equivalent level of energy is being directed towards improving the support given to young parents in order to prevent poor outcomes for them and their children.

Antenatal and postnatal support

An essential part of support for young parents is to provide easily accessible pregnancy testing, unbiased information on the options of parenthood, abortion or adoption, and speedy referral to antenatal care or NHS-funded abortion services. Denial, anxiety and fear of disapproval deter many pregnant teenagers from seeking early advice. As a result they miss out on essential antenatal care or face late abortions. Pregnancy testing by outreach nurses or trained youth workers can help reach young women most vulnerable to delays.

Youth-friendly maternity services are also important to engage young parents in antenatal and postnatal care with specialist tailored models of care proving to be very effective. One teenage antenatal service that has one-to-one midwife support and encourages buddying up between young breast feeding mothers has one of the highest breast feeding rates (66%) amongst teenage mothers in England.[25] Another organizes a special teenage antenatal session to coincide with the routine 19 week scan, at which the young women have access to a special teenage parent adviser for information on housing, benefits, education and child-care.[25] Partners are also invited and there is a young fathers' worker to provide advice and support.

Positive involvement of the father during the pregnancy is a strong predictor of involvement in the early years of the child's life. For some disadvantaged young men, the prospect of fatherhood can be a powerful catalyst to motivate them back into education or training in order to provide better for their child.

Support for education, training and employment

As well as supporting young parents to develop confident parenting skills, a major focus of the Strategy is around providing help for young parents to remain in, or return to, education and training or enter work. Activities include:

- providing one-to-one assistance to remain in mainstream school or access a specialist education unit for young parents;
- support to find a college course appropriate to the educational and confidence levels of the individual young woman;
- help with childcare costs to enable young parents to continue their own learning and development. The government's innovative 'Care to Learn' scheme provides £5175 a year per child to fund childcare for any young parent under 19 in education or training – removing the obstacle so many parents cited as the major deterrent to participation in school or college.

Sure Start Plus

One of the aims of the Strategy is to provide coordinated packages of support for young parents to ensure neither they nor their children fall through the gaps between service providers. To test out the best way of delivering this, the Sure Start Plus pilot programme was launched in 35 areas across England.

Sure Start Plus offers coordinated support to pregnant teenagers and teenage parents. It provides them with a pregnancy adviser to explore with them their options and entitlements. If they become parents then the adviser will tailor an ongoing support package to meet their individual needs, for example offering help with housing, managing finances, child-care and education.

Learning from this programme is being extracted to inform delivery of support in all local areas. What is already clear is that young parents greatly appreciate having a trusted adviser to whom they can turn for support and who will advocate on their behalf when necessary. In areas without Sure Start Plus, support packages are being developed by specialist Connexions personal advisers, or sometimes through specialist health visitors.

Supported housing

The majority of young parents are able to rely on their families for housing as well as some material and financial support. However, not all families are equipped to take on this role and young parents may need to secure alternative accommodation. Traditionally this has been poor accommodation on large estates, often away from their family and other support networks. For many this has led to isolation and obstacles, such as poor transport, making it very difficult to consider any participation in learning.

To address this, the Strategy has a goal that all under 18 lone parents who cannot live at home or with their partner are provided with supported accommodation, appropriate to their needs. For some this may be intensive support in a residential setting with a worker on site or on call 24 hours a day. For others it may be an individual flat with some shared communal space, with a part-time support worker. Some may only require the 'floating support' of an adviser to maintain an independent tenancy successfully. Six housing pilots, with different models of support, are being evaluated to help inform best practice in the future.

HOW DOES THE STRATEGY INVOLVE YOUNG PEOPLE?

From its onset the Strategy has seen consulting with and involving young people as essential to its success. Involving a broad group of young people is central to implementing the action plan. It is necessary in order to ensure that those engaged in delivering the Strategy:

- use credible approaches to awareness raising and service provision;
- communicate effectively with those groups most at risk;
- provide support services for pregnant teenagers and teenage parents that are accessible to those who need them most.

Young people have been involved in all stages and all levels of developing work around the teenage pregnancy agenda. Initially the Social Exclusion Unit talked to groups of young people and young parents, alongside consultation with professionals, in order to draw together the action plan. These young people were important in defining the problems and highlighting the areas that the strategy now targets.

Subsequently, a young people's teenage pregnancy forum has been established to feed back on the progress of the Strategy and to generate ideas for future direction.

Within local strategies, young people's participation has also been encouraged. Young people have been involved in a variety of ways, such as:

- helping develop service publicity materials;
- 'mystery shopping' inspections by young people to check that services are youth friendly;
- peer education programmes in schools;
- involvement in local youth forums and local authority scrutiny committees.

CURRENT TRENDS AND A LOOK TO THE FUTURE

Now in its fourth year, the Strategy continues to maintain a high profile, a high level of commitment inside government, and support from voluntary sector partners. Although it is still early days there are signs to suggest a positive start. The most recent figures for 2002 show a reduction of 8.6% in the under 18 conception rate since the Strategy's baseline year of 1998; eight out of the nine Government Office regions have seen declines of between 8 and 17%.[1] The proportion of young mothers in education, training or employment has also increased from 16% in 1997 to 29% in 2004.[26] Both of these indicators suggest that we are heading in the right direction.

However, the Strategy has been set over a 10 year period in recognition of the time needed to effect the behavioural and attitudinal changes required. The Strategy rests on a sound evidence base. The challenge lies in engaging the hearts and minds of all the organizations and individuals who need to work together to make the Strategy work. The Green Paper *Every Child Matters*[16] provides an exciting vision of better integrated services and professionals trained in communicating well with young people. This will help to strengthen the partnerships which local teenage pregnancy strategies have so successfully begun. However, the Teenage Pregnancy Strategy has specific actions which will need a continued focus to ensure success.

The Netherlands, which long held the accolade for the lowest levels of teenage pregnancy in Western Europe, has recently seen an increase in their rates. One Dutch expert who has worked in the area of teenage pregnancy for over 20 years attributes the rise to a loss of focus: 'We were doing so well, we took our eye off the ball' (personal communication). In the UK, at the start of the journey, it is vital that teenage pregnancy remains at the top of the agenda.

CONTROVERSIAL ISSUES AND COMMON MYTHS

In the UK the issue of teenage pregnancy attracts considerably more media interest than in other European countries. Headlines of 'sex lessons for tots' or 'morning after pills in schools' lead to polarized debate between those who believe young people should be supported to make their own informed choices and those who promote an 'abstinence only' approach. Health professionals, the media, politicians and family values campaigners all take an interest and a position; the latter groups tend to stress that teenage pregnancy is an indicator of declining moral standards in society.

Within the media coverage and high-profile debate, the majority view of parents and young people who support sex education and access to contraception is often absent. Important research evidence is frequently ignored and common myths are allowed to flourish.

Below are common questions on topical and controversial issues. (We set out the research evidence underpinning our answers in the earlier section 'The evidence base for the Strategy'.)

Does sex education encourage young people to have early sex?

There is no evidence that providing young people with sex and relationships education and contraceptive advice increases sexual activity. In contrast, there is strong research evidence showing that comprehensive school-based sex education, particularly linked to contraceptive services, is effective at delaying sexual activity and reducing pregnancy rates.

There is no strong evidence that abstinence-only programmes reduce teenage pregnancy rates.

Can young people under 16 get contraception without their parents knowing?

Health professionals can provide contraception to under 16s provided they are satisfied that the young person is competent to understand and make a choice of the treatment involved. This also applies to consent to abortion. Health professionals work within an established legal framework which includes encouraging young people to inform their parents. However, health professionals have the same duty of confidentiality to under 16s as they do to adults. A young person's request for confidentiality is respected unless there are serious child protection issues.

Doesn't the Sexual Offences Act (2003) make it illegal for teenagers to kiss or for health professionals to provide contraception to under 16s?

Under the Sexual Offences Act (2003)[27] the age of consent remains at 16 for heterosexual, gay or bisexual young people. The Act aims to protect young people from people who force them into having sex they do not want. The Act is not intended to prosecute mutually agreed sexual activity between two young people of a similar age unless there is evidence of abuse or exploitation.

Young people under 16, including those under 13, can continue to get confidential contraceptive and sexual health advice and treatment.

Health professionals can continue to provide advice and treatment to under 16s within the same legal framework and professional codes of confidentiality. The Act makes clear that anyone providing contraceptive/sexual health advice or treatment will not be guilty of facilitating any offences if they act for the purpose of:

- protecting the child from sexually transmitted infection, or
- protecting the physical safety of the child, or
- preventing the child from becoming pregnant, or
- promoting the child's emotional well-being by the giving of advice.

This covers not only health professionals, but anyone who acts to protect a child, for example teachers, Connexions personal advisers, social care professionals, teenage magazine advice columnists, parents, other relatives or friends.

Won't access to contraception in schools just increase the problem?

There is no evidence that improving young people's access to contraception increases sexual activity or teenage pregnancy rates. In contrast, there is strong evidence that linking school-based SRE with contraceptive advice services is effective at reducing pregnancy rates. The aim of school-based health services is to make it easier for young people to get one-to-one professional advice and support not solely about contraception but on a range of health, relationship or emotional issues that may be troubling them. Schools with on site services report significant benefits to pupils. In their 2002 report *Sex and Relationships Education in Schools*,[20] OFSTED recommended better access to individual advice for pupils and cited a school-based drop-in as an example of good practice.

The decision to have a school-based service, and the content of the service, rests with the governing body of the individual school, in consultation with parents, pupils and the school community.

Won't supporting teenage parents encourage more young people to get pregnant?

Early parenthood can be an indicator of many complex issues in a young person's life. There is no evidence that young people deliberately get pregnant to obtain benefits or local authority housing.

Teenage parents and their children are at greater risk of poor health and social outcomes which adversely affect them, their families and the wider community. Providing support to teenage parents through education and training, childcare and supported housing will increase their opportunities of financial independence and help to break the cycle of poverty and deprivation.

Doesn't sex education and the provision of contraception undermine the role of parents?

Research shows that the vast majority of parents support both SRE in schools and the provision of contraception to teenagers, including under 16s.

Parents play a key role in reducing the rate of teenage pregnancy. Research shows that in families where sexual issues are talked about openly and without embarrassment, young people are more likely to have sex later and to use contraception when they become sexually active. Most parents believe there would be fewer teenage pregnancies if parents talked more to their children about sex and relationships issues. However, almost half of young people say they have received nothing or not a lot of information from their parents.

WHAT RESEARCH QUESTIONS STILL NEED ANSWERS?

Key questions being addressed by the Teenage Pregnancy Unit's research programme include:

● What is the impact of growing up in rural and seaside resorts on the sexual behaviour and life chances of young people?

● What are the attitudes and behaviours of black and minority ethnic young people in relation to sexual activity, contraceptive use and teenage pregnancy?

● What is black and minority ethnic young people's experience of teenage parenthood?

● What are the educational experiences of pregnant young women and young mothers of school age?

● What are the long term consequences of teenage births for mothers, fathers and their children?

In addition, we need to know the following:

● What are the most effective ways of improving communication about sex and relationships between young people and their parents?

● What is the best way of professionals working with young people to ensure early identification and support to young women most at risk of early pregnancy?

● What are the links between unprotected sex and other risk-taking behaviour such as drinking, particularly binge drinking and drug use?

Key sources of further information and help

- **Health Development Agency:**
  www.hda-online.org.uk. The HDA is a key information resource on the evidence base for what works in preventing teenage pregnancy and supporting teenage parents. Their evidence briefing 'Teenage pregnancy and parenthood' can be accessed through their website.
- **Royal Colleges:** organizations for healthcare professionals providing representation and support, education and information, including on sexual health issues.

Royal College of General Practitioners
www.rcgp.org.uk
Royal College of Nursing www.rcn.org.uk
Royal College of Midwives www.rcm.org.uk
- **Teenage Pregnancy Unit:** www.teenagepregnancyunit.gov.uk. Regularly updated news regarding the Teenage Pregnancy Strategy. Source of guidance documents, research reports, statistical updates, teenage pregnancy-related events.

References

1. National Statistics. Health Statistics Quarterly, No. 24. London: The Stationery Office; Winter 2004.
2. Social Exclusion Unit. Teenage pregnancy. London: Social Exclusion Unit; 1999. Online. Available: http://www.socialexclusionunit.gov.uk
3. UNICEF. A league table of teenage births in rich nations. Innocenti Report Card No.3. Florence, Italy: UNICEF; 2001. Online. Available: http://www.unicef.icdc.org
4. Kiernan K. Transition to parenthood: young mothers, young fathers – associated factors and later life experiences. Discussion paper WSP/113. London: London School of Economics; 1995.
5. HM Chief Inspector of Prisons. Thematic review of young prisoners. London: Home Office; 1997.
6. Berthoud R. Teenage births to ethnic minority women. Population Trends 2001; 104:12–17.
7. Hobcraft J, Kiernan K. Childhood poverty, early motherhood and adult social exclusion. CASE paper 28. London: London School of Economics; 1999.
8. Ermisch J, Pevalin D. Who has a child as a teenager? ISER Working Paper 2003–30. Colchester: Institute for Social and Economic Research, University of Essex; 2003.
9. Health Education Authority. Young people and health. London: HEA; 1999.
10. British Market Research Bureau International. Evaluation of the Teenage Pregnancy Strategy. Tracking survey. Report of results of nine waves of research. London: BMRB; October 2003. Online. Available: http://www.teenagepregnancyunit.gov.uk
11. Blair T. Foreword. Social Exclusion Unit. Teenage pregnancy. London: Social Exclusion Unit; 1999.
12. Scottish Executive. Enhancing sexual wellbeing in Scotland: a sexual health and relationships strategy. Proposal to the Scottish Executive. Edinburgh: Scottish Executive; 2003.
13. National Assembly for Wales. Strategic framework for promoting sexual health in Wales. Cardiff: National Assembly for Wales; 2000.
14. Department of Health, Social Services and Public Safety. Teenage pregnancy and parenthood. Strategy and action plan 2002–2007. Belfast: DHSSPS, Northern Ireland Executive; 2002.
15. Swann C, Bowe K, McCormick G, Kosmin M. Teenage pregnancy and parenthood: a review of reviews. Evidence briefing. London: Health Development Agency; 2002. Online. Available: http://www.hda-online.org.uk/evidence
16. Department for Education and Skills. Green Paper. Every child matters. London: DfES; 2003. In: DfES. Every child matters: the next steps. London: DfES; 2004. (Sets out vision and plans.) Online. Available: www.dfes.gov.uk/everychildmatters
17. Department of Health. National Service Framework for children and young people. (Forthcoming: development of this NSF was announced in 2001. See: www.dh.gov.uk.)
18. Stone N, Ingham R. Factors affecting British teenagers' contraceptive use at first intercourse: the importance of partner communication. Perspectives on Sexual and Reproductive Health 2002; 34(4):191–197.
19. Department for Education and Skills. Sex and relationship education guidance. Guidance: curriculum and standards. Head teachers, teachers and school governors. London: DfES; 2000. Online. Available: http://www.dfes.gov.uk/sreguidance/sexeducation.pdf
20. OFSTED. Sex and relationships education in schools. London: OFSTED; 2002.
21. Teenage Pregnancy Unit. Best practice guidance on the provision of effective contraception and advice services. London: TPU; 2000.

22. Royal College of General Practitioners. Getting it right for teenagers in your practice. London: RCGP; 2002.

23. Royal College of General Practitioners. Confidentiality and young people: a toolkit for general practice, primary care groups and trusts. London: RCGP; 2000.

24. The Department of Health on behalf of the Teenage Pregnancy Unit. The Independent Advisory Group on Teenage Pregnancy Annual Report 2002–2003. 4YP (8.1). London: DOH; 2003.

25. Teenage Pregnancy Unit and Royal College of Midwives. Teenage parents: who cares? A guide to commissioning and delivering maternity services for young parents. London: Department of Health; 2004.

26. Office for National Statistics. Labour force survey. Household dataset: spring quarter 2003. London: ONS; 2003.

27. Sexual Offences Act 2003. London: HMSO.

Chapter **9**

Sexually transmitted infections

Susan Laverty and R. Nicholas Pugh

SUMMARY OVERVIEW AND LINKS TO OTHER TOPICS

Sexually transmitted infections (STIs) and human immunodeficiency virus (HIV) are rising rapidly, and the genitourinary medicine (GUM) services to treat them are in decline: the result is a crisis. In this chapter we explore the root causes of this crisis, analyse the changing trends in rates of STI transmission, discuss the impact of sexual health inequalities, and examine the evidence for effective interventions for improving the sexual health of the population.

STIs show increasing rates of incidence and those infections thought to be a thing of the past (such as syphilis) are re-emerging. At the end of 2002, nearly 43 000 people in England were HIV positive. STIs can have serious health consequences and people living with HIV can have many health, social and economic problems.

Inequalities feature throughout: in particular, sexual ill health affects women, men who have sex with men, young adults, and black and minority ethnic groups disproportionately.

The first *National Strategy for Sexual Health and HIV*[1] in 2001 signalled government recognition of the epidemic of sexual ill health, and aims to improve prevention and services.

Action should focus on providing good quality services and promoting sexual health with a range of methods, settings and specific target groups, but there is a lot still to be learnt about effective prevention and take-up of services.

As teenage pregnancy is another facet of sexual health, and alcohol and drugs have an impact on sexual behaviour, Chapter 8 'Teenage pregnancy', Chapter 10 'Alcohol use and misuse' and Chapter 11 'Drug use and misuse' are highly relevant to this topic. Chapter 14 'Helping individuals to change behaviour' is also relevant to sexual behaviour, and Chapter 13 'Tackling inequalities in health' addresses issues about inequalities raised in this chapter.

SEXUALLY TRANSMITTED INFECTIONS AND HIV

Sexually transmitted infections (STIs) are diseases which are passed to other people through sexual contact – not only penetrative heterosexual sex, but also oral and anal sex. All of us, regardless of our sexual identity, whether we are heterosexual, bisexual, gay or lesbian, are susceptible to these infections if we do not practise safe sex.

The main STIs are:

- HIV
- gonorrhoea
- *chlamydia*
- genital warts
- genital herpes simplex
- syphilis.

Hepatitis B can also be sexually transmitted.

These infections are important not only because they can result in unpleasant symptoms but because they can lead to serious long term health damage, and in many cases people are not aware that they are infected. Therefore people may be late in seeking treatment, or indeed never seek help at all and unwittingly pass infection on to others.

HIV

Discovered in the 1980s, HIV stands for human immunodeficiency virus. It can be spread through:

- unprotected sex (including heterosexual and homosexual practices);
- direct blood contact (including needles, blood transfusions and other blood products);
- from mother to baby.

HIV infection can result in acquired immune deficiency syndrome (AIDS) which represents the late stages of infection when the body's natural defence system is seriously weakened (immunodeficiency). This stage is characterized by certain diseases and opportunistic infections.

Although HIV and AIDS cannot be cured, the advent of new antiviral treatments now means that people can live a long time with the condition.

Why are sexually transmitted infections an important public health issue?

In its third report for the session 2002–2003, the House of Commons Health Select Committee described sexual health in England as being in crisis. The committee's chairman talked of being frankly shocked and appalled by some of the evidence: 'the whole sexual health service seems to be a shambles'. Alarmed by rapidly increasing rates of STIs and appalled by the spiralling decline in genitourinary medicine (GUM) services nationally, the committee called for action.[2]

PART OF A WIDER PICTURE

Examining changing rates of STI transmission alone will not explain the current crisis in sexual health or the implications for public health. STIs have to be examined within the broader context of sexual health and, importantly, other socio-economic factors and behaviour choices. When we look at STI rates in young people, the links with teenage pregnancy, alcohol use, deprivation and social exclusion become clear. Examination of reported outbreaks of syphilis demonstrates the complex links between STI transmission and sexual preference and behaviour, and also, in some cases, links with drug misuse.

INCREASING RATES OF INFECTION

Dramatically increasing rates of infection, the re-emergence of STIs that we thought were a thing of the past, and the HIV epidemic have served to refocus attention on sexual health and sexual health services. Over the last decade the rates of STIs have increased dramatically across Europe:

- Gonorrhoea rates rose by 92% in France in 1998 and by 154% in Sweden between 1995 and 2000.[2]

- Syphilis outbreaks have recently been reported in the Netherlands, Ireland, France and Norway.[2]

- Between 1996 and 2001, syphilis rates in England increased by 500% (from 116 to 696 cases), with notable outbreaks in London, Manchester and Brighton.[3–5]

- Gonorrhoea and *Chlamydia* infection rates soared in the same period.[2]

- At the end of December 2002, nearly 43 000 people had been diagnosed as HIV positive in England.[2]

VARIATION IN SERVICES

The number of visits to GUM departments in England has doubled over the last decade, now standing at over 1 million per year.[1] Provision of sexual health services across England is characterized by huge variation in services and unacceptable delays in access. One survey of GUM clinics found delays of up to 1 week for urgent appointments and 4 weeks for routine appointments.[6]

COSTS TO THE INDIVIDUAL AND SOCIETY

Poor sexual health and STIs are costly to both the individual and society. Consequences of STIs include:

- pelvic inflammatory disease
- infertility

- ectopic pregnancies
- cervical and other genital cancers
- viral hepatitis
- chronic liver disease
- liver cancer.

For people living with HIV the personal costs are high. Many are unable to work and battle with social isolation and discrimination on a daily basis.

Since society carries the cost, preventing poor sexual health would release finite resources. The average lifetime treatment costs for an HIV positive individual is calculated at between £135 000 and £181 000; preventing a single onward transmission saves between £500 000 and £1 million in terms of health benefits and treatment costs.[1]

HEALTH INEQUALITIES

The public health importance of STIs has to be seen not only in the context of the burden of disease and associated costs, but within the context of the broader determinants of health and health inequalities. Good sexual health is not distributed evenly across the population; inequalities exist. The burden of sexual ill health falls disproportionately on women, men who have sex with men, young adults, and black and minority ethnic groups.[7,8] Tackling sexual health inequalities is but one aspect of tackling health inequalities across society, requiring the same attention to the broader determinants of health, and commitment to social justice.

In other chapters of this book inequalities are discussed in a separate section. But as inequalities are a fundamental feature of the whole epidemiological picture of STIs and HIV, we address the issue throughout this chapter.

HOW IS SEXUAL HEALTH ADDRESSED IN NATIONAL POLICY?

In 1999, *Saving Lives: Our Healthier Nation*[9] drew attention to the public health significance of declining sexual health and rising rates of STIs, promising the introduction of a national strategy for sexual health. The launch of the first *National Strategy for Sexual Health and HIV* in 2001[1] signalled a government re-priority in the face of an epidemic of sexual ill health. The strategy promises better prevention, better services and better sexual health, as set out in Box 9.1.

WHAT IS THE CURRENT PICTURE AND WHAT ARE THE TRENDS IN STI TRANSMISSION?

We shall examine current trends in transmission of STIs in terms of the implications for certain populations, including young people, men, women and people from black and minority ethnic groups.

Box 9.1   National Strategy for Sexual Health and HIV[1,10]

The national strategy, published in 2001, aims to:

- reduce the transmission of HIV and STIs, with a national goal of achieving a 25% reduction in the number of newly acquired HIV infections and gonorrhoea infections by 2007;
- reduce the prevalence of undiagnosed STIs and HIV (setting a national standard that all GUM services should offer an HIV test to clinic attendees on their first screening for STIs);
- reduce unintended pregnancy rates, setting a national standard that women who meet the legal requirements should have access to an abortion within 3 weeks of the first appointment with the referring doctor;
- improve health and social care for people living with HIV;
- reduce the stigma associated with HIV and STIs.

YOUNG PEOPLE

In the UK, young people aged 19–24 years experience STIs disproportionately. Since 1995 the rates of *Chlamydia* and gonorrhoea in this age group have increased (see Fig. 9.1). In 2002 in England, Wales and Northern Ireland:[11]

- young women accounted for 72% of all female *Chlamydia* diagnoses and 66% of gonorrhoea diagnosed in GUM clinics;
- young men accounted for 53% of all male *Chlamydia* and 40% of gonorrhoea diagnoses;
- only 10% of new HIV diagnoses were in people aged 16–24.

Chlamydia

Rising rates of *Chlamydia* infection give particular cause for concern. In 2002, genital *Chlamydia* infection was the most common STI diagnosed in GUM clinics, with over 82 000 diagnoses made in England, Wales and

Figure 9.1   STIs in young people 1996–2002. New cases of uncomplicated *Chlamydia*, gonorrhoea and genital warts in 16–24 year olds in the UK. (Reproduced with permission from Health Protection Agency 2003.[11])

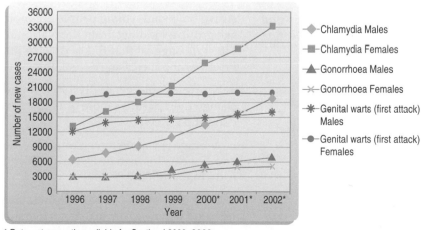

* Data not currently available for Scotland 2000–2002

Northern Ireland. *Chlamydia* infection does not show symptoms in up to 70% of female and 50% of male cases, so it is likely that these figures under represent the true prevalence of the disease.

Increasing awareness of *Chlamydia* in the general population through publicity such as the 'Sex Lottery Campaign' and 'Come Clean' as well as more sensitive laboratory testing methods may account, in part, for the increasing incidence.[11]

Identifying and treating *Chlamydia* infection is important because undiagnosed infection can result in serious problems, such as pelvic inflammatory disease and infertility in women. The National Screening Committee[12] has endorsed screening for *Chlamydia* infection and the phased rollout of a national *Chlamydia* screening programme began in 2003.

A particular concern raised by the Health Select Committee was the continuing use of insensitive tests for *Chlamydia* in many areas. In response, the government pledged increased funding to enable laboratories to switch to a more sensitive method of testing (Nucleic Acid Amplification Tests).[13]

Gonorrhoea

In 2002, nearly 25 000 cases of uncomplicated gonorrhoea were diagnosed in GUM clinics in England, Wales and Northern Ireland. Between 2001 and 2002, diagnoses of gonorrhoea increased by 8% in men and 10% in women, with the highest rates seen amongst men aged 20–24 and women aged 16–19.[11] Overall, the majority of reported cases were in men, with a preponderance of these infections acquired as a result of sex between men.[11]

Gonorrhoea infection tends to be concentrated in urban, deprived areas and among certain population groups, such as homosexual and bisexual men, young women and some black ethnic minority groups. This reflects the geographical distribution of these groups and their sexual networks.[14]

Of particular concern is the increasing resistance to antimicrobial drugs used to treat gonorrhoea infection, especially in some parts of the country such as Yorkshire and Humberside and the East Midlands.[11] In 2002, 20% of cases showed resistance to first line antimicrobial drugs, compared to 11% in 2001. As a result, transmission of infection is more likely and so are the complications associated with infection.

Sexual attitudes and knowledge

As we have said, young people are more predisposed to STIs than older age groups. Findings from the National Survey of Sexual Attitudes and Lifestyle suggest that this is due, in part, to changing trends in sexual practices and increasing sexual diversity:[15]

● Young people generally have higher numbers of sexual partners, change their partners more often than older people, and have more concurrent partners.

● Average age at first intercourse has declined from 21 years for women and 17 years for men in 1990 to 16 years for men and women born in the early to mid 1980s.

● Over 20% of 15–24 year old men and 15% of 15–24 year old women reported having a concurrent partnership in the last year.

Further factors in explaining rising STIs in young people include:

- Sexual aptitudes, including negotiating skills. Often young people do not have the knowledge or skill to negotiate safe sexual relationships, including condom use. For example, a lifestyle survey undertaken with school age young people in Walsall in 2000 found that their knowledge of HIV and its transmission was sketchy; only 77% of pupils aged 14–15 knew that HIV could be transmitted by having sex without using a condom, compared with 82% of the wider population.[16]

- Likelihood of seeking help for health problems (health seeking behaviour) and the accessibility of user friendly sexual health services;

- Alcohol use is associated with risky sexual behaviour. Binge drinking has increased amongst young women, increasing their vulnerability to sexual exploitation. A Social Exclusion Unit report showed that after uncontrolled drinking, 1 in 7 older teenagers go on to have unsafe sex and that 40% of 13–14 year olds were drunk when they experienced first intercourse.[17]

STIs in young people are not the only challenge. Ignorance and risky behaviour can have profound personal and social consequences. The UK has one of the highest rates of teenage conceptions and pregnancy in Europe (See Ch. 8 'Teenage pregnancy'). Unplanned pregnancies increase the risk of poor social, economic and health prospects in both mother and child.[1]

The provision of coordinated sexual health services for young people, including access to sexual and relationship education, GUM and family planning services, has been recognized as a priority in the *National Strategy for Sexual Health and HIV*.[1] As a result the Department of Health has funded the provision and evaluation of pilot one-stop sexual health services and primary care youth services.

WOMEN
Human papilloma virus
Genital warts

Genital warts are the most commonly diagnosed viral STI in the UK. There are nearly 100 different types of human papilloma virus (HPV), but only a few are associated with genital warts. There was a 2% increase in the number of cases of genital warts in the UK between 2001 and 2002: 53% of the approximately 70 000 diagnoses in 2002 were in men, and 47% in women. This varies across the country; for example, genital wart infection in women living in Walsall increased by approximately 30% (about 150 cases to about 200 cases).[16] The highest rates of infection in women are in the 16–19 and 20–24 age groups.[11]

Cervical cancer

HPV infection in women is especially significant because certain types of the virus are associated with cervical cancer. Fortunately, this includes only a small number out of the 100 or so different types of HPV.

Approximately 20% of women in their twenties have HPV infection but the natural history of the infection is poorly understood. In most cases the infection disappears naturally although smoking and immuno-suppressive illnesses, for example AIDS, seem to impair this. Whilst the majority of infections, even with high risk HPV types, do not result in cervical cancer, close to 100% of cervical cancers are found to have HPV. Consequently, there has been an interest in HPV testing as a way of finding out which women might be at most risk from cervical cancer. However, questions remain about the predictive value of HPV testing and this and other issues are being evaluated in several pilot projects across England.[18]

HIV

Rates of HIV infection in women are rising:[2]

- In 2002, 1993 of the 3152 heterosexually acquired new HIV diagnoses in the UK were in women.

- The male:female ratio for all new infections diagnosed in 1985–1986 was approximately 14:1, whereas in 2000–2001 it was about 1.7:1.

The largest increase has been seen in women from sub-Saharan Africa, many of whom are of childbearing age.[11] The prevalence of HIV in women giving birth in inner London was 0.53% in 2002, compared to 0.06% in the rest of England. The highest prevalence of 2.47% is in women from sub-Saharan Africa.[11]

This has several public health implications. A priority need is the provision of accessible and user friendly health services with requisite health promotion inputs for what is often a marginalized group. Prevention of further transmission within communities and to future children is also important. The difficulties and challenges of undertaking effective sexual health promotion within fragmented migrant communities have been well documented.[19]

Antenatal screening

HIV

Since the 1990s there has been an increase in the recorded number of births to HIV positive women, from 130 reports in 1994 to over 300 in 2000.[2] A national study of HIV in pregnancy and childhood estimates that by the end of June 2003, 3576 children had been born to HIV infected mothers in the UK, 28% of whom were known to be infected, while 48% were known to be uninfected, with the HIV status of the remainder unresolved or unreported.[11]

Since 1999, women in England have been offered and recommended universal antenatal screening for HIV. Antenatal testing benefits both mother and child. Detecting infection in the mother means that she can be offered appropriate treatment and advice about her own health and that of her unborn child. The use of antiretroviral treatments, Caesarean section, and the avoidance of invasive procedures significantly reduce transmission of infection to the baby.[20] In addition, antenatal screening affords the opportunity for sexual health promotion.

Since 1999, the detection rate of HIV in pregnancy has increased, with a concomitant reduction of transmission from mother to child of HIV infection from 19% of those exposed in 1997 to 8% of those exposed in 2002.[11]

Other infections

Syphilis and the blood borne virus hepatitis B are also included in the antenatal screening programme.

If a mother infected with hepatitis B transmits infection to her baby there is a high risk that the baby will become a chronic carrier of the infection, with the attendant risk of developing chronic liver disease or liver cancer later in life. Screening for hepatitis B infection allows early detection in the baby and an opportunity to offer immunization, which prevents infection in 90–95% of cases.

In September 2003 the Department of Health issued standards and good practice guidance for screening for infectious diseases in pregnancy.[21]

Women who have sex with women

Women who have sex with women (WSW) is a term describing sexual behaviour, whilst lesbian is a term denoting sexual identity. In the debate regarding sexual health and STI transmission, this is an often overlooked group.

A recent editorial in the medical press has highlighted the fact that such women form a group with particular risk profiles and health needs.[22] Most lesbians have a history of sex with men and subsequently have been exposed to many of the same sexual health risks as heterosexual women. For example, it is often assumed that WSW are not at risk of contracting HPV and do not need cervical smears. Yet one study found that one in five women who have never had heterosexual intercourse had HPV infection.[23] Transmission of syphilis by orogenital sex between women has been described[22] and an estimated 10% of women with exclusively female partners have a history of STIs.[24]

Whilst findings from the National Survey of Sexual Attitudes and Lifestyle[15] suggest that sexual diversity is more commonplace, homophobia and its resultant stigma and isolation still exist for many gay men and women. Some studies suggest that these groups may be more susceptible to mental health problems, including increased risk of deliberate self-harm, suicide, depression and anxiety disorders.[25,26] This warrants recognition by healthcare planners and providers. Good sexual health services should be underpinned by a holistic approach to health, which recognizes the implications of sexual orientation and ensures access to appropriate services. For example, an evaluation of our local GUM service in Walsall highlighted the need for better connections with our local mental health service, particularly for individuals with HIV infection.[27]

MEN

Two important infections relating to men's sexual health are HIV and syphilis. HIV continues to be the most important STI in terms of associated mortality, morbidity and costs to society. Syphilis, once considered to be an infection on the wane, is re-emerging. Both infections are strongly associated with the gay and bisexual community, conventionally described as men who have sex with men (MSM).

HIV

The HIV epidemic continues unabated in the UK:[11]

● To the end of 2002 a cumulative total of 56 000 HIV diagnoses have been made in the UK since the beginning of the epidemic: 53% have been in the MSM population with 32% acquired heterosexually.

- The estimated prevalence of diagnosed HIV infections in adults increased between 2001 and 2002 by 20% to 34 300, and undiagnosed HIV infections increased by 17% to 15 200.

- The number of new HIV diagnoses has almost doubled from nearly 3000 in 1998 to about 5500 in 2002.

In contrast, since the introduction of effective antiretroviral therapies in the mid 1990s, the number of deaths and AIDS diagnoses has declined, remaining relatively constant since the late 1990s (see Fig. 9.2).[4]

There are two key epidemiological trends contributing to this picture: heterosexually acquired infections and infection in MSM groups.

Heterosexual transmission

The rapid increase in the number of new HIV diagnoses is due largely to infections acquired heterosexually. Since 1999, the number of new HIV diagnoses in heterosexuals has exceeded that in the MSM population: over 3000 heterosexually acquired new HIV diagnoses were made in 2002. This represents a greater than three-fold increase since 1996. An estimated 50% of all HIV infections acquired heterosexually are currently undiagnosed.[11]

Infections likely to have been acquired in Africa accounted for three quarters of the heterosexually acquired infections diagnosed in the UK in 2002. In the early years, infections acquired in Eastern Africa, particularly Uganda, predominated. Since 1999, more infections have been acquired in South Eastern Africa, especially Zimbabwe. Infections acquired heterosexually in Asia, Latin America and the Caribbean continue to rise but remain low relative to infections acquired in Africa.[11] Increasing numbers of women account for these heterosexually acquired infections (see section on 'Women' above).

Since 1998, HIV infection acquired in the UK in heterosexual people has risen: 275 cases in 2002 compared to 147 cases in 1998.[11] It is thought that many of these individuals were probably infected through partners who acquired their infections outside Europe.

Transmission in MSM

Despite health promotion activity and antiretroviral therapy, there is little evidence that transmission rates for HIV in MSM are declining. Indeed, the incidence of HIV infection appears to be rising. Between 1995

Figure 9.2 HIV and AIDS diagnoses and deaths in the UK 1993–2002. Numbers will rise for recent years as further reports are received. (Reproduced with permission from Health Protection Agency 2003.[11] HIV/AIDS reports received by end of June 2003.)

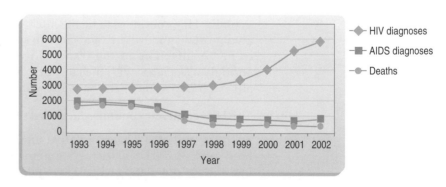

and 2001, the annual incidence of HIV infection in MSM attending GUM clinics was 2–3%. In 2002, this figure increased to 3.5%. The highest incidence is in London and in men aged 35–44 years, at an estimated 6%.[11]

Sexual behaviour is clearly a major factor in determining the incidence of HIV. Survey data in 2000 shows that MSM reported increases in unprotected anal intercourse with both regular and casual partners compared to 1995.[28] The reasons behind these changing behaviours are unclear. It may be that the advent of antiretroviral therapy, the fact that HIV infection is no longer seen as a 'death sentence', and the expanding sexual market places, for example saunas and internet chat rooms, are significant factors. However, more research is needed into changing sexual behaviours, risk taking and sexual attitudes in MSM in the UK.[29]

MSM remain the population group with the greatest number of HIV infected patients seen for care. In 2002, of all patients receiving care for HIV infection:[11]

- 46% (nearly 14 000) were MSM;
- 41% (about 12 500) were heterosexual;
- 3% (nearly 900) were injecting drug users.

There is little difference in the uptake of antiretroviral treatment between exposure groups.[11]

Syphilis

Annual diagnoses of syphilis increased by a staggering 500% (from 116 to 696 cases) between 1996 and 2001.[2] In 2002, 1095 cases in men and 137 cases in women were reported by GUM clinics in England, Wales and Northern Ireland. Of concern is the increasing association of syphilis infection and HIV infection in certain populations, particularly MSM. Co-infection (having more than one infection at the same time) increases the risk of transmission and co-infection with syphilis and gonorrhoea in this group is often a marker of high-risk sexual behaviour: 58% of syphilis diagnoses in males were in MSM. Unlike other STIs, syphilis is more prevalent in older age groups.

Recent resurgence of the disease has been associated with a number of outbreaks:

- In 1997, a Bristol outbreak was associated with heterosexually acquired infection, commercial sex work and 'crack' cocaine use.

- More recent outbreaks in London, Brighton and Manchester [3,4] have centred on the MSM population, some of whom had concurrent HIV infection.

- The London outbreak has been the largest reported to date, with over 1000 cases between April 2001 and September 2003: 256 were in heterosexual men and over 800 were in MSM, 46% of whom were co-infected with HIV.[11]

- In 2002, Walsall experienced a stark increase in cases of syphilis in MSM, from a background figure of 1–2 cases a year, to over 50 cases by the end of 2003. Outbreak measures were required.[30]

The publication in 2002 of guidelines for managing outbreaks of STIs at a local, regional and district level bears testimony to the increasing public health risks posed by such outbreaks.[31]

Why is syphilis on the increase and why such marked outbreaks?

The introduction of routine testing for syphilis in HIV infected individuals may have led to more cases of syphilis being recognized in MSM than in other groups who did not have routine syphilis testing.[32] However, similar outbreaks of syphilis have been reported in Western Europe and the USA. Many share common characteristics, including high levels of concurrent HIV infection and high rates of partner change. Especially worrying is the increased levels of risk taking and unsafe sex with partners of unknown HIV status, which feature heavily in these outbreaks.

The reasons behind these changing behaviours are not yet fully understood but the following factors may play a part.

● The advent of effective therapy for HIV infection is thought to have altered people's perception about the risks involved in unsafe sex.

● Contracting HIV is no longer associated with terminal illness.

● The expansion and increasing diversity of sexual market places, including cruising grounds, saunas and internet chat rooms facilitate partner exchange.[11] One study amongst MSM attending a sex resort found that those using the internet to seek sex partners were at a slight increased risk of acquiring and transmitting STIs.[33]

PEOPLE FROM BLACK AND ETHNIC MINORITY GROUPS

In the UK, people from black and ethnic minority groups are disproportionately affected by poor sexual health.

● In 2002, in England and Wales, black ethnic groups, mainly black Caribbean, accounted for 55% and 44% of uncomplicated gonorrhoea cases in heterosexual men and women respectively.

● Between 2001 and 2003 almost half of the syphilis cases reported to the London Enhanced Laboratory Surveillance System were in black or black British ethnic groups.

● The number of new HIV diagnoses acquired in Africa in heterosexual black African groups continues to rise.[11]

However, infection in black African adults born in the UK remains low, suggesting low levels of onward transmission within the UK.

These patterns of infection have implications for prevention and health promotion. We need to understand more about the travel and mixing patterns of black African migrant communities. In addition, we need to develop culturally sensitive health promotion interventions.

OTHER GROUPS

Finally, we need to consider briefly two other groups of people: injecting drug users and people who travel abroad.

| HIV and injecting drug users | Approximately 1 in 28 injecting drug users in contact with services in London and about 1 in 500 outside London were HIV positive in 2002. Rates of infection in this group have not changed significantly since 1994.[11] |

| Travel and STI | Expansion in global travel has had a significant impact on the epidemiology of STIs. Foreign travel allows access to increased numbers of partners and the opportunity to engage in novel sexual networks, including commercial sex. Travel to Thailand, Africa and the Caribbean has been linked to HIV, syphilis and gonorrhoea infections in heterosexual men.[11] The epidemiology of HIV in the UK is increasingly influenced by travel patterns and migration.[2] |

WHAT CAN WE DO ABOUT STIs AND HIV?

| THE HEALTH SERVICE ROLE | Whilst the health service cannot deliver good sexual health in isolation, it does have an essential role to play. To date, sexual health services, including GUM and family planning services, have been under resourced in terms of finance, staff and facilities. More generally, these services have developed in isolation, lacking coherent integration at a local level, with insufficient coordination with primary care services. *The National Strategy for Sexual Health and HIV*[1] has called for a new model of working, placing patients at the centre of services, which should be provided at three levels (see Table 9.1). |

Table 9.1   New model for sexual health services[1]

Level	Provider	Services
One	Primary care/GP	• Sexual history and risk assessment • STI testing for women • STI assessment and referral for men • HIV testing and counselling • Pregnancy testing and referral • Cervical cytology screening • Hepatitis B immunization • Contraceptive services
Two	Specialist primary care teams/joint services between primary care and specialist services	• Intrauterine device insertion • Testing and treating STIs • Vasectomy • Contraceptive implant insertion • Partner notification • Invasive STI testing for men
Three	Specialist clinical teams	• Sexual health service needs assessment • Clinical governance requirements • Outreach prevention and contraception services • Specialized infections management and coordination of partner notification • Highly specialized contraception • Specialized HIV treatment and care

PREVENTING STIs AND HIV – WHAT WORKS?

The importance of viewing STIs in the broader context of sexual health has been stressed throughout this chapter. Measures for preventing STIs and HIV have to be considered in the context of sexual relationships, practices and beliefs. In other words, STI prevention is an integral part of sexual health promotion.

What is sexual health promotion?

The World Health Organization states that:

> Sexual health is a state of physical, emotional, mental and social well being related to sexuality. Sexual health requires a positive and respectful approach to sexuality and sexual relationships, as well as the possibility of having pleasurable and safe sexual experiences, free of coercion, discrimination and violence.[34]

In 2003 the Department of Health produced a toolkit for effective sexual health promotion with clear objectives (see Box 9.2).[35]

Sexual health promotion in practice

A diverse range of approaches and methodologies are used in sexual health promotion activity across wide ranging settings.

Media and the internet

National and local media campaigns via the press, radio or internet serve to raise public awareness and can be particularly useful in reaching certain groups.

The increased use of the internet, especially amongst MSM groups, for making sexual contacts has led some to argue that its potential for promoting safe sexual relationships should be exploited more fully.[33] The advantages of internet-based sexual health promotion aimed especially at young people is increasingly recognized. The Healthy Schools programme 'Wired

---

Box 9.2   Objectives of sexual health promotion[35]

Awareness raising

- Increasing the awareness of the interrelationships between sexual, emotional and mental health and the need for professionals to build this into their practice
- Promoting awareness of sexual health issues and the importance of positive sexual and emotional relationships

Information and education

- Increasing access to sexual health information, support and advice for adults and young people regardless of age or ability

Development of services and service providers

- Increasing access to the whole range of sexual health services, including contraception and abortion services, HIV and STI testing, psychosexual and sexual health support

Skills and capacity-building in individuals and communities

- Enabling particularly vulnerable individuals, groups and communities to take greater control over their sexual health
- Offering individuals, groups and communities opportunities to gain key relationship skills, including negotiation, communication and assertiveness skills

for health' website (www.wiredforhealth.gov.uk), aimed at both teachers and young people, includes sexual and relationship education messages.

Community development

Community development approaches allow targeted efforts with specific groups and marginalized communities. For example, in Walsall, the Men's Health Project offers support and advice to men infected with HIV and has been instrumental in outreach health promotion and health screening in venues used by MSM. Walsall Teaching Primary Care Trust currently commissions outreach health promotion services for local commercial sex workers from SAFE, a non-government specialist health provider. The project adopts a holistic approach to health promotion and harm reduction, enabling access to GUM, drug, midwifery, vaccination, housing and social services.[16]

Sex and relationship education

The importance of sex and relationship education (SRE) in formal and informal settings is gaining wide recognition.

The 1996 Education Act[36] has consolidated previous legislation on the subject. It stipulates that the SRE elements in the National Curriculum Science Order across all key stages are mandatory for all pupils of primary and secondary age. More recently, non-statutory guidance[37] has enabled schools to deliver SRE as part of Personal, Social and Health Education (PSHE) and Citizenship, in a healthy school context.[38] In its report, the Health Select Committee[2] highlighted the importance of SRE and emphasized the need to improve relationship education, engage boys and young men more fully in SRE, and develop easily accessible information resources for children, teachers and parents.

Many further education colleges, tertiary colleges and universities undertake sexual health promotion activities, working through the students' union, disseminating information and condoms.

More innovative approaches include using theatre, arts projects, creative writing and photography projects in education. Introduced to support the implementation of the national Teenage Pregnancy Strategy, *It Opened My Eyes* is a good practice guide for using theatre in education to deliver SRE.[39]

The need to 'normalize' discussions about sex and mainstream sexual health promotion activity underpins recent attempts to broaden the settings used for such approaches. The use of workplace settings, pubs, retail outlets and even hairdressers and faith groups are examples of ways in which this is being tackled.[35]

(Chapter 8 'Teenage pregnancy' also discusses sex and relationship education, media campaigns and sexual health services.)

What works in STI prevention?

A key function of the Health Development Agency (HDA) is the development and update of an evidence base around the effectiveness of public health interventions. Boxes 9.3 and 9.4 summarize the findings from two HDA briefings which are relevant to preventing STIs and promoting good sexual health.[40,41]

Box 9.3   Summary of Health Development Agency review of effectiveness of HIV prevention[40]

The review focuses on priority populations for the sexual transmission of HIV in the UK, including men who have sex with men, African communities, commercial sex workers and people with HIV. Injecting drug use and mother-to-child transmission are not included.

The review covers voluntary counselling and testing with all populations but does not cover the role of condom effectiveness, post-exposure prophylaxis (preventive antiviral drug treatment *after* potential HIV infection), treatment of STIs or male circumcision in reducing the sexual transmission of HIV.

Men who have sex with men

● Community-level interventions involving peers and opinion leaders may be effective in influencing sexual risk behaviours.

● Cognitive behavioural group work involving sexual negotiation and communication skills training can be effective.

● Approaches should be set in broad context and address factors at the personal level (e.g. knowledge and skills) and the structural level (e.g. discrimination towards gay men).

● There is a question about how these findings can be generalized to UK-based non-white, non-educated men. It is suggested that interventions should be targeted to specific sub-populations, for example, black gay men.

Commercial sex workers

● There is some evidence that peer-led interventions delivered at the community level can be effective in influencing the sexual risk behaviours of commercial sex workers.

HIV counselling and testing

● There is some evidence that HIV counselling and testing can influence sexual risk behaviour in couples where one is HIV positive and the other is not. It may also influence the following groups of people who learn that they are HIV positive: injecting drug users, heterosexual men and sexual health clinic attenders.

● The effects of being diagnosed as HIV negative are not clear; some suggest that it may lessen the sense of risk and lead to possible increased risk behaviour.

● Evidence suggests, therefore, that voluntary counselling and testing should be targeted only at high risk individuals who are likely to test positive.

WHAT ARE THE GAPS IN CURRENT KNOWLEDGE?

While the evidence base for sexual health and STI and HIV prevention is growing, it still remains patchy, with limited research in some areas. *The National Strategy for Sexual Health and HIV*[1] and the Health Development Agency's *Evidence Briefing*[29] have highlighted areas for further research, including:

● links between drugs, sex and alcohol and the identification of effective interventions;
● better understanding of the sexual networks and health seeking behaviour of priority groups, including MSM, commercial sex workers and African communities;
● impact of life-prolonging antiviral treatment for HIV on behaviour and risk taking;
● impact of ethnicity, deprivation and other socio-economic factors on sexual health;

Box 9.4   Summary of Health Development Agency review of effectiveness of STI prevention[41]

The review covered partner notification, health promotion and educational interventions.

Partner notification

● Partner notification is the process whereby sexual contacts of a patient diagnosed with an STI (the index patient) are told of their potential exposure to infection. This process is effective in detecting STIs in these sexual contacts. Provider referral (where third parties, usually health advisers from GUM clinics, notify partners) is more effective than patient referral (where the index patients tell their partners themselves).

● Patient referral is less costly and in some circumstances it may be appropriate to offer the patient the choice.

● Potential harms associated with partner notification include domestic violence. More investigation is needed in this area.

Health promotion and education – features of effective approaches

Effective approaches should:
● be based on theoretical models of behaviour change;
● provide basic, accurate information about risks of unprotected sex;
● be multifaceted, including skills and attitude development and motivational aspects required to ensure behaviour change. Information is not enough;
● incorporate skills training, for example condom use;
● develop programmes appropriate to target audience in terms of age, gender, sexual experience and culture;
● use peer educators, especially for adolescent audiences;
● emphasize condom use rather than abstinence;
● be of appropriate duration: it takes time and multiple activities to alter long established sexual risk-taking behaviour.

● men's health seeking behaviour and identification of new ways of engaging young men;
● effectiveness of new models of care for improving sexual health outcomes – for example, one-stop shops;
● barriers preventing access to services;
● improving and evaluating the uptake of health screening services in non-specialist settings, especially for *Chlamydia*;
● evaluation of sociopolitical interventions, such as legislation and work on equality.

CONTROVERSIAL ISSUES

The present Labour administration is Britain's first government to tackle sexual health head on, with the launch of the national strategy in 2001,[1] as we have discussed. We have also referred to the 2003 parliamentary report,[2] which described a crisis in sexual health services delivery. This delivered an additional £11 million for England's sexual health services and further incentives were announced for GUM clinics, new *Chlamydia* tests, improved contraceptive services in poorer areas and so on.

However, there are problems. STIs are generally not perceived as killing people and neither are they implicated in blocking beds. Headlines about sexual behaviour abound but do not command the same attention that we associate with coronary heart disease or cancer. Not surprisingly then, there has been no announcement of a National Service Framework for sexual health. The intention is for government to handle sexual health within existing priority frameworks, but only later within local delivery plans (LDPs). The latter dictate the prioritization of new money. Sexual health will not feature prominently in LDPs outside London. Since LDPs are 3-year plans, a vacuum in funding will arise until their later review. This is a pity, since there is a danger that the strategy and the parliamentary report will lose their impact with time. Massive investment is needed *now* (at the time of writing in 2004) to stem the tide of unchecked increases in STIs and to turn around the grossly under resourced services.

There are other disappointments. For example, sex and relationship education has not been made a statutory part of the National Curriculum, despite being recommended by the parliamentary report.[37]

However, the overriding concern is that of significant funding. Sustained and increased funding is going to be required for years to come. In the meantime, there needs to be clarity of leadership from the centre, and an array of resource-dependent performance targets to make things happen locally.

Key sources of further information and help

- **Department of Health:** www.doh.gov.uk. The Department of Health issues news, publications and statistics, policy and guidance.
- **Health Development Agency:** www.hda-online.org.uk. The national authority on what works to improve people's health and reduce health inequalities. It gathers evidence and produces advice for policy makers, professionals and practitioners, working alongside them to make practice evidence-based.
- **Health Protection Agency:** www.hpa.org.uk. The Health Protection Agency (HPA) is a national organization for England and Wales, established in 2003. It is dedicated to protecting people's health and reducing the impact of infectious diseases, chemical hazards, poisons and radiation hazards. It brings together the expertise of health and scientific professionals working in the areas of public health, communicable disease, emergency planning, infection control, laboratories, poisons, and chemical and radiation hazards.

- **Sigma Research:** www.sigmaresearch.org.uk. A social research group specializing in the behavioural and policy aspects of HIV and sexual health. It also undertakes research and development work on aspects of lesbian, gay and bisexual health and well-being.
- **Terrence Higgins Trust:** www.tht.org.uk. The leading HIV and AIDS charity in the UK and the largest in Europe. It was one of the first charities to be set up (in 1982) in response to the HIV epidemic and has been at the forefront of the fight against HIV and AIDS ever since.
- **Wired for Health:** www.wiredforhealth.gov.uk. A series of websites managed by the Health Development Agency on behalf of the Department of Health and the Department for Education and Skills. It provides health information that relates to the National Curriculum and the National Healthy School Standard for a range of audiences.

References

1. Department of Health. The national strategy for sexual health and HIV. London: DoH; 2001.
2. House of Commons Health Select Committee. Sexual health: third report of the session 2002–2003. London: The Stationery Office; 2003. Online. Available: http://www.publications.parliament.uk/pa/cm200203/cmselect/cmhealth/cmhealth.htm
3. Communicable Disease Surveillance Centre (CDSC). Increased transmission of syphilis in Brighton and greater Manchester among men who have sex with men. Commun Dis Rep CDR Wkly 2000; 10:383–386.
4. CDSC. Syphilis transmission among homosexual and bisexual men in London and Manchester. Commun Dis Rep CDR Wkly 2001; 11(27).
5. Doherty L, Fenton KA, Jones J, et al. Syphilis: old problem, new strategy. BMJ 2002; 325:153–156.
6. Djuretic T, Catchpole M, Bingham J S, et al. Genitourinary medicine services in the United Kingdom are failing to meet the current demand. International Journal of STD and AIDS. 2001; 12(9):571–572.
7. Lacey C, Merrick D, Bensley D, et al. Analysis of the socio-demography of gonorrhoea in Leeds, 1989–93. BMJ June 14 1997; 314:1718–1719.
8. Hughes G, Catchpole M, Rogers P, et al. Comparison of risk factors for sexually transmitted infections: results from a study of attenders at three genito-urinary medicine clinics in England. Sexually Transmitted Infections 2000; 76:262–267.
9. Department of Health. Saving lives: our healthier nation. London: The Stationery Office; 1999.
10. Department of Health. The national strategy for sexual health and HIV. Implementation action plan. London: DOH; 2002.
11. Health Protection Agency. Annual report: HIV/AIDS and other sexually transmitted infections in the UK in 2002. London: HPA; 2003. Online. Available: http://www.hpa.org.uk
12. Department of Health, Social Services and Public Safety Northern Ireland, The National Assembly for Wales, The Scottish Executive, The Department of Health. Second report of the UK National Screening Committee. London: Department of Health; 2000. Online. Available: www.nsc.nhs.uk/pdfs/secondreport.pdf
13. Department of Health. Government response to the health select committee's third report of session 2002–03 on sexual health. London: The Stationery Office, 2003. Online. Available: http://www.doh.gov.uk
14. Hughes G, Andrews N, Catchpole N, et al. Investigation of the increased incidence of gonorrhoea diagnosed in genitourinary medicine clinics in England 1994–6. Sex Transm Infect 2000; 76(1):18–24.
15. Johnson A, Mercer C, Erens B, et al. Sexual behaviour in Britain: partnerships, practices, and HIV risk behaviours. Lancet 2001; 358:1835–1842.
16. Director of Public Health. Sexual health in Walsall. The 2003 annual report of the Director of Public Health Medicine. Walsall: Walsall Teaching Primary Care Trust; 2003.
17. Social Exclusion Unit. Teenage Pregnancy. London: Social Exclusion Unit; 1999. Online. Available: http://www.socialexclusionunit.gov.uk
18. NHS Cervical Cancer Screening Programme. Fact sheet: human papilloma virus. Online. Available: http://www.cancerscreening.nhs.uk/cervical/hpv.html
19. Chinouya M. Zimbabweans in England. Building capacity for culturally competent health promotion. In: MacDonald T. The social significance of health promotion. London: Routledge; 2003.
20. Mercey D. Antenatal HIV testing has been done badly in Britain and needs to improve. BMJ 1998; 316:241–242.
21. Department of Health. Screening for infectious diseases in pregnancy. Standards to support the UK antenatal screening programme. London: DOH; 2003. Online. Available: www.doh.gov.uk/antenatalscreening/
22. Hughes C, Evans A. Health needs of women who have sex with women: health care workers need to be aware of their specific needs. BMJ 2003; 327:939–940.
23. Marazzo J. Genital human papillomavirus infection in women who have sex with women: a concern for patients and providers. AIDS Patient Care STDs 2000; 14:447–451.
24. Bauer G, Welles S. Beyond assumptions of negligible risk: sexually transmitted diseases and women who have sex with women. American Journal of Public Health 2001; 91:1282–1286.
25. Skegg K, Nad-Raja S, Dickson N, et al. Sexual orientation and self-harm in men and women. American Journal of Psychiatry 2003; 160:541–546.
26. Bailey J. Homosexuality and mental illness. Archives of General Psychiatry 1999; 56:883–884.
27. Laverty S, Pugh RN, Joseph AT. The crisis in sexual health and developing genitourinary medicine services: lessons from a primary care trust. International Journal of STD and AIDS; forthcoming 2005.
28. Hickson F, Reid D, Weatherburn P, et al. Time for more. Findings from the National Gay Men's Sex Survey 2000. London: Sigma Research; July 2001.
29. Health Development Agency. Evidence briefing: HIV prevention: a review of reviews assessing the effectiveness of interventions to reduce the risk of sexual transmission. London: HDA; 2003. Online. Available: http://www.hda.nhs.uk/evidence
30. Pugh RN, Laverty S, Simms I, et al. Syphilis clusters in Walsall: case profiles and public health implications. Communicable Disease and Public Health 2004; 7:36–38.
31. Public Health Laboratory Service. Communicable Disease Surveillance Centre, Medical Society for the Study of Venereal Disease, Association of Genitourinary Medicine, Public Health Medicine Environment Group. Guidelines for managing outbreaks of sexually transmitted infections at a local, district or regional level: an outbreak plan; 2002.

32. Clinical Effectiveness Group (Association for Genitourinary Medicine and the Medical Society for the Study of Venereal Diseases). UK national guidelines on the management of early syphilis. London: Association for Genitourinary Medicine and the Medical Society for the Study of Venereal Diseases; 2002. Online. Available: http://www.mssvd.org.uk/CEG/ceguidelines.htm

33. Mettey A, Crosby R, DiClemente R, et al. Associations between internet sex seeking and STI associated risk behaviours among men who have sex with men. Sexually Transmitted Infections 200; 79:466–468.

34. WHO. Gender and reproductive rights. Glossary. WHO; 2002. Online. Available: http://www.who.int/reproductive-health/gender 2003.

35. Department of Health. Effective sexual health promotion: a toolkit for primary care trusts and others working in the field of promoting good sexual health and HIV prevention. London: DOH; 2003. Online. Available: http://www.doh.gov.uk

36. Education Act 1996. London: HMSO.

37. Department for Education and Employment. Sex and relationship education guidance. DfEE 0116/2000.

London: Department for Education and Employment; 2000. Online. Available: http://www.dfes.gov.uk/sreguidance/sexeducation.pdf

38. Department of Health. National Healthy School Standard. Website publication. Online. Available: http://www.wiredforhealth.gov.uk

39. Sawney F, Sykes S, Keene M, et al. It opened my eyes. Using theatre in education to deliver sex and relationship education. A good practice guide. London: Health Development Agency; 2002. Online available: http://www.hda-online.org.uk/search.

40. Ellis S, Barnett-Page E, Morgan A, et al. HIV prevention: a review of reviews assessing the effectiveness of interventions to reduce the risk of sexual transmission. London: Health Development Agency; 2003. Online. Available: http://www.hda.nhs.uk/evidence

41. Ellis S, Grey A. Prevention of sexually transmitted infections (STIs); a review of reviews into the effectiveness of non-clinical interventions. London: Health Development Agency; 2004. Online. Available: http://www.hda.nhs.uk/evidence

Chapter 10

Alcohol use and misuse

Richard Velleman and Lorna Templeton

SUMMARY OVERVIEW AND LINKS TO OTHER TOPICS

Alcohol is a 'social lubricant', a depressant drug, and one of the most popular and socially acceptable legally consumed drugs in the world today. Consumption in the UK has been steadily increasing since the 1950s; binge drinking, and drinking by young people and women, is of particular concern.

We define *alcohol misuse* as any use of alcohol that causes problems for either the drinker or anyone else. Alcohol misuse leads to enormous problems, affecting people in all socio-economic groups, with great economic and human cost, and serious impact on families and communities. The reasons why people develop alcohol-related problems are complex, linked to individual characteristics, family environment, life experiences, social norms and culture, and the availability and price of alcohol.

In terms of national policy, alcohol is a comparatively neglected area (especially compared with drugs); a long-awaited alcohol harm reduction strategy for England was not published until 2004,[1] although Scotland, Wales and Northern Ireland[2,3,4] developed strategies some years previously. Alcohol also features in other national strategies such as National Service Frameworks.

Possible intervention strategies include education about 'sensible drinking'; controlling the supply of alcohol; providing treatment services (including early and brief interventions); reducing the negative effects of alcohol; and working with children, families and communities affected by alcohol misuse. There are many unhelpful stereotypes surrounding alcohol misusers, and much we do not yet know about the most effective ways to reduce alcohol-related harm.

Cigarettes, alcohol and drugs are all 'drugs' so Chapter 11 'Drug use and misuse' and Chapter 4 'Smoking' are both useful to read alongside this one. Poor mental health may also be associated with alcohol misuse (see Ch. 12 'Mental health and mental health promotion').

As health inequalities feature in alcohol misuse, and lifestyle changes are important for prevention and treatment, Chapter 13 'Tackling inequalities in health' and Chapter 14 'Helping individuals to change behaviour' are also relevant.

WHAT IS ALCOHOL MISUSE?

Alcohol has pervaded human society over many millennia and continues to do so into the present century. There are numerous debates and controversies about the use and the misuse of alcohol, and how society and individuals can best respond, many as yet unresolved.

Alcohol is a depressant drug and is one of the most popular and socially acceptable legally consumed drugs worldwide, alongside nicotine and caffeine. Alcohol has a clear impact on the brain, altering mood and emotion, affecting coordination and reaction times, and impacting on our ability to assess situations such as risk-taking behaviour. Although alcohol is a sedative, it is often assumed to be a stimulant. This is partly an effect of social conditioning (if people expect to act in a more uninhibited fashion when they drink, then they do), and partly because the sedative effects of alcohol act first and faster on the higher brain functions, which are the ones which tend to inhibit people's behaviour.

In many ways, alcohol can be described as a 'social lubricant'. Key reasons for its consumption include: to enjoy the taste, to celebrate, to accompany food, to show hospitality, to feel more relaxed and have less inhibitions in social groups, to de-stress after work or to forget about worries and their accompanying negative emotions.

However, sometimes this 'lubrication' gets out of hand: sometimes people drink too much. What constitutes 'too much' has been a matter of debate for many years. Some people define 'too much' in terms of quantity and/or frequency (see Box 10.1), while others argue that 'too much' needs to be seen within a context: hence drinking even a very small

Box 10.1   Recommended sensible drinking limits

Benchmarks for sensible drinking were set by a government working group in 1995.[5]
They are:

- men: not more than 3–4 units (see 'What is a unit?' below) a day, with some days of abstinence;
- women: not more than 2–3 units a day, with some days of abstinence.

Further guidance is:

- Heavy sessional drinking (a binge) and intoxication should be avoided, but if it occurs, alcohol should be avoided for 48 hours to allow full recovery. (A *binge* is defined both as drinking at least twice the daily guidelines in one day, and drinking in order to get drunk).

- The risk of coronary heart disease in men over 40 years and postmenopausal women may be reduced by drinking 1 to 2 units a day.

- Women who are pregnant or planning a pregnancy are advised to drink no more than 1–2 units once or twice a week, and to avoid intoxication. (More recent advice from the Royal College of Obstetricians and Gynaecologists suggests that intake in pregnancy should not exceed 1 unit a day.[6])

These benchmarks replaced previous guidelines based on weekly consumption, because of concerns that occasional sessions of heavy drinking (drinking all the week's units in one go) were more harmful to health than the same amount spread out. The weekly guidelines were:

- low to moderate drinking – men: up to 21 units a week; women: up to 14 units a week;
- hazardous or risky drinking – men: 21–50 units a week; women: 14–35 units a week;
- dangerous or harmful drinking – men: 50+ units a week; women: 36+ units a week.

What is a unit?

Units are a convenient way of expressing the amount of alcohol in different drinks. In the UK, one unit is defined as 8 g alcohol. One unit is roughly equivalent to:

- one small pub measure of spirits[a]
- one small glass of wine
- half a pint of beer.

But care needs to be taken in estimating the number of units in larger measures or stronger drinks. Examples:

- One bottle (700 ml) of 12% wine = 8 units;
- One large can (440 ml) of extra strong (9%) lager or special brew = 4 units;
- One medium (175 ml) glass of 12% wine = 2 units;
- One pint of normal strength (3–3.5%) beer, lager or cider = 2 units;
- One large (50 ml) measure of spirits (40%) = 2 units[a];
- One bottle (275 ml) of 'alcopop' (5.5%) = 1.5 units;
- One measure (50 ml) of sherry, port or fortified wine (17–20%) = 1 unit.

[a] Pub measures of spirits vary across the UK. In England and Wales, one small pub measure provides 1 unit; in Scotland 1.25 units; in Northern Ireland 1.5 units.

amount might be seen as 'too much' in a devout Muslim gathering or in a Northern Ireland teetotaller group; whereas drinking rather more might be seen as acceptable during a stag night party.

Most people who consume alcohol do so in moderation and usually have no problems, but others use alcohol in ways that cause problems for themselves or other people. Over the years there have been many attempts to define alcohol misuse, with terms such as problem drinking, alcoholism, alcohol dependence syndrome (ADS), alcohol-related problems, social drinking, normal drinking, controlled drinking, and so on being used.[7(pp. 3–9)]

In this chapter we define *alcohol misuse* as any use of alcohol that causes problems for either the drinker or anyone else. These problems might be because the drinkers regularly consume quantities of alcohol which put their health at risk; or because they drink less but choose to drive, putting themselves above the legal limit; or because they drink inappropriately (e.g. during the working day) and meet with disciplinary problems at work; or because their drinking causes problems for their children or spouse.

WHAT CAUSES ALCOHOL MISUSE?

The huge number of theories about the cause of alcohol misuse can be subsumed into three main types, according to whether the cause is attributed to:

- individuals (their genetics, their personality, they have a 'disease' etc);
- their social groups (effects of peer groups, influence of the family etc); or
- societal and cultural conditions (social deprivation, per capita consumption of alcohol in society, the café society, social acceptability of heavy drinking or intoxication etc).

Most of these theories have been around for a very long time.[8,9]

There is some evidence to suggest that most of these theories hold up for some of the people, some of the time; but no one theory is backed by strong evidence that it alone holds the key to understanding alcohol misuse. In this section we outline some of the major ideas in these three groupings.

INDIVIDUAL CAUSES

Three types of 'individual cause' theories have emerged, which presume that people start to misuse alcohol for one of the following reasons:

- They *have* something that others do not have (e.g. a disease, an allergy to alcohol, an addictive personality).

- They *do not have* something that others have (e.g. an internal control mechanism, or an ability to monitor their own alcohol consumption and hence self-regulate).

- There are individual intrapsychic reasons for drinking to excess (e.g. they want to escape from negative feelings, or to gain in self-confidence, or to behave in ways that they would not normally allow themselves to).

Of all of these individual ideas, the 'disease' model is the most widespread, especially in the USA, and still also in the UK. The basic idea is that there is something about some people such that when they drink alcohol, they become unable to control their intake. This is a longstanding idea, stretching back to Greek times.[8] It gained popular backing with the rise of the Alcoholics Anonymous movement in the USA in the 1930s and scientific respectability with the work of Jellinek who wrote extensively about 'the disease concept of alcoholism' in the 1960s.[10]

Over the past 30 years the view of alcoholism as a disease has become increasingly difficult to maintain, as evidence has mounted that almost all the fundamental tenets of this view are incorrect.[11] However, popular acceptance of the disease model is still extremely strong, fuelled by tabloid coverage of sports and entertainment 'stars' who have adopted disease model approaches to overcome their alcohol or drug problems.

This disease model has also been linked with the 'genetic cause' view. Although research in this area is difficult, it is clear there is some genetic influence in problem drinking. This genetic link, however, only seems to apply to a small percentage of problem drinkers, and it is still uncertain precisely what might be genetically transmitted. Furthermore, what the genetic linkage shows is that some individuals might be *more vulnerable* to developing an alcohol problem, not that they *certainly would* develop one.

SOCIAL GROUP CAUSES

These theories suggest that people start or continue to misuse alcohol through learning from, or being pressurized by, other people to behave in these ways. Major theories here are:

- modelling from parents;
- unstable home environment;
- peer modelling or peer pressure;
- the influence of other people (e.g. at work).

Again, there is some evidence supporting all of these theories.[7,12]

SOCIETAL AND CULTURAL CAUSES

Many ideas have been put forward to try to explain the divergence across different countries in both per capita consumption and number and type of alcohol-related problems,[13,14,15] including in the *National Alcohol Harm Reduction Strategy: Interim Analytical Report*,[15] which was published prior to the Strategy itself, and analyses the available current evidence of the impact of alcohol use and misuse in the UK today. (This text is a key source for much of the information contained in this chapter.)

A highly influential theory which arose in the 1960s and 1970s suggested that:

- the number of alcohol-related problems in any society was proportional to the amount drunk generally within that society;
- this amount itself was directly related to:
  - the price of alcohol (the cheaper alcohol was in real terms, the more people would drink it) and
  - its availability and accessibility (the more outlets there were, and the easier it was to purchase alcohol, the more likely people would be to do so).

There is very strong evidence to corroborate these suppositions.[15]

These theories have led to a far greater emphasis being placed on more general health promotion information being made available, and on attempts to increase people's knowledge about how much they are drinking (see section below, 'What can we do about alcohol misuse?').

CURRENT VIEWS ON WHAT CAUSES ALCOHOL MISUSE

Although the disease model has remained one of the dominant models, particularly in the USA, over the last decades more complex models have emerged which seek to go beyond the relatively simplistic search for single causes. Of particular note are Orford's 'excessive appetites' ideas;[8] Davies' 'myth of addiction';[16] and Heather and Robertson's cognitive behavioural model.[11] The Strategy Unit's *Interim Analytical Report* summarizes well the complexity involved in looking at a more macro, societal, level.[15(pp. 114–125; 152–156)]

Interestingly, most of these more recent ideas have focused on either the individual and/or the societal, with only a small amount of work looking in more depth at the social group models.[17–19]

WHY IS ALCOHOL MISUSE AN IMPORTANT PUBLIC HEALTH ISSUE?

Alcohol misuse causes enormous problems which are likely to increase as alcohol consumption increases, with great economic and human cost, and serious impact on families and communities.

PROBLEMS CAUSED BY ALCOHOL MISUSE

Alcohol misuse causes immense problems at all levels of society:

- problems for individuals (such as with their health, finances, employment, housing and social lives);
- problems for their families (violence, finance, housing and the general effects on health, coping, relationships, family dynamics and so on caused by the day-to-day stress of living with someone with an alcohol problem);
- problems for society more generally (including crime, alcohol-related violence and disturbances, absenteeism and sickness, and costs to the NHS and criminal justice systems).

The impact of alcohol misuse is summarized in Figure 10.1.

Health impact

Across the world (including in the UK) alcohol consumption is the third highest risk factor in terms of disease burden (after tobacco and high blood pressure). High alcohol consumption is linked to a huge range of medical conditions, including:

- heart disease, strokes and high blood pressure;
- cancer;
- gastrointestinal problems;
- liver, pancreas and kidney diseases;
- obesity;
- mental health difficulties;
- problems with fertility.[20]

Annually, there are estimated to be between 20 000 and 40 000 alcohol-related deaths in England and Wales, amounting to over 75 000 years of

Figure 10.1   The impact of alcohol misuse.

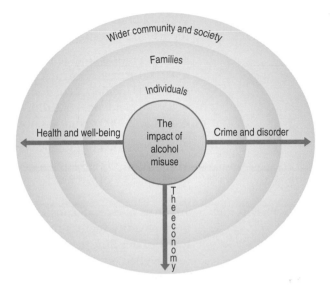

life lost prematurely that can be attributable to alcohol consumption, and up to 1000 suicides.

The rising impact of alcohol misuse on health is illustrated in the Chief Medical Officer of Health for England's annual report for 2001.[21] It showed that there have been dramatic increases in deaths due to alcohol-related liver cirrhosis over the last 30 years of the twentieth century. Especially worrying was the increase amongst younger people aged 35–44, where there was a significant eight-fold rise in deaths amongst men, and a six-fold increase amongst women. Even amongst 25–34 year olds there was a three-fold rise in the death toll over the 30 years. This contrasts starkly with other European countries where liver cirrhosis death rates are broadly falling.[21]

Drinking whilst pregnant brings potential problems for mothers and their unborn children. The most serious of these is fetal alcohol syndrome (FAS), in which a range of characteristics may be seen in babies whose mothers drank heavily whilst pregnant (although the exact level and degree of drinking, and when in the pregnancy it might occur, is disputed). Problems for babies include facial and growth disfigurement, brain damage and a range of behavioural problems. However, serious problems can occur for babies and mothers at much lower levels of consumption than those required to create FAS, with low birth weight being particularly likely in mothers who drink more heavily. These problems are all exacerbated by other factors, including age, nutrition, drinking history, other health problems and socio-economic status.

The impact of alcohol misuse on accident and emergency (A&E) departments has been given particular prominence in recent years, with some figures suggesting that one third of all attendances at A&E departments (and hence a third of the costs) are alcohol-related. Alcohol misuse is a factor in nearly 75% of A&E attendances between midnight and 5 a.m., particularly at weekends.

Crime and disorder

Alcohol is strongly linked with crime and disorder. In the Strategy Unit report[15] figures suggest that each year in the UK there are:

- over a million incidences of alcohol-related crime;
- 80 000 arrests for drunk and disorderly behaviour;
- 360 000 incidences of domestic violence where alcohol is a factor;
- 85 000 incidences of drink driving;
- nearly 20 000 sexual assaults where alcohol is a factor.

Around a third of violence between partners is influenced by alcohol. The number of prisoners with alcohol problems is also high: about 66% of men and 33% of women.

A GROWING PROBLEM

In terms of overall consumption, the amount consumed in the UK has been steadily increasing since the 1950s. Although we drink less than many of our European partners, consumption in many of those countries has levelled off or fallen, whereas UK consumption has been increasing. Recent estimates suggest that, if present trends continue, the UK will overtake France in the consumption league in 2007.[22]

The majority of the UK public (over 90%) drink alcohol at some level. More than half are drinking within current UK recommended guidelines (see Box 10.1), at perceived 'healthy' levels, and at levels that may incur health benefits.

However, the level and impact of the drinking of the rest of the population is of growing concern in the following areas:

- what people drink;
- how much they drink and how frequently;
- how many people are drinking at more harmful levels;
- the range and level of negative effects of alcohol consumption.

A particular pattern of drinking, *binge drinking* (see note in Box 10.1), is becoming prominent in the UK, a pattern akin to other Northern European countries particularly amongst men and young people generally. Young people, and young women in particular, are drinking more than ever and more than their peers in other European countries. Furthermore, there is concern about the minority of people who do not curb their consumption, leading to a host of other problems that negatively affect the lives of individuals, communities and the UK as a whole.

IMPACT ON THE ECONOMY

There are positive economic impacts of the production, distribution and sale of alcohol. The drinks industry has an estimated total value of at least £30 billion, equivalent to 5.8% of all consumer expenditure. It creates around a million jobs in the UK, and has a particular impact in the leisure and tourism sectors. The Chancellor receives about £7 billion annually in revenue from alcohol.

However, the negative economic impact of alcohol use and misuse is estimated to be 2–5% of UK gross national product, and to be well in excess of £20 billion.[8] For example, the Strategy Unit estimated that alcohol costs society around:[15]

- more than £7 billion to the criminal justice system (includes costs to the police, probation service, prisons and courts) and in disorder;
- nearly £2 billion in terms of health (incorporating costs to inpatient, outpatient and emergency care, GP and other primary care, and specialist services);
- over £6 billion in terms of impact on the workplace and productivity (includes absence due to illness, inability to work and premature death).

These costs are all underestimates, in that they exclude all the human and health costs and emotional impact on family members, victims of alcohol-related crimes, and others.

THE IMPACT ON FAMILIES AND COMMUNITIES

Further work is needed to quantify the economic impact in terms of cost to families and social networks, but the impact of alcohol problems on families and communities is unquestionable. For every person with an alcohol problem (not necessarily dependence) it is suggested that there are, on average, two close family members negatively affected by the situation. This means that there may be anything up to 10 million family members in the UK affected in this way – including up to a million children.

The range of problems experienced by families includes poor physical and psychological health, relationship problems, poor parenting, domestic violence, unsafe sex and unplanned pregnancy, as well as an impact on education, employment, finances and social life, often accompanied by a range of negative emotions such as shame, guilt, fear, anger and embarrassment.[23] The range of problems experienced by communities includes crime and antisocial behaviour, street drinking and homelessness, truancy and delinquency, and neglected neighbourhoods.

These problems, of course, are very much the same problems experienced by alcohol misusers themselves.

The impact on children

Children can have a particularly hard time as a result of someone in their family (usually a parent) having an alcohol problem.[18,24,25] They often take on responsibilities that are beyond their years, thus affecting their education and peer relationships. Children can be deprived of their childhood, as they may be too ashamed to bring friends home, or unable to go out with friends because they have to care for a sibling or drunken parent. Experiencing or witnessing physical, verbal and sexual abuse are realities for many children, with the drinking also affecting family holidays and celebrations such as Christmas and birthdays.[26] Children are usually the innocent, but harmed, bystanders of domestic violence, experiencing problems with family attachment, aggression or withdrawal, sleep problems, fear and a wish for safety.[27] Many children affected by problem drinking within the family environment will reach the attention of social services; there is evidence that between one and two thirds of child protection cases involve alcohol.[28]

How children are affected by parental problem drinking can vary, with gender and development being particular areas of variation.[24] Increasingly, research provides evidence of the impact of parental substance misuse on child welfare at both emotional and physical level and of the effects on child–parent attachment across the life cycle.[18] On the other hand, research[29] is also showing that some children are resilient, and that there are a range of factors which increase the chances of a child becoming resilient, even if they live with a parent with a serious alcohol problem. These 'protective' factors include a positive relationship with a key and stable adult (for example the other parent, a grandparent or someone outside the family), shared family activities and affection, and engagement with outside activities (sports, culture, religion) or with a positive peer group.

Far less is known about the continued impact of parental drinking when these children are adults, when many will have families of their own. One major study[29] found that whilst some children were still suffering when they were older because of their childhood experiences, many seemed able to survive their ordeals without such high levels of negative effects. Other studies have shown problems continuing into adulthood.[30]

HOW IS ALCOHOL MISUSE ADDRESSED IN NATIONAL POLICY?

NATIONAL POLICIES ON ALCOHOL MISUSE

Although there has been a national drugs strategy (see Ch. 11 'Drugs') in place in England and Wales for at least a decade, and national alcohol strategies for Scotland since 2002, Wales since 1996 and Northern Ireland since 2000,[2,3,4] it was not until 2004 that a long-awaited national alcohol harm reduction strategy for England was finally published.[1] Prior to that, many commentators and workers within the alcohol field had felt that the continuing lack of such a national strategy for England underlined the policy neglect at the heart of government, and made the job of developing coherent treatment and prevention initiatives very problematic, and that the focus for attention (and hence resources) had been far more on the drugs field (see Ch. 11 'Drugs').

The main features of the new strategy for England[1] are summarized in Box 10.2.

On publication, the strategy was greeted with muted praise by commentators. Its final appearance was welcomed, but there was concern over significant gaps, and a call for more urgent action to boost treatment and counselling services for people experiencing drink problems. The authors of this chapter mirror this view and also regret the fact that there is little mention of the needs of children and families of those with a drink problem, although the serious effects on them had been underlined in the Strategy Unit's *Interim Analytical Report*.[15]

OTHER NATIONAL POLICY INITIATIVES

Some other policy initiatives and laws have been developed to try and combat particular issues relating to alcohol misuse:

● Alcohol has been identified as an important (or at least contributory) issue within many of the recent Department of Health National Service Frameworks (e.g. for cancer, coronary heart disease, mental health, older people).[31–34]

Box 10.2   *Alcohol Harm Reduction Strategy for England* 2004: summary of key features[1]

The report sets out the government's strategy for tackling the harms and costs of alcohol misuse in England. The aim of this strategy is to prevent any further increase in alcohol-related harms in England.

The report states that the vast majority of people enjoy alcohol without causing harm to themselves or to others – indeed they can also gain some health and social benefits from moderate use. But for others, alcohol misuse is a very real problem. The Strategy Unit's interim analysis estimated that alcohol misuse is now costing around £20 billion a year. Binge drinking and chronic drinking patterns are particularly likely to raise the risk of harm.

The strategy is intended to provide a strong base for where government should intervene and lead, whilst recognizing that responsibility for alcohol misuse cannot rest with government alone. Importantly, the strategy sets out a new cross-government approach that relies on creating a partnership at both national and local levels between government, the drinks industry, health and police services, and individuals and communities to tackle alcohol misuse.

The strategy sets out four key areas for action.

Better education and communication

Measures are aimed at achieving a long term change in attitudes to irresponsible drinking and behaviour, including:

- making the 'sensible drinking' message easier to understand and apply;
- targeting messages at those most at risk, including binge and chronic drinkers;
- providing better information for consumers, both on products and at the point of sale;
- providing alcohol education in schools that can change attitudes and behaviour;
- providing more support and advice for employers; and
- reviewing the code of practice for TV advertising to ensure that it does not target young drinkers or glamorize irresponsible behaviour.

Improving health and treatment services

The strategy proposes a number of measures to improve early identification and treatment of alcohol problems.

Combating alcohol-related crime and disorder

The strategy proposes a series of measures to address the problems of those town and city centres that are blighted by alcohol misuse at weekends.

Working with the alcohol industry

The strategy will build on the good practice of some existing initiatives (such as the Manchester Citysafe Scheme) and involve the alcohol industry in new initiatives at both national level (drinks producers) and at local level (retailers, pubs and clubs).

Making it all happen

Making it happen will be a shared responsibility across government. Ministers at the Home Office and the Department of Health will take the lead; the government will measure progress regularly against clearly defined indicators and will take stock in 2007.

- There have been policy developments in terms of licensing law, with the new Licensing Bill[35] having been approved by both Houses of Parliament in 2003 with a transitional period to enable the switch from the existing licensing system to the new regime, and expected to be in effect by early 2005. The main changes are to liberalize opening (and closing) hours to try to reduce the binge drinking which is caused by speedy 'drinking up' at closing times, and to stagger closing times so as to reduce alcohol-related disturbances caused by all licensed premises turning intoxicated patrons onto the streets at the same time. These changes have been significantly controversial, with many fearing an increase, not a decrease, in alcohol-related city centre disturbances.

● There has been policy debate about the blood alcohol level at which it is illegal to drive, with many arguing for a reduction from the UK level of 80 mg of alcohol in 100 ml of blood to the level adopted in the majority of EU countries. At the time of writing, in May 2004, four of the 15 EU member states have an 80 mg limit, nine have a 50 mg limit, one has 40 mg and one has 20 mg. Spain will shortly lower its limit from 80 mg to 50 mg.

INTERNATIONAL POLICY

There is also an international dimension to alcohol policy. In 1995, the European Conference on Health, Society and Alcohol adopted the European Charter on Alcohol.[36] This charter sets out 10 strategies that provide the framework for implementing the World Health Organization (WHO) European Alcohol Action Plan (EAAP), which was adopted by the WHO Regional Committee for Europe in 1992.[37] In 1999, the Regional Committee agreed a second phase of the EAAP, to span the period 2000–2005.[38]

However, while alcohol has long been an important part of the agenda of WHO in Europe, its place in EU health policy has been much less clear. Instead, legislation about alcohol issues has generally been left within the remit of agricultural or industrial policy, and as such there has been little coherent drive to ensure an overall EU-wide approach to tackling alcohol problems.

DO HEALTH INEQUALITIES FEATURE IN ALCOHOL MISUSE?

There are two answers to this question. The first is that alcohol misuse and alcohol-related problems seem to affect people from all walks of life, all socio-economic groups, and all socio-cultural populations. Given the ubiquity of alcohol misuse, it is not possible to predict confidently who is more likely to drink excessively and/or develop problems as a result of their alcohol consumption. As the Strategy Unit concluded from the evidence it reviewed,[15] problem drinking is a result of the interaction of a large number of individual and external factors and characteristics working together: age, gender, family background, culture, price, availability and advertising are some examples. The factors identified as more likely predictors of alcohol problems fell into five main categories: individual characteristics; family environment; life events and experiences; social norms and culture; and the market (see Table 10.1).[15]

On the other hand, there are also some marked health inequalities. These occur in two ways.

● There is a large effect of economic cushioning. At any given level of excessive alcohol consumption, the negative effects are greater if people are poorer.
● There are also some specific effects of inequalities. It is suggested that the following are all areas where health inequalities may feature:[39]

Table 10.1 Predictors of alcohol problems[15]

Individual characteristics	Family environment	Life events and experiences	Social norms and culture	The market
• Personality type • Perception of risk • Genetics • Age and sex • Occupation • Geography • Ethnic minority status	• Parental divorce • Relationship with parents and their drinking behaviour • Children in care • Children with multiple problems	• A reaction to stress or trauma (include violence) • Relationship breakdown	• Drinking culture (North versus South European) • Other aspects of culture, e.g. design of pubs, concept of 'buying in rounds', workplace etiquette • Other influences, e.g. friends, acceptance, searching for a relationship, social trends, social norms and image (e.g. portrayal in media)	• Supply driven, e.g. fall in production and distribution costs, rise in service costs, licensing, branding of alcohol and pubs, 'product innovation' (e.g. alcopops) • Demand driven, e.g. people have more disposable income, change in lifestyle, increase in leisure time and travel, increased age for marriage and starting a family

– sex, with women experiencing greater negative effects at any given level of consumption;

– socio-economic status, as above, with poorer people experiencing greater negative effects;

– age, with greater effects for both young and elderly people;

– ethnicity, where some minority ethnic groups may drink more, such as the Irish, Sikh men, and black men and women in the Midlands;

– location, with more alcohol misuse in areas of social deprivation.

(See Ch. 13 'Tackling inequalities in health'.)

WHAT CAN WE DO ABOUT ALCOHOL MISUSE?

There is a range of approaches to intervention at both community and individual level.

DO NOTHING?

One approach is to do nothing. Drinking patterns change with age, and it seems likely that most young people (about whom there is currently most concern) will naturally reduce consumption as they grow older. Generally, when people finish their education, move into the employment sector and start to settle down with families of their own, consumption sharply reduces.

Furthermore, many people (not just young ones) recognize for themselves when their drinking is becoming excessive, take steps to reduce it, and overcome any associated problems; longitudinal studies suggest that large numbers of people seem able to overcome their drinking without resort to formal help. For example, one study of alcohol use and misuse in men throughout their life span (from 20 to 70–80 years) found that whilst the mortality rate was higher than that seen in other populations, alcohol misuse was not as progressive as previously thought, nor could it be assumed that those with a higher level of social disadvantage, a family history of alcohol problems, or the earliest onset of an alcohol problem, would have the most problems when older.[40]

A RANGE OF INTERVENTION AND TREATMENT STRATEGIES

Many commentators would argue that, although many people do sort out their problems for themselves, there is still a need to provide a range of interventions to reduce excessive alcohol consumption and deal with the numbers of people with problems. The Strategy Unit[15] concurred, concluding that a range of intervention/treatment strategies was required, and identifying four categories of intervention (summarized in Table 10.2).

The Strategy Unit acknowledges that 'the inter-relationships between service providers are complex, the system is difficult for users to navigate and some users pass repeatedly through the system'.[15(p. 138)] We would agree with this, but we would add to this complexity by suggesting that a fifth category of intervention is required, that focuses on the needs of children, families and communities affected by alcohol misuse. Although the Strategy Unit's *Interim Analytical Report*[15] acknowledges the impact that alcohol has on families and communities, it ignores these elements when it comes to look at useful interventions, and gave them little attention in the final Alcohol Harm Reduction Strategy for England.[1]

Table 10.2   Four categories of intervention with alcohol misuse[15]

Category	Agencies responsible for action	Key messages/interventions
Education	• Education system • Employment sector • Social services • Sure Start • Connexions	• Sensible drinking messages • Advertising, product labelling etc. • A need to focus on young people • Working with schools and workplaces
Supply	• 'The industry' – includes licensing, pricing, customs and producers	• Price • Availability • Other factors (includes design of pubs and bars)
Treatment	• NHS primary care • Hospital (including A&E) • Specialist treatment agencies (includes residential services) and self-help organizations	• Prevention • Identification (includes screening) • Treatment (includes brief interventions, residential and self-help organizations and the need to follow-up)
Safety	• Police • Courts • Probation • Prisons • Child protection service • Youth justice board	• Prevention • Identification • Enforcement (includes arrest referral schemes, alcohol-free zones and drink driving initiatives) • Need to follow-up and promote rehabilitation

CONTROL ALCOHOL AVAILABILITY

One approach is to control the amount of alcohol within a community, possibly via government control. There is a long history of government control measures, with the UK system of licensing laws perhaps the best known, which in the past sought to restrict the number of outlets selling alcohol. In other countries (such as within Scandinavia) alcohol can only be purchased from a limited number of government liquor stores. These measures are often associated with lower per capita consumption but with greater binge drinking.

Other control mechanisms include increasing taxation, restrictions on advertising, greater enforcement of the law (for example on underage purchasing, or selling to intoxicated people), and national media campaigns.

COMMUNITY INITIATIVES

Another way is through community initiatives. In Victorian times these showed themselves in the rise of temperance organizations, but nowadays the focus is on promoting 'sensible drinking' guidelines, minimizing harm from alcohol and preventing alcohol misuse by young people.

Promoting 'sensible' drinking

The public health concept of developing an agreed 'alcohol unit' system, developing sensible and safe drinking guidelines and encouraging people to limit their own drinking has emerged (see Box 10.1). Despite campaigns to raise public awareness of the benefits of such guidelines and associated government policies that set targets to reduce alcohol consumption (such as the White Paper *The Health of the Nation*[41]), it is clear that, so far, the hoped-for results have not been achieved.

Harm minimization

A second community intervention approach is to focus on reducing the negative effects of alcohol consumption, as opposed to the consumption itself. Examples of such initiatives (mainly locally developed) include:

- the requirement to use safety glasses (which shatter without leaving sharp shards of glass and hence reduce 'glassing' injuries) in order to obtain a nightclub licence;
- 'doorsafe' schemes which train door staff to deal with drunken customers in ways which minimize violent incidents;
- 'designated driver' schemes (hence reducing problems of drinking and driving).

Prevention of alcohol misuse by young people

A third approach is to try to prevent alcohol problems and alcohol misuse by intervening with young people before they start drinking. However, a recent systematic review looking at the prevention of alcohol misuse in young people found that 'no firm conclusions about the effectiveness of prevention interventions in the short and medium term were possible'.[42](p. 397) One USA approach, the Strengthening Families Programme, was found to have the most promise and the best evidence for its effectiveness in the longer term, but these findings need replication. This approach has recently been implemented (but not rigorously evaluated) within the UK.[43]

THERAPEUTIC APPROACHES

Where prevention and 'natural' reduction of alcohol misuse as people age has not 'worked', a wide range of therapeutic approaches are in use.

They include psychological approaches designed to help people change their drinking behaviour, and drugs which impact upon the areas of the brain that influence the desire to drink alcohol or the experience of a 'high'.[44,45] In general, these interventions are effective.

Brief interventions are a particularly useful approach in primary care and community settings. This means providing advice and feedback, which could be as short as 5 or 10 minutes, to people drinking at hazardous levels. Brief interventions are likely to work because they have an important motivational enhancement element and are:

- acceptable (particularly to those with less severe drinking problems);
- able to be delivered opportunistically (making them particularly suitable for environments such as primary care and A&E departments);
- more cost-effective than other forms of intervention.[46]

For individuals with more severe problems, a brief intervention may be a useful first step as part of a stepped care approach.[44]

Other treatments with the strongest evidence of efficacy are those that focus on people's interactions with others. A new therapy based on this principle is social behaviour and network therapy[47] which uses people's families and other people as 'encouragers' to reduce or stop drinking.

WORKING WITH FAMILIES

Help for family members has been notoriously lacking; a family member is often seen as an add-on to treatment, someone who can help the misuser curb or stop their problematic consumption. More recent approaches have viewed the family member as someone who may need help in their own right. Whilst many family members may feel that there is nothing that can be done unless the person with the problems makes the necessary changes, there are in fact things that family members can do to improve the situation for themselves, and in turn for others in their wider community. One brief therapeutic approach along these lines has been developed and is being evaluated in the primary care and specialist settings,[48] and there are other approaches.[49]

CONTROVERSIAL ISSUES

There are many controversial issues within the alcohol field; a few currently 'hot' issues in prevention and health promotion are highlighted and briefly discussed below.

POLICY

The primary issue at present is the implementation of the national *Alcohol Harm Reduction Strategy*.[1] Does it come with enough money, and with coherent government backing? At present it is a shared responsibility across government, so agreement needs to be sought from different departments, often with differing priorities, and perhaps competing interests. Furthermore, how will the national strategy be translated regionally and locally, and is it focusing on the right issues?

Related to this is the extent to which the alcohol field should be linked with drugs. Many people worry that, if it is, it will be swallowed up;

others worry that if it is not, there will be huge duplication, with essentially similar structures being developed for both issues.

HEALTH

There is still controversy over the emerging evidence that alcohol consumption at lower levels acts as a protection against some health problems, especially coronary heart disease and stroke, particularly in the over 40s when the risk of these health problems is at its highest. In fact, the number of people believed to benefit from such protection every year is estimated to be equal to the number of annual alcohol-related deaths.

PREVENTION

The key issue here is about how best to prevent alcohol misuse. There is still a major controversy over whether we should be focusing our prevention and intervention approaches on those at most serious risk, or aiming for a whole population approach.

ADVERTISING, MARKETING, YOUNG PEOPLE AND BINGE DRINKING

The role that the alcohol production, distribution and sales industry plays in the development of harmful attitudes and behaviour is still highly controversial. The industry itself has developed the Portman Group (a consortium of major British drinks companies established to 'promote sensible drinking and reduce alcohol-related harm')[9(p. 313)] but the same industry is also responsible for developing products such as 'alcopops' and using marketing strategies which seem to focus on the growth markets of young people and women.

Similar concerns have been raised over the serious rise in binge drinking, the association of binge drinking with images of young people having fun, both on holiday and at home, and the part that the drinks industry plays in promoting such associations.[21]

COMMON MYTHS

NEGATIVE STEREOTYPES

There are many common myths in this area,[7(Ch. 9)] mainly relating to negative stereotypes about the sort of person who develops alcohol problems (such as: they are all park bench alcoholics) or the ability of problem drinkers to change their behaviour; for example:

- they always lie about how much they consume;
- one can't work with someone until they admit that they are an alcoholic;
- one can't work with someone until they have reached rock bottom;
- abstinence is the only solution;
- there's no point in trying to help an alcoholic because success is so rare;
- problem drinkers can only be helped by other people who have or have had drinking problems;
- you don't have an alcohol problem unless you drink in the mornings;
- you don't have a problem unless you drink more than your GP.

QUESTIONS THAT STILL NEED ANSWERS

The questions that still need answering focus on some key controversial issues which we have already touched on.

- How to reduce the problem? We know a lot about prevention programmes which do not work, but little about those that do. A major issue is whether or not we should be trying to reduce overall per capita consumption or focusing on at-risk groups.

- What is the effect of advertising and media representations? Should we be aiming for a ban on advertising, or for health warnings on alcohol containers?

Eric Appleby, Chief Executive of Alcohol Concern (the national agency on alcohol misuse, website www.alcoholconcern.org.uk), in writing his

Key sources of further information and help

- **Alcohol Concern:** www.alcoholconcern.org.uk. Alcohol Concern was established in 1983; it is the national agency on alcohol misuse working to 'reduce the incidence and costs of alcohol-related harm and to increase the range and quality of services available to people with alcohol-related problems'.
- **Alcohol Education and Research Council (AERC):** www.aerc.org.uk: The AERC finances projects within the United Kingdom for education and research and for novel forms of help to those with drinking problems.
- **Alcohol strategy for England:** Prime Minister's Strategy Unit: Strategy Unit project on tackling the problems associated with alcohol misuse. www.strategy.gov.uk. This has produced the *Alcohol harm reduction strategy for England*.[1] There is also an excellent interim analysis of the problems caused by alcohol,[15] available at www.pm.gov.uk/output/Page4498.asp. (See www.pm.gov.uk/output/Page5506.asp for all the Strategy Unit background papers.) There are various commentaries on the Strategy, downloadable from the Alcohol Concern website.
- **Alcohol strategy for Northern Ireland:** Northern Ireland have both a Drugs and an Alcohol Strategy. The alcohol strategy is called the *Strategy for Reducing Alcohol Related Harm*.[4]

- **Alcohol strategy for Scotland:** See the Scottish Executive's *Action Plan on Alcohol Problems*.[2] www.Scotland.gov.uk/health/alcohol
- **Alcohol strategy for Wales:** National Assembly for Wales. Wales have a combined Drug and Alcohol Strategy launched in 1996, which has now been superseded by the 2000 8-year substance misuse strategy *Tackling Substance Misuse in Wales*.[3]
- **Down Your Drink:** an online self-help programme for safer drinking. Website: www.downyourdrink.org.uk/main.php
- **Drinkline:** Tel: 0800 917 8282; Website: www.wrecked.co.uk. NHS interactive quiz providing information about drinking.
- **European network for children affected by risky environments in the family (ENCARE):** www.encare.info. A European project founded to help professionals tackle problems faced by children who live in risky family environments; the first risky environment examined relates to families where parents have problems with alcohol.
- **Health Development Agency:** Prevention and reduction of alcohol misuse: evidence briefing. London: HDA; 2002. www.hda.nhs.uk/evidence

wish list for 2004 and for the national *Alcohol Harm Reduction Strategy*,[1] said that he wanted to see:

> True understanding of the nature of alcohol problems – individual and societal – and ... a commitment to tackling the root causes. This involves a recognition that destructive drinking styles, millions of assaults and overstretched health and care services are not just about individual responsibility – crucial though it is – but about wider issues such as the attitudes and behaviour that we don't just tolerate, but actively encourage in a myriad of ways.[50](p. 2)

References

1. Prime Minister's Strategy Unit. Alcohol harm reduction strategy for England. London: The Cabinet Office; 2004. Online. Available: http://www.strategy.gov.uk or http://www.pm.gov.uk/output/Page3669.asp

2. Scottish Executive. Action plan on alcohol problems. Edinburgh: Scottish Executive; 2002. Online. Available: http://www.Scotland.gov.uk/health/alcohol

3. National Assembly for Wales. Tackling substance misuse in Wales: a partnership approach. Cardiff: National Assembly for Wales; 2000. Online. Available: http://www.wales.gov.uk/subisocialpolicy/content/direct/misuse.htm

4. Northern Ireland Department of Health, Social Services and Public Safety. Strategy for reducing alcohol related harm. Belfast: DHSS: 2000. Online. Available: http://www.dhsspsni gov.uk/publications/archived/2000/alcohol.pdf

5. Department of Health. Sensible drinking: the report of an inter-departmental working group. London: HMSO; 1995.

6. Royal College of Obstetricians and Gynaecologists. Alcohol consumption in pregnancy. London: Royal College of Obstetricians and Gynaecologists; 1999.

7. Velleman R. Counselling for alcohol problems. 2nd edn. London: Sage Publications; 2001.

8. Orford J. Excessive appetites: a psychological view of addictions. 2nd edn. Chichester: Wiley; 2001.

9. Barr A. Drink: a social history. London: Pimlico; 1998.

10. Jellinek E. The disease concept of alcoholism. New Haven, New Jersey: Hillhouse; 1960.

11. Heather N, Robertson I. Problem drinking. 3rd edn. Oxford: Oxford University Press; 1997.

12. Houghton E, Roche AM, eds. Learning about drinking. Philadelphia: Taylor and Francis; 2001.

13. Shaw S, Cartwright A, Spratley T, Harwin J. Responding to drinking problems. London: Croom Helm; 1978.

14. Babor TF, Caetano R, Casswell S, et al. Alcohol: no ordinary commodity: research and public policy. New York: Oxford University Press; 2003.

15. Prime Minister's Strategy Unit. Alcohol harm reduction project: interim analytical report. London: Strategy Unit; 2003. Online. Available: http://www.pm.gov.uk/output/Page4498.asp

16. Davies JB. The myth of addiction. Amsterdam, The Netherlands: Harwood Academic; 1997.

17. Velleman R, Copello A, Maslin J. Living with drink. women who live with problem drinkers. London: Longman; 1998.

18. Kroll B, Taylor A. Parental substance misuse and child welfare. London: Jessica Kingsley; 2003.

19. Plant M. Drinking careers: occupations, drinking habits and drinking problems. London: Tavistock Publications; 1979.

20. Donnellan C. Alcohol. Cambridge: Independence Educational Publishers; 1999 (Volume 39).

21. Department of Health. Annual report of the Chief Medical Officer of the Department of Health. London: DOH; 2003. Online. Available: http://www.publications.doh.gov.uk/cmo/annualreport2001

22. Institute of Alcohol Studies. Alcohol consumption and harm in the UK and EU. London: IAS; 2002.

23. Orford J, Natera G, Davies J, et al Stresses and strains for family members living with drinking or drug problems in England and Mexico. Salud Mental 1998; 21:1–13.

24. Cleaver H, Unell I, Aldgate J. Children's needs – parenting capacity: the impact of parental mental illness, problem alcohol and drug use, and domestic violence on children's development. London: The Stationery Office; 1997.

25. Tunnard J. Parental problem drinking and its impact on children. Research in Practice; 2002.

26. Velleman R. The children of problem drinking parents: an executive summary. Executive summary series. Executive Summary 70, 1–5. London: Imperial College Faculty of Medicine, Centre for Research on Drugs and Health Behaviour; 2002. Online. Available: http://www.med.ic.ac.uk/divisions/64/execsum70.pdf

27. Mullender A, Hague G, Imam U, et al. Children's perspectives on domestic violence. London: Sage Publications; 2002.

28. Forrester D, Harwin J. Picking up the pieces. Community Care 2002; 12–18 December: 36–37.

29. Velleman R, Orford J. Risk and resilience. London: Harwood; 1999.

30. Callingham M. The ACOA fact-finder. Addiction Today 1999 (November-December).

31. Department of Health. National Service Framework for cancer. London: Department of Health; 2000.

32. Department of Health. National Service Framework for coronary heart disease. London: Department of Health; 2000.

33. Department of Health. National Service Framework for mental health. London: Department of Health; 1999.

34. Department of Health. National Service Framework for older people. London: Department of Health; 2001.

35. Licensing Bill 2002. London: The Stationery Office; 2002. Online. Available: http://www.publications parliament.uk/pa/id200203/idbills/001/2003001.htm

36. World Health Organization. European charter on alcohol. WHO Regional Office for Europe; 1995. Online. Available: http://www.euro.who.int/about WHO/Policy/20010927_7

37. World Health Organization. European alcohol action plan. Document EUP/RC42/8. Copenhagen: WHO Regional Office for Europe; 1992.

38. World Health Organization. European alcohol action plan 2000–2005. Copenhagen: WHO Regional Office for Europe; 1999.

39. Waller S, Naidoo B, Thom B. Prevention and reduction of alcohol misuse: evidence briefing. London: Health Development Agency; 2002.

40. Vaillant G. A 60-year follow-up of alcoholic men. Addiction 2003; 98:1043–1051.

41. Department of Health. The health of the nation: a strategy for health in England. London: HMSO; 1992.

42. Foxcroft DR, Ireland D, Lister-Sharp DJ, et al. Longer-term primary prevention for alcohol misuse in young people: a systematic review. Addiction 2003; 98:397–411.

43. Marsh M, Male S. Altogether now: supporting Barnsley parents. Birmingham: AERC; 2003. Online. Available: http://www.aerc.org.uk/then follow link relating to the AERC Conference on Family Approaches to Alcohol Problems, Birmingham UK, 11th November 2003.

44. Babor TF, Del Boca FK. Treatment matching in alcoholism. Cambridge: Cambridge University Press; 2003.

45. Miller W, Wilbourne P. Mesa Grande: a methodological analysis of clinical trials of treatments for alcohol use disorders. Addiction 2002; 97:265–277.

46. Moyer A, Finney JW, Swearingen CE, et al. Brief interventions for alcohol problems: a meta-analytic review of controlled investigations in treatment seeking and non-treatment seeking populations. Addiction 2002; 97:279–292.

47. Copello A, Orford J, Hodgson R, et al. Social behaviour and network therapy: Basic principles and early experiences. Addictive Behaviours 2002; 27:345-366.

48. Copello A, Orford J, Velleman R, et al. Methods for reducing alcohol and drug related family harm in non-specialist settings. Journal of Mental Health 2000; 9:329–343.

49. Velleman R, Templeton L. Family interventions in substance misuse. In: Peterson T, McBride A, eds. Working with substance misusers: a guide to theory and practice. London: Routledge; 2002: 145–153.

50. Appleby E. Straight Talk. Editorial. London: Alcohol Concern; 2003; 4:2.

Chapter 11

Drug use and misuse

Richard Velleman and Lorna Templeton

SUMMARY OVERVIEW AND LINKS TO OTHER TOPICS

In this chapter *drug misuse* is defined as 'any use of drugs that causes problems for either the drug taker or anyone else'. This chapter focuses on illegal drugs: stimulants including cocaine, crack and ecstasy; depressants including heroin, methadone, solvents and tranquillizers; and hallucinogens including LSD, cannabis and magic mushrooms.

Most people who try drugs use them experimentally or recreationally and have no problems; others (the minority) develop problems. Drug misuse is an important public health issue because of associated health problems and risk of death, and the impact on families and the wider community, including increased crime to pay for drugs.

A survey in 2002/2003 indicated that over one third of the population aged 16–59 in the UK has 'ever' used an illegal drug, and 28% of 16–24 year olds reported that they had taken an illegal drug in the last year. Cannabis is the most popular illegal drug, with its use increasing. Amphetamines, cocaine and ecstasy are the next most commonly used, almost all in younger age groups. Inequalities feature: drug misuse is linked with high unemployment and social deprivation.

There have been national drug strategies since 1995. Evidence-based approaches focus on prevention, harm minimization and treatment, which are increasingly often provided in conjunction with the criminal justice system.

Controversies abound, particularly about what the legal status of drugs should be, and the use of methadone as a substitute drug for opiates. A great deal of research and development of effective ways to help drug misusers and their families remains to be done.

Cigarettes, alcohol and drugs are all 'drugs', so Chapter 10 'Alcohol use and misuse' and Chapter 4 'Smoking' are both useful to read alongside this one. Poor mental health may also be associated with drug misuse: see Chapter 12 'Mental health and mental health promotion'.

As health inequalities feature in drug misuse, and lifestyle changes are important for prevention and treatment, Chapter 13 'Tackling inequalities in health' and Chapter 14 'Helping individuals to change behaviour' are also relevant.

WHAT IS DRUG MISUSE?

Like alcohol (see Ch. 10), other substances have for centuries been attractive to enable people to achieve an altered state of consciousness. There are many such substances: this chapter will primarily consider three main types of drug,[1] categorized according to their main effects on the central nervous system:

- stimulants, including amphetamines, cocaine, crack, methylenedioxymethamfetamine (MDMA) known as ecstasy and its derivatives, and amyl/butyl nitrites;
- depressants, including opiates (both natural such as heroin, and synthetic such as methadone), solvents and tranquillizers;
- hallucinogens, including LSD, cannabis and magic mushrooms.

(Table 11.1 provides a list of common illegal drugs, while Gossop[2] and McBride[3] provide more detailed descriptions of drugs.)

In the past, many of these drugs had medical uses for a wide range of conditions and were generally not deemed problematic. Drugs which were formerly in use but are now highly restricted include opiates such as laudanum to provide pain relief or to treat insomnia, coughs and diarrhoea; stimulants such as amphetamines and cocaine to treat depression and help weight control;[4] and cannabis to deal with 'hysteria, anorexia nervosa, epilepsy, rheumatism, bronchial asthma, pain, glaucoma and nausea induced by chemotherapy'.[5(p. 75)] Today, many of these substances are illegal in the UK, and are controlled under the 1971 Misuse of Drugs Act.[6]

This chapter will focus on the use and misuse of *illegal* drugs.

People use drugs for a variety of reasons, in much the same way as they might choose to drink alcohol (see Ch. 10), smoke, or engage in other

Table 11.1   Common illegal drugs

Type of drug	Name of common drug	Effect on users	Class[a]/legal status
Stimulants	amphetamines	Excitement, confidence, energy	B (but A if injected)
	cocaine	A 'high', sense of well-being, confidence, alertness	A
	crack (a smokeable form of cocaine)	As cocaine, with a more intense shorter 'high'	A
	ecstasy (MDMA) and its derivatives	Alert, in tune with surroundings; sound, colour and emotions intense; may dance for hours	A
	amyl/butyl nitrite	Brief but intense 'high'/intoxication	Amyl nitrite is a prescription-only medicine; possession is not illegal but supply can be an offence
Depressants	opiates, both natural such as heroin, and synthetic such as methadone	Warmth, well-being, relaxation	A
	solvents (gases, glues, aerosols)	Slow down, relieve tension and anxiety; high doses can make drowsy	Illegal to sell gas lighter refills to under 18s, illegal to sell gases, glues and aerosols to under 18s, or to people acting for them if suspect intention of abuse
	tranquillizers	Calm down, relieve tension and anxiety; high doses can make drowsy and forgetful	Not illegal to possess but supply is illegal with Class C penalties
Hallucinogens	LSD	A 'trip' in which movement, time, objects, colours and sound may be experienced in a different way	A
	cannabis	Relaxed and talkative	C
	magic mushrooms	Similar to LSD but trip often milder and shorter	A when prepared (not illegal to possess raw)

[a] Under the Misuse of Drugs Act (1971)[6] drugs are classed into three categories (A, B and C), according to the harm they can do; Class A is the most harmful. There is a range of penalties for possession, supply and manufacture/cultivation, according to class. Penalties range from a maximum of life imprisonment and an unlimited fine for supplying/dealing a Class A drug to a maximum of 2 years in prison and unlimited fine for possession of a Class C drug.

'excessive appetitive' behaviours.[4] There have been many attempts to define drug misuse, and many terms used, such as: use, risky use, problem use, dependent use, addiction, as well as 'abuse' (which tends to be used in North America) and 'misuse' (used more commonly in the UK).

A helpful categorization is one which suggests that a person's use of substances can be:

- experimental
- recreational or
- dependent/problematic.

For the vast majority of people who try drugs, drug use will remain in the first or the first two of these categories, with problems for themselves or others less likely.

Trends in drug use have varied over time, partly helped by advances in technology which have led to the manufacture of cheap and very easily obtainable 'synthetic' drugs such as MDMA (ecstasy) and its derivatives.[4(pp. 66–67)] Routes of administration (i.e. how drugs are taken) have also changed over time, particularly between injecting and inhaling ('snorting', smoking, or 'chasing the dragon').

In this chapter we define drug misuse as we did in Chapter 10 with respect to alcohol: any use of drugs that causes problems for either the drug taker or anyone else.

WHAT CAUSES DRUG MISUSE?

A range of theories are used to try and understand drug misuse and drug problems.[7] For the most part these are the same theories as were discussed in Chapter 10 in relation to alcohol misuse:

- those which look to the individual for causation (their genetic make-up or personality, or they have a 'disease');
- those which direct attribution to social groups (the influence of others such as peers or family);
- those which consider societal and cultural conditions (such as social deprivation or the illegal nature of the drugs under discussion).

Consideration of the nature of drug misuse in Europe and the USA is dominated by the 'disease' model, linked with pharmacological theories about the reaction of the body to drugs involving phenomena such as tolerance and withdrawal. More recent developments focus on more integrative approaches, such as those integrating behavioural conditioning and learning ideas with pharmacological approaches,[8] and approaches that consider the problem more holistically in terms of social groups.[9]

WHY IS DRUG MISUSE AN IMPORTANT PUBLIC HEALTH ISSUE?

Compared to the prevalence of some issues discussed in this book, the problem of drug misuse in terms of numbers of people affected can appear quite small. However, other factors mean that it is no less of a public health concern. These factors include:

- The illegal nature of these drugs. All users of illegal drugs become offenders against the law, irrespective of whether their drug use causes other difficulties.

- The range of associated problems that drug use and misuse brings, including the impact on the users themselves, on their families and on communities. It is estimated that drug use costs UK society, in social and economic terms, between £10 and £18 billion annually.[10]

PREVALENCE OF ILLEGAL DRUG USE

The findings from the 2002/2003 British Crime Survey[11] provide probably the most up-to-date information about the prevalence and trends of drug use.

- Over one third of the population aged 16–59 has 'ever' used an illegal drug, and currently there are estimated to be about 4 million users of illicit drugs in the UK, based on figures of 12% of 16–59 year olds reporting that they had taken an illegal drug in the last year.

- An estimated 1 million people used a Class A drug in the last year, again based on figures of 3% of 15–59 year olds who had reported such use.[11]

However, drug use among young people is rising, and there is a very strong age bias in the figures above, with people in the younger age ranges reporting rates of 'ever' and 'in the last year' drug use which are two to three times higher than the overall rates. So for example:

- 28% of 16–24 year olds reported having used an illegal drug in the last year;
- about 8% said they had used a Class A drug in the last year.[11]

The National Treatment Agency estimates that about a quarter of a million people in England and Wales will develop serious problems associated with their drug use every year,[12] although this is not to say that other users and misusers of illegal drugs are exempt from causing harm to themselves and others.

Which drugs are used most?

- **Cannabis** remains the most popularly used illegal substance in the UK, and its use continues to increase. Figures from the 2002/2003 British Crime Survey[11] show that just over one quarter of 16–24 year olds and about 11% of 16–59 year olds used the drug in the last year, equating to about 3 million people.

- **Amphetamines, cocaine and ecstasy** (all stimulants) are the next most commonly used illicit drugs across the general population, each used by about 2% of 16–59 year olds. Within this group of stimulants, use of one drug or the other differs slightly according to age of user:
  - Among 16–24 year olds ecstasy and cocaine are the most favoured drugs (after cannabis), used by about 5% of that group, followed by 4% who use amyl nitrites and amphetamines.
  - Among 25–34 year olds, cocaine use stands at 4%, followed by use of amphetamines and ecstasy at 3% and amyl nitrites at 2%.

Use of drugs other than cannabis in any of the older age groups is rare.

Trends

In terms of trends, comparisons between the two British Crime Surveys of 1996 and 2001/2002 show that the rise in use of cocaine and its purer freebase form, crack, is of particular note. This is the main explanation for the overall rise in use of Class A drugs, although ecstasy use also rose significantly over this period. In contrast, overall use of amphetamines, LSD and steroids fell between these two surveys.

Use by minority ethnic groups

Illegal drug use is by no means homogeneous across all minority populations, but generally use amongst minority ethnic groups is not believed to be any higher than in the majority white population. Patterns of drug use seem to be similar, although injecting does not seem so prevalent in these groups, and there are additional drugs not usually seen amongst the overall population, such as khat, a naturally grown, cultivated stimulant which is chewed and kept in the cheek as a 'quid'. It originated in Ethiopia, and it is now used mainly by those who originate from countries where khat is cultivated: much of the lower Middle East and Africa.[13]

The minority populations remain, however, a high risk population, because drug misuse is related to greater social deprivation and social exclusion, which affects many minority ethnic communities.[13]

PROBLEMS CAUSED BY DRUG MISUSE

Figure 11.1 provides a summarized overview of problems which can result from drug misuse.

Health problems

There are strong links between drug misuse and morbidity and mortality. There are many associated potential physical problems,[14] including:

- infections: skin, septicaemia, endocarditis, hepatitis, pulmonary infections and orthopaedic infections;
- problems linked to injecting behaviour, e.g. with veins, kidneys, and transmitted diseases including HIV and those affecting the liver;
- the risk of overdose and fatality.[15]

Drug-related deaths

Each year in England there are believed to be about 1350 premature deaths linked to the misuse of drugs.[12] Drug-related deaths have been rising, with mortality particularly associated with opiate use:[16] deaths

Figure 11.1 Problems caused by drug misuse.

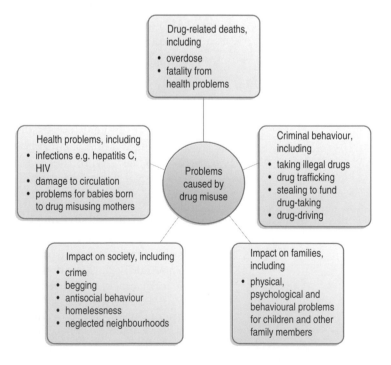

from heroin overdose doubled in the second half of the 1990s, particularly affecting both young people and those who inject their drugs.[17]

Death related to ecstasy use is rare, but it has received particular attention. This is due to the more unpredictable circumstances surrounding illness and death, and the characteristics of the victims, who are usually young people who do not fit stereotypical images of 'drug takers'.[18]

There is a range of risk factors that are most likely to be associated with overdose and death, particularly linked to opiates.[17] Some are to do with the individual, for example:

- injecting;
- simultaneous use of depressants or alcohol;
- not being in treatment;
- starting methadone treatment;
- dropping out of treatment.

Other risk factors are to do with wider issues such as the availability of prescribed drugs, the purity of the drug taken, and social situations such as homelessness.

There are a variety of strategies that can significantly reduce the risk of overdose (and potentially death),[19] including altered prescribing policies, harm reduction policies and an increased level of care during and after any time spent in prison.

Problems caused by injecting drugs

There are particular risks from injecting drug behaviour. In 1999 it was believed that about one third of the injecting drug-taking population shared needles, syringes and other equipment, though other work suggested that the rate was much higher than this at that time.[20–22]

The risks associated with injecting behaviour include:

- blood-borne viruses (such as hepatitis and HIV);
- bacterial and fungal infections;
- damage to the circulation system;
- increased risk of overdose, dependence and death.[20]

Of particular health concern in recent years has been the rise of hepatitis C infection, with more than 1 million people across the EU believed to be infected.[16] The rate of hepatitis C amongst injecting drug users is much higher than that found in the general population,[20] although estimates vary widely from 33% to 80%. Most of these will have contracted the infection through sharing needles and other equipment. Young people and those new to injecting behaviour are at greatest risk.[16]

Criminality

There is also a strong link between drug misuse and criminality.[11,16,23] We will outline three areas: trafficking, drug use and other crime, and drug-driving.

Drug trafficking

Significant resources are put into controlling drug trafficking. Figures from the Home Office show that in 2001 the overall number of drug seizures was 5% higher than the previous year.[24] Nearly three quarters of all seizures were of cannabis, but seizures of Class A drugs (especially cocaine and crack, but also heroin and ecstasy) also rose in this time, by 10%. Nevertheless, most commentators conclude that these seizures are only a small minority of the amount of drugs that successfully enter the country.

Drug use and other crime

The findings of seven studies reported by the Home Office[25] highlight the link between drug use and crime among male prisoners, with just under three quarters reporting use of drugs (mainly heroin) in the year before entering prison, a far higher percentage than in the general population.

Pre-prison levels of drug use amongst female prisoners, particularly white women, 'matched or even exceeded that of male prisoners'.[25(p. 1)] White women reported use mainly of heroin, black women reported use mainly of crack. Department of Health figures suggest that 20% of those with a probation order, 11% of convicted male and nearly a quarter of convicted female prisoners are drug dependent.[26]

Drug-driving

Drug-driving has become recognized in recent years as a danger, although it is still unclear how serious a problem it is. The exact number of those who drive whilst under the influence of drugs (other than alcohol or tobacco) is uncertain, as is the extent of risk and damage that may be being inflicted as a result.[27] What is clear is that there are detectable levels of drugs in a high percentage of driving fatalities, with pathologists demonstrating that 24% of accident fatalities had illegal drugs in their bloodstream.[27]

The difficulty with trying to estimate both the prevalence and the significance of drug-driving is the length of time drugs can remain in the body and still have an effect, and the variety and level of purity of many drugs. These factors make it hard to know at what level drug-taking can start to impair driving and other related functions. There are, however, a number of screening initiatives that are in the early stages of development and implementation.

The impact on families and communities

As with alcohol, the impact of drug use and misuse is not simply something that affects the individual. For every person who misuses drugs (i.e. has any sort of problem, not necessarily a full blown 'drug dependence') it is suggested that there are, on average, two close family members negatively affected. Hence, the current estimates of 250 000 dependent drug users in England and Wales, 1 million users of Class A drugs and 4 million drug users overall, lead to an extrapolation of anywhere between half a million and 8 million family members affected by drug misuse.

The situation for children in these families has been highlighted by the Advisory Council on the Misuse of Drugs.[28] The experiences of these children and other family members are very similar to those experienced by family members of alcohol misusers: that is, children will often suffer a range of problems, physical, psychological and behavioural, as a result of being in such a childhood environment. They often take on responsibilities that are beyond their years, thus affecting their education and peer relationships. They may be too ashamed to bring friends home, or not be able to go out with friends because they have to care for a sibling or parent under the influence of drugs. They can experience or witness physical, verbal and sexual abuse. Problem drug use can affect family holidays, and celebrations such as Christmas and birthdays.

Although many of these problems are similar to those experienced by children in alcohol-misusing families, differences when a parent misuses drugs include the illegal nature of drug use, the different modes of ingestion (watching someone snort, inject etc.), the links to crime, and the use of the home as a location for groups of people to take drugs (with drug misuse more likely to be a home-based activity); drug misuse also has links to poverty, unemployment, social deprivation.[29-32] (See also Ch. 10.)

Many children in this situation will reach the attention of social services.[32,33] The issue of 'resilience' touched on in Chapter 10 on alcohol is relevant here, too: research shows that some children are resilient, and that a range of factors increase the chances of a child becoming resilient even if they live with a parent with a serious problem.[34-37] These 'protective' factors include a positive relationship with a key and stable adult (e.g. the other parent, a grandparent, or someone outside the family), shared family activities and affection, and engagement with outside activities (sports, culture, religion) or with a positive peer group.

The growing numbers of people with drug-related problems means that the numbers of children brought up in this environment are rising. Much work needs to be done to clarify how badly these children are affected, how long any effect might last, and what steps can be taken to help children break this new intergenerational cycle of deprivation.

The range of problems experienced by communities because of drug misuse includes crime (especially acquisitive crime, i.e. stealing to fund a drug habit), begging and other anti-social behaviour, homelessness, and neglected neighbourhoods.

IS DRUG MISUSE GETTING BETTER OR WORSE?

There have been changes in patterns of drug use since 1996. Particular concerns are:

- the rising level of use among young people;
- the continued popularity of cannabis and heroin;
- rises in the use of cocaine and crack;
- the rise in hepatitis C infection;
- drug use in prisons, and the strong links to crime.

The resulting strain on resources, and the problem of access to treatment services are yet further causes for concern.

The fact that young people appear to use illicit drugs more frequently and are therefore at greatest risk of developing problems is balanced by the fact that longitudinal research suggests that people do 'grow out' of drug use and misuse; the vast majority of people who use drugs experimentally, or even recreationally, do not develop problems or are able to curb their drug use before problems get too serious. This can be seen in the great disparity between the numbers who have used drugs, and the numbers who develop serious problems, as outlined above. Most young people use drugs at a certain stage of their lives, and when they 'settle down' (stop going to clubs so frequently, start a career, start a family) the contexts within which they used drugs are no longer appropriate. The influence of context is shown most starkly in research on US soldiers returning from the Vietnam war.[38] Of those who used heroin regularly in Vietnam, only 28% continued to do so on their return to the USA; and of those, only 28% of them went on to become 'addicted' in the USA.

WHO IS AT RISK? DO HEALTH INEQUALITIES FEATURE IN THIS TOPIC?

As the Home Office puts it:

> Drug problems are most serious in those communities where social exclusion is acute, where people lack the will or the resources to control or manage drug problems. Where people are grouped together in areas of high unemployment, crime, fractured families and poor housing, drug misuse grows and its effects are magnified. Drug markets develop to serve the demand for drugs created by people who have no vision of or hope for the future.[10(p. 30)]

Everyone is at potential risk of misusing drugs and developing problems as a result. Young people, and those experiencing problems with unemployment, deprivation and social exclusion, including minority ethnic groups, are of particular concern. The 2002/2003 British Crime Survey continued to highlight the greater use of drugs amongst younger people, whilst also acknowledging that gender, ethnicity and location are factors to be taken into account.[11] Women can have particular fertility, obstetric and gynaecological problems associated with drug misuse, and babies born to drug-using mothers are at risk of harm or death.[15,39]

Broad approaches to tackling inequalities in health are relevant here (see Ch. 13 'Tackling inequalities in health').

HOW IS DRUG ABUSE ADDRESSED IN NATIONAL POLICY?

> The history of British drug policy has swung between the perception of drug use as a moral failing controllable by legal sanctions and drug use as a condition susceptible to medical treatment or other interventions albeit within a legal framework.[40(p. 217)]

In Britain, policy-making over the 60 years from the 1920s to the 1980s centred on a medical prescribing/treatment model. Practices ranged from long term maintenance prescribing of heroin or alternative drugs during the 1920s to the 1960s,[41,42] to short term reduction prescribing aiming at abstinence in the 1970s.

Prescribing was not the only plank of government policy: enforcement has always been incorporated into the system of controlling drug use in the UK,[43] but prescribing alternative drugs was the primary focus.

In the first half of the 1980s there was a shift in focus towards enforcement/punishment, exemplified by the five pronged approach of:

- reducing supplies from abroad;
- tightening controls on drugs produced and prescribed;
- making policing even more effective;
- strengthening deterrence; and
- improving prevention, treatment and rehabilitation.[44]

This was severely criticized for concentrating police attention on prosecuting very large numbers of cannabis-smoking young people, at the expense of tackling more serious drug problems. Even attempting to debate the position of 'potentially less harmful drugs' such as cannabis proved difficult. The balance between 'treatment' and a criminal justice approach has been hard to reach. The difficulty of pooling resources meant that it was problematic for local and regional bodies to adopt a more strategic and coordinated approach towards tackling drug misuse.

NATIONAL DRUGS STRATEGIES

From the mid 1990s, the policy position stabilized with the advent of a national drug strategy:[10,45,46]

- in 1995 *Tackling Drugs Together* was published;[45]
- this was followed in 1998 by a revised strategy: *Tackling Drugs to Build a Better Britain*;[46]
- this was updated again in 2002.[10]

Implementation of the strategy has been a key area of policy action, with further specific and separate strategy initiatives being developed in Scotland,[47] Wales[48] and Northern Ireland.[49] The prison service has also had a drug strategy in place since the late 1990s,[25] and there are policy initiatives at the international level, for example the EU Action Plan on Drugs 2000–2004.[50]

The 1998 drug strategy[45] had six key aims (see Table 11.2), with the three elements of prevention, treatment and harm minimization emerging (or returning to centre stage).

The most recent drug strategy,[10] whilst still working to meet these original aims, has made a particular commitment to:

- combating use of Class A drugs;
- focusing on education, prevention, enforcement and treatment;
- putting more resources into the battle against drugs;
- supporting young people;
- decreasing drugs available on the streets;
- expanding the treatment sector;
- expanding help available through the criminal justice system and improving after- and through-care services.

In addition, the government stated that they would work with those communities most affected by drug misuse and have a particular focus on reversing the trend of increasing cocaine and crack use. The *National Crack Action Plan* was launched in 2002.[52]

Table 11.2   The six key aims of the 1998 Drug Strategy[46]

Reducing the harm that drugs cause to society – communities, individuals and their families	• Prevent use amongst young people • Reduce prevalence of drugs on the street; tackling supply at all levels • Reduce drug-related crime • Reduce demand by reducing number of drug users
Preventing today's young people becoming tomorrow's problematic drug users	• Substance misuse education is part of the National Curriculum, with the majority of primary (80%) and secondary (96%) schools having drug education policies. Connexions, youth offending teams, young people treatment services (usually delivered through the Drug Action Team) and Positive Futures (a national sports-based social inclusion programme)[51] are all further initiatives designed to work with young people affected by their own or someone else's drug misuse. Substance misuse treatment has also been extended within the youth justice system • Other initiatives include the improvement and provision of drug education, a campaign to warn people of the dangers of Class A drugs, stricter penalties for dealers, improved services for parents and carers and an expansion of prevention programmes
Reducing the supply of illegal drugs	• Other strategic developments have included moves to combat the trafficking of drugs into the UK and reduce the overall supply. Cooperation and communication with police, customs etc. in the UK and with governments and similar agencies in other countries, such as across the EU and further afield (e.g. Afghanistan), along with increased penalties for the dealing and trafficking of those substances classified under the Misuse of Drugs Act[6]
Reducing drug-related crime and its impact on communities	• New treatment programmes to work with offenders – arrest referral schemes and Drug Treatment and Testing Orders • Increased efforts to move drug users from the criminal justice system and into the treatment sector – expanding arrest referral schemes, Drug Treatment and Testing Orders, prison-based treatment, increased through and after-care and extension of drug testing • Programmes through the Job Centre Plus initiative (e.g. progress2work) to help drug users find and sustain employment • Localized measures to strengthen communities affected by drug misuse • Guidance to local organizations to help in the prevention of other drug-related problems such as housing, homelessness, neighbourhood renewal
Reducing drug use and offending through treatment and support. Reducing drug-related death through harm minimization	• Expanding the treatment sector to be able to work with more drug users. This includes filling gaps in treatment, for example to work with crack and cocaine users and safe heroin prescribing to those with a clinical need for it • Ensuring people receive treatment more quickly – reducing referral and waiting times • Act to reduce the number of drug-related deaths • Maintain needle exchange schemes to reduce risks associated with death, HIV and hepatitis • Formation of the National Treatment Agency • Have more offenders accessing treatment and improving treatment provision in prisons

LEGISLATION

The Misuse of Drugs Act 1971[6] was amended in 2004,[53] making cannabis a Class C drug, and effectively decriminalizing simple cannabis possession. Cannabis is still illegal, but it became the case that most offences of cannabis possession were likely to result in a warning and confiscation of the drug, although the police still retained discretion to arrest and prosecute, especially when there were 'aggravating factors, such as smoking in a public place or repeat offending'.[54]

WHAT CAN WE DO ABOUT PREVENTION AND HEALTH PROMOTION?

There are three key areas:

- prevention
- harm minimization
- treatment.

These are discussed below; treatment includes interventions through the criminal justice system and other interventions targeted at specific groups.

One of the main drivers for change since the 1995 White Paper *Tackling Drugs Together*[45] has been Drug Action Teams (DATs), multidisciplinary cross-agency groups set up to support the implementation of *Tackling Drugs Together* and the subsequent 10 year strategy, and the creation of pooled budgets. This enabled far more coordinated efforts to be made across agency and organizational boundaries, and across these three linked areas of work.

PRIMARY PREVENTION

The usual debates about where best to focus prevention activities have also arisen in the drugs field:

- whether to focus on the whole population or to target at-risk groups;
- which of a wide range of approaches might work best:
  - information-based (providing accurate information about drugs and their dangers)
  - psychosocial (developing young people's social competence, assertiveness and ability to withstand peer pressure)
  - environmentally focused (positively affecting the environment in ways which make drug misuse become less likely, e.g. clear regulation on drug use in schools, community centres etc., encouraging drug-free school zones, restoring run down areas where drug using young people congregate)
  - school- or family-based (working with school and peer groups, strengthening parent–child communication, having parents serve as positive role models)
  - based on community norms (working with civic, religious, law enforcement and government organizations to enhance anti-drug norms in the community)
  - focused on the provision of alternatives for young people (providing alternative activities which might attract young people and which are mutually incompatible with drug use, such as extreme sports).

Particular issues have arisen over:

- whether to adopt a 'shock–horror' approach in an attempt to ensure that young people do not start using drugs;
- whether it is possible to focus on preventing *all* use (the 'Just Say No' campaign), as opposed to preventing *problematic* use, against a backdrop where significant percentages of young people are *not* 'saying no'.

Personal and social life skills approaches to prevention (including life skills education and the development of psychosocial competence) have been extremely popular across the UK. These approaches use skill building exercises to help young people increase their ability to handle social situations, and focus on decision making, problem solving, goal setting, refusal skills, effective communication and assertiveness. Approaches focusing on helping young people to recognize the outside pressures from advertising, celebrities, peers and other social influences that promote or encourage drug use have been similarly popular. Unfortunately, their popularity is not matched by their effectiveness. Two major reviews concluded that few interventions are adequately evaluated, and even those that are, do not provide enough data to draw clear conclusions.[55,56] Few studies examine longer term effectiveness, and those that do suggest that programme gains, if any, do not last long.

Work based on developing greater resilience and on integrated approaches to drug prevention in families has a slightly better evidence base. Although these approaches have been used less frequently in the UK, there is a developing evidence base that they can be effective.[57–59]

HARM MINIMIZATION

A great deal of effort has been put into reducing the harm that drug misuse causes in both individuals and communities. In broad terms, the basic techniques for harm reduction projects and programmes are now known, and there is substantial research and practical evidence to indicate their successful implementation and impact.[60] The techniques include a focus on:

- reducing the harm that drugs cause as opposed to attempting to reduce the drug use itself (for example providing clean injecting equipment so that injectors can inject more safely);
- opportunistically providing further services when people are attending for a service anyway (for example, when people attend to pick up injecting equipment, providing information on safer injecting practices and on AIDS and safer sexual practices, and providing condoms);
- introducing harm reduction approaches to drug education initiatives aimed at young people, based on the logic of acknowledging that because many young people *will* try drugs it is important to give them information about drug use and less hazardous ways of using them.[41]

Another example of harm minimization is the attempt to reduce acquisitive crime (often carried out to fund drug purchase) by diverting drug misusers into treatment. Further development has been the formation of Crime and Disorder Reduction Partnerships (CDRPs), which exist alongside or have integrated with DATs, and have as part of their remit the task of tackling drug problems and associated criminal and antisocial behaviour.

TREATMENT   Formal treatment for drug misusers has existed for many years, though until relatively recently services tended to be few and far between, medically based, and able to see only a small number of addicts (normally those with problems associated with opiates). In the 1980s, as drug use and problems started to escalate, many non-statutory (often incorrectly termed 'voluntary') agencies were set up and more residential services were developed.

Gradually, a more integrated treatment system started to emerge, involving a wider range of other services and greater interaction between non-statutory drug agencies and the specialist statutory sector. There was also a more multidisciplinary ethos, and the numbers of people with drug problems who could be seen rose greatly. By the 1990s, newer statutory services were also emerging: Community Drug Teams (CDTs) were being established (some of them later to become Community Drug and Alcohol Teams), and the involvement of primary care was starting to become much more important. By the early 2000s, a key aim of most statutory CDTs was to support GPs and other primary care workers in their work with drug misusers (this supportive interaction is termed 'shared care'), but the extent to which primary care feels this is part of its core role remains an issue for debate.[61]

Similarly, the growing realization that drug use in prisons was a major problem led to the development of services concentrated on the prison sector: the CARAT (counselling, assessment, referral, advice and throughcare) schemes. The realization that a huge amount of crime occurred in order to fund drug use meant that it became imperative to wean people off illicit drugs, as opposed to simply recycling them through overcrowded prisons or probation services. This led to the DTTO scheme (Drug Treatment and Testing Orders) where people could opt to enter a treatment programme and undergo regular drug testing as opposed to having a custodial sentence.

In 2001, attempts were made to integrate all of these initiatives by the creation of the National Treatment Agency (NTA), a special health authority whose main task is to 'improve the availability, capacity and effectiveness of treatment for drug misuse in England', particularly for the quarter of a million or so people who are at risk of developing serious problems.[10,62] Similar organizations have been put in place by the Scottish Executive and the Assemblies of Wales and Northern Ireland. The NTA has developed initiatives to ensure coordinated action and high standards, including the production of *Models of Care*,[63] a national framework to oversee the commissioning of adult treatment, and *QuADS*[64] – organizational standards for alcohol and drug treatment services – to ensure minimum and good practice standards for treatment provision.

There is one caveat to this positive story of the development of services. Services for drug users tend to be individualistic, based on pharmacological interventions, and oriented particularly towards opiate users. More recent moves have started to recognize the need to:

- target users of other drugs such as cocaine/crack;
- target specific user groups such as minority ethnic groups (*Models of Care*[63] contains specific guidance for working with these groups), young people and women;
- offer more non-pharmaceutically oriented treatments; these could be offered in tandem with medications;
- move to a more holistic way of working that includes the children and family members of drug misusers.[65]

Amongst the alternatives to pharmaceutically oriented treatments which could be offered are ones with increasing evidence for their efficacy: these tend to be approaches based wholly or partly on cognitive behavioural theory,[49] including relapse prevention, cue exposure and motivational interviewing.[66,67]

Does treatment work?

Underpinning the development of services is the realization that whilst many people with major drug problems can and do 'grow out' of it and 'get better' by themselves, many others do so, or do it faster, with the help of treatment agencies: basically, treatment works.

The evidence for this has proved overwhelming. Clearly, not everyone succeeds in overcoming their drug problems. But a number of longitudinal studies have shown that many do.[68] There have also been four large treatment outcome studies in the drug field, some including alcohol as well, which provide clear evidence that treatment of drug problems is effective.[69–71] The government itself is clear that treatment works; the *Updated Drugs Strategy* states that 'for each £1 spent, an estimated £3 is saved in criminal justice costs alone'.[10]

Interventions through the criminal justice system

For those who are identified through the criminal justice system there is a range of options, classed together as 'coercive treatment'.[26] There are those who argue against enforced treatment, stating that it is unethical and an excessive form of social control,[26] but the main benefits of enforced treatment seem to be:

- the increased access to treatment for a high risk group of drug users who may not otherwise receive help;
- that coercion can improve retention in treatment programmes (although not necessarily success);
- the obvious knock-on social and economic benefits of diversion from the criminal justice system and into treatment.

Interventions through the criminal justice system can be implemented as an alternative to further progression through the system at three key points: arrest, court and prison.

Interventions at arrest

Arrest referral schemes, run by partnerships between the police, drug agencies and DATs, exist in all England and Wales police forces. They offer the opportunity for intervention at a far earlier stage than might otherwise happen; an evaluation in three areas found that almost half of those seen had not previously received any treatment.[26] When arrested, the arrestee has the option of being referred into treatment, where the provision of advice/information, prescribing and counselling are all possible.

The interim report of the first national evaluation concluded that the schemes 'are making a substantial contribution to engaging drug-driven criminals in treatment and contributing to reductions in drug use and crime'.[72]

Interventions at court   Court diversion is implemented via drug treatment and testing orders (DTTOs), an alternative to sentencing. Although this is offered as coercive treatment, offenders do have the option to remain in custody instead, receiving standard punishments and imprisonment. The treatment on offer is varied, including substitute medication, counselling and residential treatment. Early pilots suggested that DTTOs 'will make a substantial contribution to reducing drug-driven crime and net considerable savings for society'.[73]

There is much work to be done to further explore and resolve issues such as non-compliance and early completion:[74] having the order revoked and dropping out of treatment are common outcomes, and the longer term impact of DTTOs requires further investigation. Evaluation of DTTOs brings its own challenges, as regional variations exist according to the history and availability of treatment for drug misusers.

Interventions in prison   Drug use does reduce during and after time in prison,[25] with a number of strategies contributing to this positive downward shift, both in drug-taking and offending behaviour. An international review of the literature[25] found that the most beneficial forms of treatment were those involving cognitive behavioural therapy, 12-step abstinence-based programmes and methadone prescription.

Again, there is still much to be done. For example, there has been a call to reform women's prisons, linked to the high rates of serious problems experienced by female prisoners, with over 75% believed to be addicted to drugs (particularly crack and heroin) and/or alcohol.[75]

INTERVENTIONS ORIENTED TOWARDS OTHER TARGET GROUPS

The government has outlined specific initiatives and targets to focus on drug use amongst young people (see Table 11.2 and the 2002 strategy).[10] Part of the thinking behind this, and the strategy as a whole, has been in terms of integrated services and therefore funding: 'To drive forward the integration of young people's substance misuse services within the wider provision of services for young people, a pooled budget simplifying the way these services are funded will be piloted in 25 areas from April 2003. If the pilot succeeds pooled budgets will be rolled out nationally from April 2004.'[10(p. 24)] The pilots did succeed and this system was implemented nationally. Other options for intervention with drug misusers include self-help groups (such as Narcotics Anonymous and Cocaine Anonymous, which follow the Alcoholics Anonymous 12-step model)[76] and complementary therapies such as acupuncture, biofeedback, electrostimulation, herbal medicine and hypnotherapy.[77]

Finally, as touched on above, the interventions provided for people who misuse drugs are very individually oriented. There have been calls for a greater focus on interventions that take more account of the context of people's lives, and especially involve individuals' families.[65,78]

CONTROVERSIAL ISSUES

The many controversial issues in the drugs world tend to fall into two main categories: those related to the illegality of drug use, and those related to the provision, planning and commissioning of treatment services.

CONTROVERSY ABOUT LEGAL STATUS

Perhaps the most topical controversial issue at the time of writing (2004) surrounds the declassification of cannabis[54] from Class B to Class C in the classification of the Misuse of Drugs Act (1971)[6] following advice from the Advisory Council on the Misuse of Drugs (ACMD). Whilst not committing the government to any firm decision either way in terms of the legalization or decriminalization of cannabis, the penalties for possession and supply are significantly reduced, with arrest for simple possession now extremely unlikely.

This move has been welcomed by many, enabling people to use cannabis for medical conditions such as multiple sclerosis without fear of arrest, and enabling the police to concentrate more on drugs that many consider to be far more dangerous.

On the other hand, others see this as a 'slippery slope' towards legalization, and as sending a very confusing message out to young people ('it is illegal, but if you take it we will not arrest you'). They fear this will mean that more people will use the drug, and will then move on to using other substances (see the 'gateway' myth below).

The situation with cannabis, of course, is just part of a wider debate about whether illegal drugs should be legalized or their use decriminalized. The biggest problem in this area for politicians in recent years has been the impossibility of entering into a debate without being accused of dangerous and immoral behaviour simply by raising the issues. It is to be welcomed that the possibility of such a debate seems a bit nearer.

CONTROVERSY ABOUT TREATMENT

Controversial issues related to treatment include:

- whether services are too focused on opiates;
- whether the provision of substitute medication (especially methadone) is a good or a bad thing;
- whether there should be more widespread prescribing of heroin as a substitute medication;
- the place of non-pharmacological interventions in current treatment services.

We will look at two issues in more depth: substitute prescribing, and injecting centres.

Substitute medication

When opiate users seek help, they will often be prescribed substitute medication. The expected pattern is the 'phased withdrawal of the original preparation' with the 'administration for a prolonged period of a less harmful form of substitute drug'.[79] The reason why opiate misusers receive prescribed substitute drugs when stimulant misusers do not is simply because such substitutes exist for opiates, and do not (yet) for stimulants. The most common substitute drugs prescribed are methadone (usually in oral preparation) and more recently buprenorphine (Subutex and Temgesic).

In many ways, the provision of methadone and other substitute preparations is a harm minimization technique: it removes people from the illicit market, ensures that there is basic quality control over the substances that they ingest, takes them away from risky environments (they get their drugs from the chemist, not the dealer), and makes other dangerous activities such as injecting less likely. On the other hand, those who wish people to stop using drugs altogether see providing drugs to people who are already drug-dependent as acting irresponsibly, with drug workers as state-employed drug dealers maintaining people in drug dependency.

Methadone has the strongest evidence base to support its continued widespread use.[80,81] Whilst further research is needed, the evidence base to support an expansion of use of buprenorphine as a viable alternative to methadone is growing.[80,82,83]

Perhaps the most controversial substitute medication is heroin (diamorphine) itself, in intravenous form. It is a rare treatment option worldwide, with one review concluding that the practice is 'controversial, expensive yet promising so much'.[84] It is best suited to long term heroin users who have not responded to other, more traditional forms of treatment.[85]

Interestingly, although substitute drugs are recommended in conjunction with counselling as the central process, often the counselling does not happen. So people argue that if drug misusers come simply to obtain free drugs and have no intention of engaging in counselling or other therapeutic activities, they should be discharged. Others argue that simply engaging people in using unadulterated drugs hugely reduces the risk of overdose, and getting into a regular routine of taking drugs safely keeps people from acquisitive crime, makes them live more safely, and keeps open the possibility of further treatment.

Most commentators who agree with the provision of substitute drugs argue that their provision should be linked with good associated practices, such as supervised consumption, urine testing, regular check-up visits, and shared care with primary care colleagues.[83]

Moves to reduce risks associated with injecting behaviour

A key aim of treatment is to reduce the rate of and risks associated with injecting behaviour. As we have said, injecting drug users pose a particular threat to themselves especially if needles and other equipment are shared. Needle exchanges, which have existed in the UK for about 20 years, have been fundamental in trying to achieve this aim, particularly by reducing rates of HIV and hepatitis infection.

A relatively new public health concept to further reduce risks, particularly the risk of overdose, is medically supervised injecting centres:[85,86] 'to enable the consumption of pre-obtained drugs under hygienic, low-risk conditions … supervision and consequent speed of response in the event of overdose'.[85] These centres have been established in parts of Europe, but not so far in the UK. There has not been enough evaluation of their effectiveness, though the work that has been done in Europe is positive.[19,85]

COMMON MYTHS

There are too many myths to go into all of them in detail. We will briefly consider three, but in fact all of them really utilize the same myth: that there is something so magically scary about 'addiction' that when people are 'addicted' they somehow behave in completely different ways than they did before; and that drugs somehow 'make' people addicted, and hence out of control.

All drug use leads to addiction

This myth suggests that all drugs are the same, and that all people are the same: hence if anyone takes any drug, they will become addicted. This completely ignores the point that whether a drug is legal or illegal is not decided using any objective criteria. All drugs that are currently illegal in the UK were legal in the past, and most legal drugs in the UK are illegal in some other cultures. It is not even clear what constitutes a 'drug' in the first place: if it is any substance which causes an effect on the human brain, then most substances we currently use in cooking might come into that category. The differences between someone who becomes ecstatic when tasting a delightful food, and someone who becomes ecstatic when ingesting a 'drug' are not as clear cut as some would wish.

Some drugs act as a gateway to others

This idea is prevalent in arguments relating to cannabis: even if the drug itself is not very dangerous, it acts as a gateway drug so people who take it are more likely to go on to use other, more dangerous, substances. Evidence to back up this assertion usually takes the form of showing that most (or even all) heroin addicts report that they used cannabis before they 'progressed' to heroin. But most (or even all) heroin addicts would also report that prior to becoming 'addicts' they had parents, drank coffee, ate toast, drank alcohol, and so on. The thing that makes cannabis different to coffee or alcohol in this example is that coffee and alcohol are legal in this culture and period in history, and cannabis is not. In one way, that is the biggest single argument for legalizing cannabis, rather than for retaining it as an illegal substance.

Once an addict, always one

This myth suggests that due to the mystical properties of addiction, once a person has succumbed to being addicted they can never cease to be so. Whereas there is probably some truth in the idea that any area where a person has developed a problem is an area where they may be at risk in the future, there is no evidence for the 'once an addict' myth; in fact, the evidence is in the opposite direction. The study of returning addicted Vietnam soldiers outlined above[38] shows very clearly that the large majority of people addicted in one context simply do not remain or become addicted in a different context.

WHAT DON'T WE KNOW ENOUGH ABOUT YET?

There are many questions where we do not know the answers. In many ways, the most interesting questions are still the most fundamental:

- We still do not know how to prevent drug use effectively, or how to stop drug use for some people turning into drug misuse and drug problems.

- We still do not know how best to engage people who simply and understandably want access to free drugs, moving them into more wide ranging treatments which would enable them to live lives not dominated by drug misuse and dependence.

- We still do not know what is the best way to intervene with people who really *do* want to stop their drug use: helping people quit a dependency is very difficult, and although success rates are good, it is still the case that for many people getting over a drug misuse problem is a long haul.

- Drug misuse affects many people other than the person who takes the drugs. Yet services for family members and for communities affected by drug misuse are very few and far between.[78] A key question is how we can ensure that strategies are developed and implemented which will help the families and wider communities affected by drug misuse.

- Finally, it is still the case that most help for drug misusers is highly individualized, even if they access psychological as well as pharmacological services. People live in social contexts (families, friendship networks, work and housing environments), and yet our treatments largely ignore that. A really interesting question is how to help treatment services recognize this and move out of their safe, individualized confines to help drug users deal with the wider world that they need to inhabit.

Key sources of further information and help

- **Cross-government national drug strategy website** for drug prevention and treatment professionals and others interested in the drug strategy: www.drugs.gov.uk. There are similar strategies for Scotland, Wales and Northern Ireland: www.scotland.gov.uk/library/documents-w7/tdis-00.htm, www.wales.gov.uk/subisocialpolicy/content/direct/misuse.htm, www.nics.gov.uk/drugs/pubs/strat.pdf
- **DrugScope:** www.drugscope.org.uk. The UK's leading independent centre of expertise on drugs.
- **Drug and Alcohol Findings:** www.drugandalcohol findings.org. A journal which summarizes evidence about the effectiveness of interventions to

treat, prevent or reduce drug and alcohol problems. It is produced in the UK by a partnership of leading national charities dealing with drugs and alcohol: DrugScope, Alcohol Concern and the National Addiction Centre.
- **European Monitoring Centre for Drugs and Drug Addiction (EMCDDA):** www.emcdda.eu.int. The Centre was set up to provide the European Community and its Member States with 'objective, reliable and comparable information at European level concerning drugs and drug addiction and their consequences'. It provides statistical, documentary and technical information on drugs in Europe.

(Continued)

Key sources of further information and help (continued)

- **Health Development Agency:** www.hda-online. org.uk. The national authority on what works to improve people's health and reduce health inequalities. It gathers evidence and produces advice for policy makers, professionals and practitioners, working alongside them to get evidence into practice. See especially: *Health Promotion in Young People for the Prevention of Substance Misuse*, 1997,[55] available online at http://www. hda-online.org.uk/html/research/effectiveness reviews/ereview5.html
- **Health Education Board for Scotland:** www.hebs.scot.nhs.uk. See its Working Paper *Drug education: approaches, effectiveness and implications for delivery.*[56]

- **National Treatment Agency (NTA):** www.nta.nhs.uk. The NTA aims to increase the availability, capacity and effectiveness of treatment for drug misuse in England. See also the Scottish Executive's Drug Misuse Information – Scotland (www.drugmisuse.isdscotland.org/eiu/ eiu.htm), the Welsh Assembly's Social Justice and Regeneration section (www.wales.gov.uk/ subisocialjustice/content/grants/guide2-sjr-e.htm# DATF) and the Northern Ireland Assembly's Health Promotion Agency for Northern Ireland (www. healthpromotionagency.org.uk/Work/ Drugs/menu. htm).

References

1. Donnellan C, ed. Drug misuse. Cambridge Independence; 2001 (Volume 2).
2. Gossop M. Living with drugs. Aldershot: Ashgate Publishing; 2000.
3. McBride A. Some drugs of misuse. In: Petersen T, McBride A, eds. Working with substance misusers: a guide to theory and practice. London: Routledge; 2002.
4. Orford J. Excessive appetites: a psychological view of addictions. 2nd edn. Chichester: Wiley; 2001.
5. Johnson BA. Cannabis. In: Glass IB, ed. The international handbook of addiction behaviours. London: Routledge; 1991.
6. Misuse of Drugs Act 1971. London: HMSO.
7. Bennett P. Behavioural and cognitive behavioural approaches to substance misuse treatment. In: Petersen T, McBride A, eds. Working with substance misusers: a guide to theory and practice. London: Routledge; 2002.
8. Stolerman IP. Behavioural pharmacology of addiction. In: Glass IB, ed. The international handbook of addiction behaviours. London: Routledge; 1991.
9. Gabe J, Bury M. Drug use and dependence as a social problem: sociological approaches. In: Glass IB, ed. The international handbook of addiction behaviours. London: Routledge; 1991.
10. Home Office. Updated drug strategy 2002. Home Office Drugs Strategy Inspectorate. London: HMSO; 2002.
11. Condon J, Smith N. Prevalence of drug use: key findings from the 2002/2003 British Crime Survey. Home Office Findings 229. London: Home Office; 2003.

12. National Treatment Agency, London. Background. www.nta.nhs.uk/about/background.htm January 2004.
13. Fountain J, Bashford J, Winters M, et al. Black and minority ethnic communities in England: a review of the literature on drug use and related service provision. London: National Treatment Agency and the Centre for Ethnicity and Health; 2003.
14. Day E, Crome IB. Physical health problems. In: Petersen T, McBride A, eds. Working with substance misusers: a guide to theory and practice. London: Routledge; 2002.
15. Farrell M. Physical complications of drug abuse. In: Glass IB, ed. The international handbook of addiction behaviours. London: Routledge; 1991.
16. Aujean S, Murphy R, King L, Jeffery D, eds. Annual report on the UK drug situation 2001. EMCDDA and Drugscope; 2001.
17. Best D, Man LH, Zador D, et al. Overdosing on opiates. Drug and Alcohol Findings 2000; 4:4–19(Part I).
18. Gowing LR, Henry-Edwards SM, Irvine RJ, et al. The health effects of ecstasy: a literature review. Drug and Alcohol Review 2002; 21:53–63.
19. Best D, Man LH, Zador D, et al. Overdosing on opiates. Drug and Alcohol Findings 2001; 5:4–18(Part II).
20. Department of Health. Hepatitis C – guidance for those working with drug users. London: Department of Health; 2001.
21. Bennett G, Velleman R, Barter G, et al. Gender differences in sharing injecting equipment by drug users in England. AIDS Care 2000; 12:77–87.

22. Bennett G, Velleman R, Barter G, et al. Low autonomy in injecting is a risk factor for sharing injecting equipment. Addiction Research 2000; 8:81–93.

23. Hammersley R, Marsland L, Reid M. Substance use by young offenders. Home Office Findings 192. London: Home Office; 2003.

24. Corkery JM, Airs J. Seizures of drugs in the UK 2001. Home Office Findings 202. London: Home Office; 2003.

25. Ramsay M. Prisoners' drug use and treatment: seven studies. Home Office Findings 186. London: Home Office; 2003.

26. Summers Z. Coercion and the criminal justice system. In: Petersen T, McBride A, eds. Working with substance misusers: a guide to theory and practice. London: Routledge; 2002.

27. Cross government drug strategy website: www.drugs.gov.uk/NationalStrategy/ Communities/Toolkits/DrivingRoadSafety

28. Advisory Council on The Misuse of Drugs (ACMD). Hidden harm: responding to the needs of children of problem drug users. The report of an inquiry by the Advisory Council on the Misuse of Drugs. London: HMSO; 2003.

29. Velleman R, Bennett G, Miller T, et al. The families of problem drug users: the accounts of fifty close relatives. Addiction 1993; 88(9):1275–1283.

30. Kroll B, Taylor A. Parental substance misuse and child welfare. London: Jessica Kingsley; 2003.

31. Barnard M, McKeganey N. The impact of parental problem drug use on children: what is the problem and what can be done to help? Addiction 2004; 99(5):552–559

32. Cleaver H, Unell I, Aldgate J. Children's needs – parenting capacity. London: The Stationery Office; 1999.

33. Murphy J, Jellinek M, Quinn D, et al. Substance abuse and serious child mistreatment: prevalence, risk, and outcome in a court sample. Child Abuse and Neglect 1991; 15(3):197–211.

34. Gilligan R. Promoting resilience: a resource guide on working with children in the care system. London: BAAF; 2003.

35. Newman T. Promoting resilience: a review of effective strategies for child care services. Centre for Evidence-based Social Services, Exeter, England and Barnardos; 2002.

36. Rutter M. Psychosocial resilience and protective mechanisms. American Journal of Orthopsychiatry 1987; 57(3):316–331.

37. Werner E. Risk, resilience and recovery: perspectives from the Kauai longitudinal study. Development and Psychopathology 1993; 5:503–515.

38. Robins L, Davis D, Wish E. Detecting predictors of rare events: demographic, family and personal deviance as predictors of stages in the progression towards narcotic addiction. In: Straus S, Babigian H, Roff M, eds. The origins and course of psychopathology: methods of longitudinal research. New York: Plenum; 1977.

39. Hepburn M. Drug use and women's reproductive health. In: Petersen T, McBride A, eds. Working with substance misusers: a guide to theory and practice. London: Routledge; 2002.

40. Blank M. A suitable case for treatment: an introduction to British drug policy. In: Petersen T, McBride A, eds. Working with substance misusers: a guide to theory and practice. London: Routledge; 2002.

41. Velleman R, Rigby J. Harm-minimisation: old wine in new bottles? In: South N, ed. Drugs, crime and criminal justice. Volume 1 of the International Library of Criminology, Criminal Justice and Penology. Aldershot: Dartmouth Publishing Company; 1995:225–228. (Reprinted from International Journal on Drug Policy 1990; 1(6):24–27.)

42. MacGregor S, Ettorre B. From treatment to rehabilitation – aspects of the evolution of British policy on the care of drug takers. In: Dorn N, South N, eds. A land fit for heroin? Drug policies, prevention and practice. London: Macmillan; 1987.

43. Stimson G. British drug policies in the 1980s. In: Heller T, Gott M, Jeffery C. Drug use and misuse: a reader. Chichester: John Wiley; 1987:118–125.

44. Home Office. Tackling drug misuse: a summary of the government's strategy. 2nd edn. London: HMSO; 1986.

45. Home Office, Department of Health and Department for Education. Tackling drugs together: a strategy for England 1995–1998. London: HMSO; 1995.

46. Home Office. Tackling drugs to build a better Britain. The Government's ten-year strategy for tackling drugs misuse. London: HMSO; 1998.

47. Scottish Executive. Tackling drugs in Scotland: action in partnership. Edinburgh: Scottish Executive; 1999.

48. The National Assembly for Wales. Tackling substance misuse in Wales: a partnership approach. Cardiff: The National Assembly for Wales; 2000.

49. Northern Ireland Executive. Drugs strategy for Northern Ireland. Belfast: Northern Ireland Office; 1999.

50. European Union. EU Action Plan on Drugs 2000–2004. EU; 1999.

51. Home Office Drugs Strategy Directorate. Cul-de-sacs and gateways: understanding the Positive Futures approach. London: Home Office; 2003. Online. Available: http://www.drugs.gov.uk

52. Home Office Drugs Strategy Directorate. Tackling crack – a national plan. London: Home Office; 2002. Online. Available: www.drugs.co.uk.

53. Misuse of Drugs Act 2004. London: HMSO.

54. See www.drugs.gov.uk/NationalStrategy/ CannabisReclassification

55. Health Development Agency. Health promotion in young people for the prevention of substance misuse. Health promotion effectiveness reviews. Summary bulletin 5. London: HDA; 1997. Online. Available: http://www.hda-online.org.uk/html/research/ effectivenessreviews/ereview5.html

56. Health Education Board for Scotland. Drug education: approaches, effectiveness and implications for delivery. HEBS working paper number 1. Edinburgh: Health Education Board for Scotland; 2003. Online. Available:

http://www.hebs.org.uk/topics/topiccontents.
cfm?topic= drug&TxtTCode=167&TNav=1

57. Spoth R, Guyll M, Trudeau L, et al. Two studies of proximal outcomes and implementation quality of universal preventive interventions in a community–university collaboration context. Journal of Community Psychology 2002; 30(5):499–518.

58. Spoth RL, Redmond C, Shin C. Randomized trial of brief family interventions for general populations: adolescent substance use outcomes 4 years following baseline. Journal of Consulting and Clinical Psychology 2001; 69(4):627–642.

59. Kumpfer K. Strengthening America's families: exemplary parenting and family strategies for delinquency prevention. US Department of Justice; 1999. Online. Available: http://www.strengtheningfamilies.org/html/review.html

60. Stimson GV. Harm reduction in action: putting theory into practice. International Journal of Drug Policy 1998; 9(6):401–409.

61. Strang J. Service development and organization: drugs. In: Glass IB, ed. The international handbook of addiction behaviours. London: Routledge; 1991.

62. National Treatment Agency. Purpose and principles. London; NTA. Online. Available: http://www.nta.nhs.uk/about/purpose.htm (accessed 26 January 2004).

63. National Treatment Agency. Models of Care for the treatment of drug misusers. Part 2: full reference report. London: NTA; 2002.

64. Alcohol Concern/Standing Conference on Drug Abuse (SCODA). QuADS. Quality in alcohol and drug services: organisational standards for treatment in alcohol and drug services. London: Alcohol Concern/SCODA; 1999.

65. Velleman R, Templeton L. Family interventions in substance misuse. In: Peterson T, McBride A, eds. Working with substance misusers: a guide to theory and practice. London: Routledge; 2002.

66. Davies M, Petersen T. Motivationally based interventions for behaviour change. In: Petersen T, McBride A, eds. Working with substance misusers: a guide to theory and practice. London: Routledge; 2002.

67. Miller WR, Rollnick S. Motivational interviewing: preparing people to change addictive behaviour. New York: Guilford Press; 1992.

68. Raistrick D. Career and natural history. In: Glass IB, ed. The international handbook of addiction behaviours. London: Routledge; 1991.

69. Franey C, Ashton M. The grand design: lessons from DATOS. Drug and Alcohol Findings 2002; 7:4–19.

70. Gossop M, Marsden J, Stewart D. NTORS from the inside. Drug and Alcohol Findings 1999; 2:17.

71. Gossop M, Marsden J, Stewart D, et al. The National Treatment Outcome Research Study (NTORS): 4–5 year follow-up results. Addiction 2003; 98(3):291–303.

72. Ashton M. Arrest referral tackles drug-driven crime. Drug and Alcohol Findings 2003; 8:14.

73. Ashton M. Treatment and testing orders should make a substantial dent in drug-related social costs. Drug and Alcohol Findings 2001; 5:11.

74. National Audit Office. The drug treatment and testing order: early lessons. London: HMSO; 2004.

75. Leader. Lives lost in jail. Observer. 8 August 2004. Online. Available: http://www.observer.guardian. co.uk/leaders/story 9 February 2004.

76. Wells B. Self-help groups. In: Glass IB, ed. The international handbook of addiction behaviours. London: Routledge; 1991.

77. White A, Ernst E. Complementary or alternative medicine for substance misuse. In: Petersen T, McBride A, eds. Working with substance misusers: a guide to theory and practice. London: Routledge; 2002.

78. Velleman R, Templeton L. Alcohol, drugs and the family: results from a long running research programme within the UK. European Addiction Research 2003; 9:103–112.

79. Madden JS. Detoxification, pharmacotherapy and maintenance: drugs. In: Glass IB, ed. The international handbook of addiction behaviours. London: Routledge; 1991.

80. National Treatment Agency. Prescribing services for drug misuse treatment in England. Research into practice: briefing no. 2. 2003; 2. London: NTA. Online. Available: http://www.nta. nhs.uk/publications/ research_briefing2.htm 5 February 2004.

81. Ashton M. Injectable methadone maintenance suitable for more severely affected heroin addicts. Drug and Alcohol Findings 2001; 5:14.

82. Ling W, Huber A, Rawson RA. There is an alternative: buprenorphine maintenance. Drug and Alcohol Findings 2002; 7:27–30.

83. Merrill J. Medical approaches and prescribing: drugs. In: Petersen T, McBride A, eds. Working with substance misusers: a guide to theory and practice. London: Routledge; 2002.

84. Ashton M, Witton J. Role reversal. Drug and Alcohol Findings 2003; 9:16–23.

85. Strang J, Fortson R. Commentary: supervised fixing rooms, supervised injectable maintenance clinics – understanding the difference. BMJ 2004; 328:102–103.

86. Wright NMJ, Tompkins CNE. Supervised injecting centres. BMJ 2004; 328:100–101.

Chapter **12**

Mental health and mental health promotion

Linda Seymour and Elizabeth Gale

SUMMARY OVERVIEW AND LINKS TO OTHER TOPICS

Mental health is a particularly challenging public health topic: complex, difficult to define and measure, and hard to be clear about how to promote positive mental health and measure the effectiveness of interventions. This chapter provides a guide through a thorny undergrowth of opinions and facts.

There are helpful models of positive mental health, identifying factors that make people more at risk of, or protect them from, mental health problems. Useful frameworks for mental health promotion are discussed, and we provide an overview of how mental health is addressed in national policy including the *National Service Framework for Mental Health*.[1] We look at trends in prevalence and how these may be measured. Inequalities feature, both as a cause and a consequence of poor mental health. Reviews of evidence lead to a number of suggestions about how best to improve individual and collective mental health and well-being.

The most controversial issue in mental health promotion is the development of robust evaluation frameworks. The chapter ends by identifying some of the many myths and unanswered questions in this field.

As there is a clear association between mental ill health and deprivation, Chapter 13 'Tackling inequalities in health' is highly relevant to any consideration of mental health promotion. Chapter 6 'Physical activity' is especially relevant as exercise is one of the most effective ways to promote and protect the mental health of adults.

Also relevant to mental health are Chapters 2, 3, 4 and 5 – covering heart disease, diabetes, smoking and obesity – as all these health problems are more prevalent in people with mental health problems.

WHAT IS MENTAL HEALTH?

Mental health problems are common and widely misunderstood. At any one time, one adult in six suffers from mental health problems of varying severity.[2] Other research suggests that one person in four will experience some kind of mental health problem in the course of a year.[3] A survey of children and young people's (aged 5–15) mental health found that the proportion of children and adolescents with any mental disorder was greater among boys than girls across the age range: 11% compared with 8%.[4]

But how can we define 'mental health'? It is a contested concept, described in a variety of different but complementary ways. The terminology used includes:

- psychological well-being
- psychosocial health
- psychosocial well-being
- wellness
- well-being
- positive mental health
- emotional health.

Some useful models of mental health are summarized in Table 12.1.[5–8]

Definitions of positive mental health are still under debate but there has been a movement away from a focus solely on individual attributes, such as coping skills or resilience, to one which incorporates environmental and social conditions[9–11] recognizing that the risk of mental illness is influenced by a range of socio-economic, interpersonal and hereditary factors.[12]

These differing models and definitions of mental health illustrate an array of individual and environmental risk and protective factors – those which put people at greater risk of mental ill health and those which protect them from it – although why a particular risk factor should result in poor mental health outcomes for one individual and not another is as yet unknown.

Table 12.1   Models of mental health

Model	Description
The deficit model	Only the absence of an objectively diagnosable disease equates to the existence of mental health
The positive holistic model[5,6]	Health as a state of physical, social and mental well-being; within this, mental health is closely aligned with, and interdependent on, a broader health and social context
The six-dimensional model[7]	Mental health is multifaceted with six dimensions: • affective • behavioural • cognitive • sociopolitical • spiritual • psychological
The mentally healthy individual model[8]	The mentally healthy individual is someone who can: • develop emotionally, creatively, intellectually and spiritually • initiate, develop and sustain mutually satisfying personal relationships • face problems, resolve them and learn from them • be confident and assertive • be aware of others and empathize with them • use and enjoy solitude • play and have fun • laugh, both at themselves and at the world

A useful definition of mental health is that used by the World Health Organization: 'Mental health is a state of well-being in which the individual realises his or her own abilities, can cope with the normal stresses of life, can work productively and fruitfully and is able to make a contribution to his or her community'.[13]

Consequently, anyone has the capacity for good mental health, regardless of whether they have a diagnosed mental health problem.

What all these models of mental health acknowledge is the extent to which mental health is entrenched within wider social and economic relationships.

WHAT CAUSES POOR MENTAL HEALTH?

Just as mental health is embedded within social relationships, so also are the risk and protective factors for mental health. These are rooted in links between individuals and their social contexts as well as individual responses to those social relations.

RISK FACTORS

The strength of evidence on risk and protective factors for mental health varies. Risk factors for poor mental health are myriad and include:[14]

• family history of psychiatric disorder
• violence

- childhood neglect
- family breakdown
- unemployment.

Gender

Gender has a significant impact on risk and protective factors for mental health.[15] For example poor mental health in men is reflected in rates of suicide that are four times as high as those for women.[16] In women, however, poor mental health emerges in increased risks for depression and anxiety, eating disorders and self-harm.[17]

Life events

Life events that increase risk include bereavement, physical illness, relationship breakdown, job insecurity, long term caring and moving into residential care. Loss of a loved one, financial strain and long term caring are risk factors across the life cycle and especially in later life.[18]

Socio-economic factors

There are well documented links between social inequalities and increased incidence of a range of mental health problems. A review among children and young people aged 5–15 identified an association between socio-economic circumstances and increased prevalence of mental disorder. For example, about one fifth of children in families without a working parent had a mental disorder, more than twice the proportion among children with at least one working member of the family.[4]

A review of the published evidence on links between social position and common mental disorders found that prevalence was more marked amongst socially disadvantaged populations. More consistent associations were with unemployment, less education and low income or material standard of living. Occupational social class was the least consistent marker.[19]

Mental health problems are associated with socio-economic disadvantage. Among people aged 60–74 living in private households in UK, the likelihood of having a neurotic disorder increased in both sexes as income fell. Among women in this age group, the prevalence of a neurotic disorder such as anxiety or depression was around three times as common among those with a weekly household income of under £200 as it was among those with a weekly household income of £500.[20]

Racial factors

Mental health is not simply a characteristic of individuals. Whole schools, organizations, neighbourhoods and communities – including faith communities, ethnic communities and communities of identity – can feel marginalized, fearful, insecure, excluded, unable to influence decisions, or unable to participate fully. Perceptions of racial discrimination are a significant factor in the poor health of black and minority ethnic groups, over and above socio-economic factors.[21]

A study in Camberwell, South London, based on contact with psychiatric services over a 10 year period, found that the incidence of schizophrenia in non-white ethnic minorities increased significantly as the proportion of such minorities in the local population fell.[22,23] These findings add weight to the importance of social factors as an important explanation for the increased rate of schizophrenia among British-born ethnic minorities. These could include reduced protection against stress and life events due to isolation and fewer social networks. People from ethnic minorities may be more likely to be singled out or to be more vulnerable when they are in a small or dispersed minority.

PROTECTIVE FACTORS

Psychological protective factors for mental well-being include feeling respected, valued and supported, together with a sense of hopefulness about the future.[24,25] These psychological characteristics are influenced by wider socio-economic factors, for example parenting, schools, employment, housing and financial security. They also influence how individuals respond to stressful or traumatic life events. However, social and economic factors which support warm, affectionate parenting and strong child/carer attachment are particularly significant.[26]

A framework developed by the Health Education Authority emphasized the importance of social and environmental factors in determining mental health.[27] In addition to genetic inheritance the three key areas influencing mental health were identified as:

- beneficial economic and cultural structures
- sound social networks and social inclusion
- robust emotional resilience.

WHAT IS MENTAL HEALTH PROMOTION?

There are several models of mental health promotion within the literature; they are closely associated with the definitions of mental health we have described previously.

Current frameworks for mental health promotion no longer concentrate only on the prevention of mental illness; rather, enhancing a sense of well-being or promoting positive mental health is also seen as a key goal.[14]

A common approach is to take a broad public mental health focus which goes beyond targeting the individual, with, for example, community interventions about building social capital or structural interventions that widen participation in education. In recognition of the importance of the physical and social environment to the mental health of individuals, the concept of the public mental health also extends to enhancing the mental health of organizations and communities with a view to fostering a mentally healthy society.[28]

FRAMEWORKS FOR MENTAL HEALTH PROMOTION

Two frameworks, summarized in Table 12.2, are particularly useful.[10,27]

Neither of these frameworks represents hierarchies and the actions described are key elements of interventions which operate in parallel. Action at these interdependent levels should work to reduce the risk factors that undermine positive mental health, for example social alienation, stress or emotional abuse; and to enhance those factors which promote mental health, such as environmental quality, self-esteem and social participation.

Social capital

One of the most useful theoretical models with relevance to mental health promotion, especially for communities, is the concept of social

Table 12.2   Frameworks for mental health promotion

Health education authority[27]	McDonald and O'Hara[10]
Three levels to reduce risk factors and increase protective factors by: ● strengthening individuals (e.g. fostering coping and life skills) ● strengthening communities (e.g. developing support networks, improving neighbourhood environments, anti-bullying strategies) ● reducing structural barriers to mental health (e.g. reducing discrimination; facilitating access to meaningful employment)	Three levels of action: ● the micro level – individuals ● the meso level – groupings such as the family and peer group ● the macro level or wider systems which can impact on people's lives – such as governments, formal religions and large and influential companies

capital. Developed by Putnam,[29] social capital is a model which represents prosperity engineered through the development of healthy neighbourhoods and social networks.

The four main tenets are:

● community networks;
● civic engagement/participation in the community networks;
● local identity, solidarity, and equality within the community;
● trust developed through norms of reciprocity.

Trust and altruism seem to be the most important concepts, as people perform activities which help others, with no immediate reward but in the belief that in the longer term they or their families will benefit. Research on social capital looks beyond individual interventions to develop more embracing structural initiatives. (Readers should visit www.hda.nhs.uk/sarpnet for reports on the evaluation of the Nottingham Social Action Research Project.)

WHY IS MENTAL HEALTH AND ITS PROMOTION AN IMPORTANT PUBLIC HEALTH ISSUE?

By any yardstick mental health problems impose an enormous burden on individuals, on families and on society. The economic and social costs of mental health problems in England are estimated to be £77.4 billion.[30] This equates to:

● £12.5 billion for care provided by the NHS, local authorities, privately funded services, family and friends;
● £23.1 billion in lost output in the economy caused by people being unable to work (paid and unpaid);
● £41.8 billion in the human costs of reduced quality of life, and loss of life, amongst those experiencing a mental health problem.

The costs of mental health problems to businesses and to individuals dwarf the sums of money used for treatment. Approximately 39% of working age adults with a mental health problem, for example, have no job. That figure represents a loss to the economy of £9.4 billion and is one third again as much as the £6.5 billion the NHS spent on mental health services in 2002.

HOW IS MENTAL HEALTH ADDRESSED IN NATIONAL POLICY?

Since the late 1990s a range of policy initiatives have been introduced at national and local level. Policies have been informed by an acknowledgement that mental distress is shaped by a wealth of life experiences such as poverty, unemployment, poor educational attainment, bad housing, trauma, racism and abuse. They have at their core the aim of tackling inequalities and ensuring that the needs of the individual are addressed with respect and understanding of diversity.

A First Class Service in 1998[31] explained how NHS standards would be set, delivered and monitored. A key ingredient of this change programme was the development of National Service Frameworks (NSFs).

NATIONAL SERVICE FRAMEWORKS (NSFs)

The National Service Framework for Mental Health[1] was one of the first NSFs. It aimed to set national standards that would eliminate variations in quality of, and access to, services. Service models for promoting mental health and treating mental illness were also defined. It set standards that addressed the design and delivery of services, needs of people with severe and enduring mental health problems, needs of carers and prevention of suicide.

Standard One of the NSF concentrated on mental health promotion, aiming to ensure that health and social services promote mental health and reduce the discrimination and social exclusion associated with mental health problems. These services are required to promote mental health for all, working with individuals and communities; and to combat discrimination against individuals and groups with mental health problems and promote their social inclusion. Guidance to support implementation of Standard One was published in 2001 by the Department of Health.[14]

The NSF for mental health focused exclusively on the mental health needs of working age adults up to 65. It touched on the needs of children and young people, but not in any detail; a dedicated NSF for children and young people is still in process. (Readers should visit www.doh.gov. uk/nsF/children for up-to-date information on developments in the children's NSF.)

An NSF addressing the needs of older people, including those with mental health problems, was published in 2001.[32] Standard Eight of this NSF focused on the promotion of health and active life in older age with the stated aim to extend the healthy life expectancy of older people. The NHS, with support from councils, is tasked with promoting the health and well-being of older people through a coordinated programme of action.

These NSFs provide clear policy drivers for the promotion of mental health and well-being for people at different stages of the life cycle. Not

OTHER NATIONAL POLICIES

Mental health in specific population groups

only existing users of mental health services, but also whole populations and communities, are potential targets for mental health promotion interventions, initiatives and programmes.

More specific guidance has also been published which addresses the mental health needs of women,[15] people who are deaf[33] and black and minority ethnic communities.[34,35]

Suicide prevention

A national suicide prevention strategy was published in 2002[36] which set out a range of actions to support reductions in suicide incidence. One of the key goals is to promote mental well-being in the wider population. The strategy is not a one-off document: it is a coordinated set of activities that will take place over several years, and it will evolve as new priorities and new evidence on prevention emerge. The strategy will be delivered by the National Institute for Mental Health in England (NIMHE) and as one of its core programmes will be subject to annual review. Updated versions of the strategy will be published regularly.

Other policies across UK countries

Across the UK there have been parallel policies on mental health and its promotion. In Scotland the *National Programme for Improving Mental Health and Well-Being* has identified mental health promotion as a key objective.[37] In Northern Ireland a 5-year strategy and action plan for promoting mental health was launched in 2003.[38] Wales has a national service framework on mental health that includes standards on promoting social inclusion and empowering service users and their carers.[39]

Social exclusion policy

The cross-cutting theme of social inclusion also impacts on mental health promotion. The Social Exclusion Unit has been coordinating a consultation exercise on what more can be done to improve employment opportunities and social networks for people with mental health problems. Readers should visit www.socialexclusionunit.gov.uk for up-to-date information and developments.

This review signals a general recognition across government that effective promotion of mental health will only be delivered in partnership and is not solely the remit of mental health services.

PREVALENCE AND TRENDS IN MENTAL HEALTH

Anyone can experience a mental health problem. On average one person in four will experience some kind of mental health problem in the course of a year. However, a much smaller number of people will be diagnosed with a serious and enduring mental health problem.

This leads us to consider definitions of mental health problems (in contrast to the definitions of positive mental health we considered earlier). Despite the controversy surrounding definitions and the usefulness of the term 'mental illness', mental health problems today still remain largely in the province of psychiatry, and hence are usually discussed in medical terms. Psychiatrists subdivide the different kinds of mental health disorders in several different ways.

- *organic* (identifiable brain malfunction) versus *functional* (not due to simple structural abnormalities of the brain);
- *neurosis* (severe forms of normal experiences) versus *psychosis* (severe distortion of a person's perception of reality);
- ICD–10 Classification, which lists major groups of disorders in related families, e.g. mood disorders, including depression and manic depression.[40]

The majority of mental health problems, especially those classified as neurotic disorders such as depression and anxiety, do not result in hospital admissions. They do, however, have a significant impact on the overall health and well-being of individuals, families, communities and organizations. Anxiety and depression are among the commonest reasons for consulting general practice. For people from more deprived areas, incidence rates are around twice as high as rates in the least deprived areas.[41,42]

IS MENTAL HEALTH GETTING BETTER OR WORSE?

In mental health promotion the outcomes are far broader than a reduction in the prevalence of medically defined mental health disorders or a decrease in suicide rates. However, this is generally how the effectiveness of mental health promotion is measured and therefore what we have to use when looking at trends in prevalence.

There is no clear picture on whether the prevalence of mental health problems is increasing. On the one hand the problem seems to be getting worse. The World Health Organization has estimated that by 2020 depression will be the second biggest killer worldwide, after coronary heart disease.[13] However, in the UK recent data on suicide rates have shown a slight decrease.[20] There was an overall decrease among women of all ages and among older men. The rates of suicide among young men, one of the highest risk groups, have shown a slight decrease since the late 1990s.

What does seem clear is that mental health is not purely an individual concept, entirely the result of genetic or neurological predisposition. Rather, mental health is determined within a broader social context. Consequently, mental health problems are inextricably linked to broader social and economic trends. Logically then, promotion of mental health must also look beyond the individual and this raises the challenge of how to identify and measure trends in community mental health.

DO HEALTH INEQUALITIES FEATURE IN MENTAL HEALTH?

The inequalities targets in the NHS Plan[43] require health and social care services to consult with, engage and involve communities, addressing the psychological and emotional impact of deprivation and exclusion. This also means a greater focus on quality of life indicators that measure the impact on how people feel. The agenda for public services and regeneration could have a huge impact on the mental and emotional well-being of individuals and communities.

Health inequalities are both a cause and a consequence of poor mental health. We show this in discussing the links with physical health and socio-economic deprivation.

LINKS BETWEEN MENTAL AND PHYSICAL HEALTH

Mental health may be central to all health and well-being because how we think and feel has a strong impact on physical health. There is a growing body of research that demonstrates the impact of mental health on physical health.

Much of the research in this area is concerned with how the social environment acts on biology to cause disease.[44] What has been called *stress biology* looks at the relationship between chronic stress and the nervous, cardiovascular and immune systems, influencing cholesterol levels, blood pressure, blood clotting and immunity. Chronic anxiety, insecurity, low self-esteem, social isolation and lack of control over work appear to undermine mental and physical health. Perceived low control beliefs, such as powerlessness and fatalism, accounted for more than half the mortality risk for people of low socio-economic status.[45]

Research in many countries has reliably confirmed that psychiatric patients have high rates of physical illness, much of which goes undetected and results in increased rates of chronic morbidity and mortality.[46–48]

● People who use mental health services, in particular those with a diagnosis of schizophrenia or bipolar disorder (characterized by swings between depression and excessive cheerfulness and activity), are at increased risk for a range of physical illnesses, including coronary heart disease, diabetes, infections and respiratory disease. They are almost twice as likely to die from coronary heart disease as the general population and four times more likely to die from respiratory disease.[49–51]

● A study of people with severe and enduring mental illness living in the community found that they had rates of other physical problems such as obesity, high blood pressure and respiratory problems significantly higher than in the general population.[52]

● A person with schizophrenia can expect to live 10 years less than someone without a mental health problem and much of this excess mortality is caused by physical health problems.[53]

● A prospective survey of the lifestyle of 140 people with schizophrenia also found that their diet was unhealthy (low in fibre and high in fat), they took less exercise than the general population, and had significantly higher levels of cigarette smoking.[53] Smoking-related fatal disease is much more common among people with schizophrenia than in the general population.[54]

(For further information on heart disease, diabetes, smoking and diet see Chs 2, 3, 4 and 5.)

LINK WITH SOCIO-ECONOMIC DEPRIVATION

We have already discussed how socio-economic factors impact on mental health, and that anxiety and depression are far more common in deprived areas.

The Acheson Report on inequalities in health[55] describes how the overall improvement in health outcomes in the 1970s and 1980s did not benefit people from disadvantaged groups. The subsequent implementation guidance[56] emphasized the strong associations between socio-economic deprivation and poor physical and mental health and the role of services in improving the lives of vulnerable individuals and communities.

However, a recent survey of people with mental health problems showed that there were also inequalities in their access to general health services and information and to health promotion services and information. This increased the inequalities of health further for an already vulnerable group.[57]

(See also Ch. 13 'Tackling inequalities in health'.)

WHAT CAN WE DO ABOUT PREVENTION AND HEALTH PROMOTION?

The models of mental health promotion we described earlier highlight the range of possible interventions which could promote mental health and provide a framework for developing them. But first we look at underlying principles and the issue of measuring effectiveness.

KEY PRINCIPLES

The key unifying principle for all the models of mental health promotion is the need to deliver interventions which aim to reduce identified risk factors for mental health or enhance identified protective factors for mental health. This can apply to individuals or communities, and delivery within key settings and structures.

Effective mental health promotion interventions have been described as those which include the following approaches:[58]

- The intervention aims to influence a combination of several risk or protective factors.
- It involves the social network of the target group.
- It intervenes at a range of different times rather than once only.
- It involves a combination of intervention methods.

Prevention and promotion programmes should be context and objective specific:[22] one size does not fit all and programmes that might work with a certain group or in a particular setting may not necessarily transfer to different groups or settings. This fact highlights the need to involve people who are the targets of interventions in their design and sometimes in their delivery.

MEASURING MENTAL HEALTH PROMOTION EFFECTIVENESS

Thinking about mental health promotion interventions raises the question of how to measure mental health, and what indicators to use to ascertain progress and outcomes of programmes. As a rule there has been a focus on measures to detect mental ill health (we have already commented on the tendency to use suicide rates as an indicator of mental health) and on negative symptoms such as sadness, anxiety or pessimism.

Tools to measure mental health

There are a number of well validated instruments designed to measure *positive* aspects of mental health in individuals.[59] These include the Psychological Well-being Scale, the Sense of Coherence Scale, the Affect Balance Scale and the Affectometer. Key elements of these tools include:

- agency – a sense of control over one's destiny
- capacity to learn, grow and develop
- feeling loved, trusted, understood and valued
- interest in life
- autonomy
- self-acceptance and self-esteem
- optimism and hopefulness
- resilience

Quality of life indicators

Quality of life indicators developed by the Audit Commission are relevant, at least in part, to mental health outcomes for individuals and communities.[60] They include:

- the percentage of people satisfied with their neighbourhood as a place to live;
- quality and amount of natural environment;
- cultural, recreational and leisure services available;
- opportunities to participate in local planning and decision making;
- percentage of people who consider that their neighbourhood is getting worse;
- percentage of respondents concerned about noise;
- area of parks and green open spaces per 1000 head of population.

Indicators of social capital

Finally, indicators are emerging which explore the relationship between social capital and health. These include formal and informal social networks, group membership, generalized trust, reciprocity and civic engagement. Readers can visit www.statistics.gov.uk/social capital for more information on defining and measuring social capital.

In areas where neighbourhood renewal programmes are well developed, or where community strategies are in process of implementation, some of the following indicators are coming into more common use:

- feeling safe
- trusting unfamiliar others
- participation
- influencing local decisions
- believing the local neighbourhood is improving
- access to social support
- employment
- meaningful activity
- support for parents.

Outcome measures for interventions that promote mental health can be drawn from some or all of these indicators. For example, interventions that facilitate the capacity to learn – an individual indicator – may also include measures of participation – a social capital indicator.

HOW MIGHT MENTAL HEALTH PROMOTION WORK AT A COMMUNITY LEVEL?

The social environment and regeneration

At a community level, initiatives which aim to tackle inequalities and regenerate deprived communities will benefit from a greater awareness of how factors combine cumulatively to increase mental health risks for individuals living in deprived localities. For example, Local Strategic Partnerships, Neighbourhood Renewal and Community Safety Partnerships can all contribute to achieving suicide reduction targets.

Research on social capital and inequality suggests that how individuals and communities feel – levels of trust, tolerance and participation – may be a critical factor in determining health.[61–65] For example, one study found that of trust in friends, family and community, only lack of trust in community predicted psychological distress. In other words, the extent to which people believe that unfamiliar others are trustworthy was an important factor determining levels of distress.[66]

Community interventions which focus on building social capital or structural interventions that widen participation in education offer opportunities for promoting the health of communities.[67,68]

Green spaces

Access to green, open spaces has important benefits for mental and physical health.[69–71] Reducing inequalities in access to green spaces and developing accessible local green spaces, for example community gardens, should be included as part of a stronger recognition of the impact of the environment on health, especially mental health and quality of life. The Communities Plan *Sustainable Communities: Building for the Future*[72] sets out a long term programme of action for delivering sustainable communities in both urban and rural areas. The plan offers a new approach to how we build and what we build.

Health promoting schools

One of the most well evaluated community interventions to promote mental health is health promoting schools.[73,74] School health promotion initiatives that make changes to the school's environment and attempt to involve parents and the wider community provide a more effective framework within which to promote mental health than those that use a curriculum-based approach only.

There is evidence suggesting that a health promoting schools approach can have an impact on aspects of mental and social well-being such as self-esteem and bullying which have previously proved difficult to influence.

There is also evidence that stress management and life skills training in schools have a positive impact in interventions addressing psychological aspects of health.

HOW CAN WE BEST HELP INDIVIDUALS?

Parenting programmes

There is evidence to suggest that the origins of many common mental health problems lie in infancy and childhood. A number of reviews have identified parenting as a prime public health issue.[75,76] Parenting has been found to be the single largest variable implicated in health outcomes for children, notably accident rates, teenage pregnancy, substance misuse, truancy, school exclusion and under-achievement, child abuse, employability, juvenile crime and mental illness.[77/8]

Parenting programmes attempt to impart information, awareness or skills on aspects of parenting. The basic aim is to improve parent–child interactions and so enhance factors known to be protective for the mental health of children, parents and families. The evidence suggests that such programmes can make a significant contribution to the mental health of mothers on outcome measures of depression, anxiety/stress, self-esteem and relationship with partner.[75,76]

There is evidence for the effectiveness of group-based parenting education programmes for children's behaviour problems and parental mental health. The effect is sustained in the medium to long term, i.e. greater than one year.[78]

There is also evidence to suggest that group-based parenting programmes can be effective in improving the short term (up to 1 year) mental health of infants and toddlers 0–3 years including emotional and behavioural adjustment and sleep patterns.[79]

Promoting physical activity

Exercise is one of the most effective interventions to promote and protect the mental health of adults. It has been shown to prevent clinical depression, reduce anxiety and enhance mood.[80–82] It also has a positive effect on self-esteem, particularly in terms of physical self-perception; the strongest association for this positive affect is in children and middle-aged adults.[83]

Evaluation of a GP-prescribed 10 week programme of exercise showed that it significantly reduced depression and anxiety and increased quality of life and self-efficacy. Non-clinical depression scores were achieved by 68% of clinically depressed patients within 3 months.[84]

A systematic review of studies in which exercise had been used to treat clinically defined depression concluded that the evidence was strong enough to support a causal link between physical activity and reduced clinical depression.[82] The review also demonstrated that inactivity produces higher risk of subsequent depression; and that physical activity can be an effective medium for its treatment.

Evidence from meta-analysis, narrative review, epidemiological and experimental studies supports a positive relationship between physical activity and psychological well-being. Physical activity is consistently associated with positive affect and mood.[85] There is evidence to support a low-to-moderate anxiety-reducing effect of physical activity, with some studies suggesting a potentially greater effect.[86]

(See also Ch. 6 'Physical activity'.)

Positive ageing

Mental health promotion initiatives are also vital for people in later life. One in five people is aged over 60, life expectancy is growing and by 2025 20% of the population in industrialized countries will be aged 65 and over.[87] As a consequence, mental health promotion programmes have the potential to make a significant difference to the health and well-being of a large population cohort. Although there is lack of clarity about what constitutes *successful ageing* it seems evident that it involves a complex process of adaptation to physical, social, interpersonal and psychological changes that accompany ageing.[88]

Good mental health and well-being are as important for older people as for any other age group and may also confer additional benefits, because of the links between positive mental health and good physical health we have already discussed, notably in relation to reduced risk of cardiovascular disease.[89,90] Emotional well-being also protects against stroke, with sustained low mood and depression increasing the risk of stroke.[91,92]

An estimated 15% of people over the age of 65 years are experiencing depression, 5% severely.[93,94] Mild depression has been reported to be 69% higher among older people than in the general population because of less social contact and low self-esteem.[95] Elderly people from ethnic minorities may be at particular risk in suffering from dementia and depression.[96]

Targeting depression in older people

Programmes and initiatives which target depression and its impact on morbidity and mortality are especially relevant in later life because depression is a very common problem.[97] There is an association between depression and negative emotions on physical health[98,99] and increased risk of suicide.[100]

Social support has been shown to be effective in countering depression. An overview of home visits by public health nurses with all groups in Canada showed reduced levels of care required for the elderly.[101] A telephone-based support service in the USA concluded that this sort of outreach strategy was moderately effective in targeting older adults with depressive symptoms, social isolation and unmet needs.[102]

Suicide is strongly related to untreated depression and specialist services can play a positive role in identifying and preventing elderly suicide. An evaluation of one such initiative in the USA concluded that community agencies with specialized programmes for older adults showed promise.[103]

Enhancing social networks

A meta-analysis on social activity and subjective well-being found that social activity was positively and significantly related to subjective well-being.[104] The analysis found that informal activities and activities with friends were not related consistently more strongly to subjective well-being than were formal activities or those with neighbours. However, scope and frequency of social activity did have an impact on subjective well-being.

Good personal support networks, for example friendship or a confiding relationship, and opportunities for social and physical activities protect mental health and enable people at any age to recover from stressful life events like bereavement or financial problems.[105] This can be particularly effective for those in later life whose social networks may have been reduced through bereavement or relocation. Access to information and practical help can play an important role in reducing feelings of exclusion and isolation.

People with a small primary support group of three people or less are at greatest risk of mental health problems.[106] Social support reduces death rates, susceptibility to infection and depression, notably in older people.[107,108]

Walking and regular social activities are positively associated with successful ageing. Involvement in social activities provides significant protection against illness, as well as good quality of life.[109]

Reducing social isolation of older people

Systematic review evidence suggests that effective interventions to combat social isolation and loneliness among older people tend to be long term group activities that are aimed at a specific target group, include an element of participant control and utilize a multifaceted approach.[110] Causes of social isolation and loneliness were identified through the literature by questioning experts in the field and by asking older people themselves. Identified causes were:

- physical disability, e.g. loss of mobility, deterioration of eyesight, loss of hearing;
- social, e.g. bereavement, loss of home, loss of family, break-up of community;
- environmental, e.g. poor housing, lack of transport, lack of local services;
- psychological, e.g. fear of crime, fear of traffic, motivation, locus of control;
- financial, i.e. poverty.

Effective interventions were characterized by group activities that:

- targeted specific groups of participants;
- utilized more than one intervention method;
- aimed to deliver across a broad range of outcomes;
- allowed participants some level of control.

There is limited but positive evidence that self-help groups provide an effective approach to lessening the impact of loneliness and social isolation for older people.[88]

Voluntary work

Meta-analysis provides evidence that interventions that provide opportunities for older people to do voluntary work lead to improved mental health in those who volunteer. Reduced depression in older people who receive services such as visits or peer counselling from an older volunteer is also reported.[111] Nearly three quarters of the older volunteers scored higher on quality of life measures than did their non-volunteer counterparts. Nine of every ten clients counselled by older volunteers experienced greater improvement on outcome measures such as diminished depression than their average counterpart who did not receive services from an older volunteer.

Figure 12.1 provides an overview of effective interventions at community and individual level.

CONTROVERSIAL ISSUES

The most controversial issue in mental health promotion is the development of robust evaluation frameworks that can produce rigorous, good quality evidence on process, impact and outcomes of mental health promotion interventions.

Figure 12.1   Evidence-based approaches to promoting positive mental health.

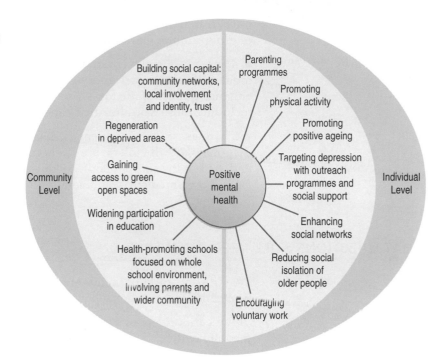

The *National Service Framework for Mental Health*[1] utilized an approach to evidence that positioned systematic reviews and randomized controlled trials at the top of a hierarchy. In our view, the complex social action research required to evaluate mental health promotion initiatives does not lend itself to this type of experimental investigation. Innovative methodologies are in development that will deliver research on a range of interventions that will be acceptable not only within mental health promotion but also in the wider research community.[112,113] In the meantime, the existing evidence on what works in mental health promotion is often open to challenge, especially within the medical establishment.

COMMON MYTHS AND QUESTIONS

There are many common myths and questions about mental health in general, but four issues stand out specifically on the promotion of mental health.

- There is still an 'us and them' perception of mental health in the public mind, despite the well known message that one in four people will have a mental health problem in any given year.

- There is a widespread assumption that only people with a diagnosis of mental illness have mental health needs. This view undermines broader mental health promotion initiatives and indeed many existing interventions and programmes are targeted only at high risk individuals or groups rather than at whole communities.

● There is a misperception that mental health promotion can prevent mental illness. In fact interventions to promote mental health aim to enhance quality of life for individuals, communities and organizations including those who already use mental health services.

● There is still a prevalent belief that people with mental illness diagnoses are all violent, are likely to commit an offence of some kind and are not the sort of people to have living next door. Public attitudes have shown no increase in tolerance towards people with mental health problems.[114]

WHAT QUESTIONS STILL NEED ANSWERS?

We still do not know enough about what works to promote mental health, for whom and in what circumstances. For example:

● A recent review of systematic reviews on interventions to promote mental health[115] drew mainly on research on at-risk populations, from countries other than the UK, using mainly experimental research methods.

● Many local initiatives and programmes to improve mental health have either not been evaluated or have used monitoring tools which are open to bias. Often these programmes are very short term and offered on a one-off basis due to resource constraints.

● Much of what we do know about what works to promote mental health has derived from research with Caucasian populations. The specific needs of black and minority ethnic communities have still to be explored and addressed.

● Most existing research has focused on interventions with individuals. Broader community or population-wide interventions have not been either conducted or evaluated. The principles of effective mental health promotion dictate that intervening at a community and structural level is essential to overall efficacy, and so this is a serious gap.

● One of the most striking omissions from existing evidence is any review of interventions that examines the mental health promoting elements of programmes to reduce inequalities. There are well documented links between social inequalities and increased incidence of a range of mental health problems.

The most pressing issues in building a credible evidence base in mental health promotion concern the development of robust evaluation tools that can be applied to a range of different programmes.[116] Once this has been done there will be a data pool which can be systematically examined and from which more compelling conclusions can be drawn.

Key sources of further information and help

- **mentality:** www.mentality.org.uk. National charity dedicated solely to the promotion of mental health, working with the public and private sector, user and survivor groups and voluntary agencies to promote the mental health of individuals, families, organizations and communities. Affiliated to the Sainsbury Centre for Mental Health.
- **Mental Health Foundation:** www.mentalhealth. org.uk. UK charity working in mental health and learning disabilities. Website provides news and information on problems, treatments and strategies for living with mental distress.
- **National Electronic Library for Mental Health:** www.nelmh.org. Specialist mental health library.
- **National NHS organizations:** providing news and information on mental health, health promotion and public health:
  - Department of Health, Social Services and Public Safety, Northern Ireland www.dhsspsni.gov.uk
  - Health Development Agency www.hda.nhs.uk/ evidence – provides evidence briefings on mental health and other topics
  - Health Scotland www.healthscotland.org.uk (formerly Health Education Board for Scotland and Public Health Institute for Scotland)
  - National Institute for Mental Health in England (NIMHE) www.nimhe.org.uk
  - Welsh Assembly www.wales.gov.uk
- **Sainsbury Centre for Mental Health (SCMH):** www.scmh.org.uk. Charity working to improve the quality of life for people with severe mental health problems. It aims to influence national policy and encourage good practice in mental health services. Affiliated to the Institute of Psychiatry, King's College, London.
- **Samaritans:** www.samaritans.org. Provide confidential emotional support 24 hours a day for people in distress or despair.

References

1. Department of Health. National Service Framework for mental health. London. HMSO; 1999. Online. Available: http://www.doh.gov.uk/mentalhealth
2. Office for National Statistics. Survey of psychiatric morbidity among adults living in private households. London: HMSO; 2000.
3. Goldberg D. Filters to care. In: Jenkins R, Griffiths S, eds. Indicators for mental health in the population. London: The Stationery Office; 1991.
4. Meltzer H, Gatward R, Goodman R, Ford T. The mental health of children and adolescents in Great Britain: summary report. London: Office for National Statistics; 2000.
5. World Health Organization. Constitution. New York: World Health Organization; 1946.
6. World Health Organization. Ottawa charter for health promotion. Ottawa: World Health Organization; 1986.
7. Tudor K. Mental health promotion: paradigms and practice. London: Routledge; 1996.
8. The Mental Health Foundation. Factsheet: What is mental health? London: Mental Health Foundation: 2000. Online. Available: http://www.mentalhealth. org.uk.
9. Rutter M. Resilience in the face of adversity: protective factors and resistance to psychiatric disorder. British Journal of Psychiatry 1985; 147:598–611.
10. MacDonald G, O'Hara K. Ten elements of mental health, its promotion and demotion: implications for practice. Society of Health Education and Promotion Specialists; 1998.
11. Secker J. Current conceptualisations of mental health and mental health promotion. Health Education Research 1998; 13(1):57–66.
12. Albee GW, Ryan-Finn KD. An overview of primary prevention. Journal of Counselling and Development 1993; 72:115–123.
13. World Health Organization. Mental health: new understanding, new hope. The World Health Report 2001. Geneva: WHO; 2001.
14. Department of Health. Making it happen: a guide to delivering mental health promotion. London. HMSO; 2001. Online. Available: http://www.doh.gov.uk/ mentalhealth
15. Department of Health. Women's mental health: into the mainstream: strategic development of mental health care for women. London: Department of Health; 2002.

16. Meltzer H, Gill B, Pettigrew M, Hinds K. The prevalence of psychiatric morbidity among adults living in private households. OPCS surveys of psychiatric morbidity in Great Britain Report 1. London: HMSO; 1996.

17. Piccinelli M, Wilkinson G. Gender differences in depression. British Journal of Psychiatry 2000; 177:486–492.

18. Milne A, Hatzidimitriadou E, Chryssanthopoulou C, Owen T. Caring in later life: reviewing the role of older carers. London: Help the Aged; 2001.

19. Fryers T, Melzer D, Jenkins R. Social inequalities and the common mental disorders: a systematic review of the evidence. Social Psychiatry and Psychiatric Epidemiology 2003; 38:229–237.

20. Summerfield C, Babb P, eds. Social trends no. 34. London: The Stationery Office; 2004.

21. Nazroo JY, Karlsen S. Ethnic inequalities in health: social class, racism and identity. ESRC research findings 10 from the Health Variations Programme. Lancaster: Lancaster University; 2001.

22. Boydell J, van Os J, McKenzie K, et al. Incidence of schizophrenia in ethnic minorities in London: ecological study into interactions with environment. British Medical Journal 2001; 323:1336.

23. Sharpley MS, Hutchinson G, Murray RM, McKenzie K. Understanding the excess of psychosis among the African-Caribbean population in England: review of current hypotheses. British Journal of Psychiatry 2001; 178 (suppl 40):60–68.

24. Pollock LR, Williams JM. Problems solving suicidal behaviour. Suicide and Life Threatening Behaviour 1998; 28(4):375–387.

25. Williams JMG, Pollock LR. Psychological aspects of the suicidal process. In: van Heeringen K, ed. Understanding suicidal behaviour. Chichester: John Wiley; 2001.

26. Fonagy P, Higgitt A. An attachment theory perspective on early influences on development and social inequalities. In: Osofsky J, Fitzgerald H, eds. WAIMH handbook of infant mental health. New York: John Wiley; 2000:521–560.

27. Health Education Authority. Mental health promotion: a quality framework. London: HEA; 1997.

28. Friedli L. From the margins to the mainstream: the public health potential of mental health promotion. International Journal of Mental Health Promotion 1999; 1(2):30–36.

29. Putnam R. The prosperous community: social capital and public life. American Prospect 1993; 13:35–42.

30. Sainsbury Centre for Mental Health. The Economic and Social Costs of Mental Illness. London: SCMH; 2003.

31. Department of Health. A First Class Service: Quality in the new NHS. London: Department of Health; 1998.

32. Department of Health. National Service Framework for older people. London: HMSO; 2001. Online. Available: http://www.doh.gov.uk/nsf/olderpeople

33. Department of Health. A sign of the times: mental health services for people who are deaf. London: HMSO; 2002.

34. National Institute for Mental Health in England. Inside, outside: mental health services for black and minority ethnic communities. Leeds: NIMHE; 2003.

35. National Institute for Mental Health in England. Celebrating our cultures: mental health promotion with black and minority ethnic communities. Leeds: NIMHE; 2004.

36. Department of Health. National suicide prevention strategy. London: HMSO; 2002.

37. Scottish Executive. National programme for improving mental health and well-being action plan 2003–2006. Edinburgh: Scottish Executive; 2003.

38. Department of Health, Social Services and Public Safety. Promoting mental health: strategy and action plan 2003–2008. Belfast: DHSSPS; 2003.

39. Welsh Assembly. Adult mental health service National Service Framework for Wales. Cardiff; Welsh Assembly; 2002.

40. World Health Organization. International Classification of Diseases (ICD). Mental and behavioural disorders (F00–F99). Geneva: WHO; 2003. Online: http//www.who.int/classifications/icd.

41. Kessler D, Lloyd K, Lewis G. Cross sectional study of symptom attribution and recognition of depression and anxiety in primary care. British Medical Journal 1999; 318:436–439.

42. Shaw I, Middleton H. Recognising depression in primary care. Journal of Primary Care Mental Health 2001; 5(2):24–27.

43. Department of Health. The new NHS: a plan for investment, a plan for reform. London: The Stationery Office; 2000.

44. Marmot M, Wilkinson R. Social determinants of health. Oxford: Oxford University Press; 1999.

45. Bosma H, Marmot MG, Hemmingway H. Low job control and risk of coronary heart disease in Whitehall II (prospective cohort) study. British Medical Journal 1997; 314:558.

46. Koran LM, Sox HC, Marton KI, et al. Medical evaluation of psychiatric patients. 1. Results in a state mental health system. Archives of General Psychiatry 1989; 46:733–740.

47. Makikyro T, Karvonen JT, Hakko H, et al. Co-morbidity of hospital-treated psychiatric and physical disorders with special reference to schizophrenia: a 28 year follow-up of the 1966 northern Finland general population birth cohort. Public Health 1998; 112:221–228.

48. Lawrence D, Holman CDJ, Jablensky AV. Preventable physical illness in people with mental illness. Perth: The University of Western Australia; 2001. Online. Available: http://www.dph.uwa.edu.au

49. Phelan M, Stradins L, Morrison S. Physical health of people with severe mental illness. British Medical Journal 2001; 322:443–444.

50. Harris EC, Barraclough B. Excess mortality of mental disorder. British Journal of Psychiatry 1998; 173:11–53.

51. Barr W. Physical health of people with severe mental illness. British Medical Journal 2001; 323:231.

52. Kendrick T, Burns T, Freeling L, et al. Randomised controlled trial of teaching general practitioners to carry out structured assessments of their long-term mentally ill patients. British Medical Journal 1995; 311:93–98.

53. Brown S, Inskip H, Barraclough B. Causes of the excess mortality of schizophrenia. British Journal of Psychiatry 2000; 177:212–217.

54. Addington J, el-Guebaly N, Campbell W, et al. Smoking cessation treatment for patients with schizophrenia. American Journal of Psychiatry 1998; 155:974–976.

55. Department of Health. Independent inquiry into inequalities in health (the Acheson report) The Stationery Office. London: 1998.

56. Department of Health. Tackling health inequalities: the results of the consultation exercise. London: The Stationery Office; 2002.

57. mentality. Not All in the Mind: The physical health of people with mental health problems. Radical mentalities briefing paper series. London: mentality; 2003.

58. Bosma MWM, Hosman CMH. Preventie op waarde geschat. Nijmegen: Beta; 1990.

59. Stewart-Brown S. Measuring the parts most measures do not reach. Journal of Mental Health Promotion 2002; 1(2):4–9.

60. Audit Commission. Quality of life: a good practice guide to communicating quality of life indicators. London: Audit Commission; 2003. Online. Available: http://www.audit-commission.gov.uk

61. Wilkinson R. Unhealthy societies: the afflictions of inequality. London: Routledge; 1996.

62. Wilkinson R. Inequality and the social environment: a reply to Lynch et al. Journal of Epidemiological Community Health 2000; 54:411–413.

63. Cooper H, Arber S, Fee L, Ginn J. The influence of social support and social capital on health. London: Health Education Authority; 1999.

64. Kawachi I, Kennedy B, Lochner K. Social capital, income inequality and mortality. American Journal of Public Health 1997; 87:491–498.

65. Kawachi I, Kennedy BP. Income inequality and health: pathways and mechanisms. Health Services Research 1999; 34:215.

66. Berry HL, Rickwood DJ. Measuring social capital at the individual level: personal social capital, values and psychological distress. International Journal of Mental Health Promotion 2000; 2(3):35–44.

67. East of England Faiths Leadership Conference. Faith in action: a report on faith communities and social capital in the East of England. Online. Available: 2003. http://www.eeflc.org.uk/faith.pdf

68. Cameron M, Edmans T, Greatley A , Morris D. Community renewal and mental health: strengthening the links. London: Kings Fund; 2003.

69. Lewis G, Booth M. Are cities bad for your mental health? Psychological Medicine 1994; 24:913–915.

70. Dalgard OS, Tambs K. Urban environment and mental health: a longitudinal study. British Journal of Psychiatry 1997; 171:530–536.

71. mentality. Nature and psychological well-being: a briefing for English Nature. London: English Nature; 2003.

72. Office of the Deputy Prime Minister. Sustainable communities: building for the future. London: ODPM; 2003. Online. Available: http://www.odpm.gov.uk

73. Lister-Sharp D, Chapman S, Stewart-Brown S, Sowden A. Health promoting schools and health promotion in schools: two systematic reviews. Health Technology Assessment 1999; 3(22):1–207.

74. Wells J, Barlow J, Stewart-Brown S. A systematic review of universal approaches to mental health promotion in schools. Oxford: Health Service Research Unit, University of Oxford, Institute of Health Sciences; 2001.

75. Barlow J, Coren E, Stewart-Brown S. Meta-analysis of the effectiveness of parenting programmes in improving maternal psychosocial health. British Journal of General Practice 2002; 52:223–233.

76. Barlow J, Coren E. Parent-training programmes for improving maternal psychosocial health. In: The Cochrane Library Issue 3: 2002. Oxford: Update Software; 2002.

77. Hoghughi M. The importance of parenting in child health. British Medical Journal 1998; 316:1545.

78. Dimond C, Hyde C. Parent education programmes for children's behaviour problems. Medium to long-term effectiveness. A West Midlands Development and Evaluation Service Report. Development and Evaluation Service. Department of Public Health and Epidemiology. University of Birmingham; 1999.

79. Barlow J, Parsons J. Group-based parent-training programmes for improving emotional and behavioural adjustment in 0–3 year old children. In: The Cochrane Library Issue 4: 2002. Oxford: Update Software; 2002.

80. Grant T, ed. Physical activity and mental health: national consensus statements and guidelines for practice. London: Somerset Health Authority/Health Education Authority; 2000.

81. Fox KR. Self-esteem, self-perceptions and exercise. International Journal of Sport Psychology 2000; 31:228–240.

82. Mutrie N. The relationship between physical activity and clinically defined depression. In: Biddle SJH, Fox KR, Boutcher SH, eds. Physical activity and psychological well-being. London: Routledge; 2000.

83. Biddle SJH, Fox KR, Boutcher SH, Faulkner GE. The way forward for physical activity and the promotion of psychological well-being. In: Biddle SJH, Fox KR, Boutcher SH, eds. Physical activity and psychological well-being. London: Routledge; 2000.

84. Darbishire L, Glenister D. The Balance for Life scheme: mental health benefits of GP recommended exercise in relation to depression and anxiety. Essex Health Authority; 1998.

85. Biddle SJH. Emotion, mood and physical activity. In: Biddle SJH, Fox KR, Boutcher SH, eds. Physical activity and psychological well-being. London: Routledge; 2000.

86. Taylor A. Physical activity, anxiety and stress. In: Biddle SJH, Fox KR, Boutcher SH, eds. Physical activity and psychological well-being. London: Routledge; 2000.

87. Kinsella K. Demographic aspects. In: Ebrahim S, Kalache A, eds. Epidemiology in old age. London: BMJ Publishing; 1996.

88. Godfrey M. Preventive strategies for older people: mapping the literature on effectiveness and outcomes. Anchor Research; 1999.

89. Hippisley-Cox J, Fielding K, Pringle M. Depression as a risk factor for ischaemic heart disease in men: population based case control study. British Medical Journal 1998; 316:1714–1719.

90. Bosma H, Marmot MG, Hemmingway H. Low job control and risk of coronary heart disease in Whitehall II (prospective cohort) study. British Medical Journal 1997; 314:558.

91. Jonas BS, Mussolino ME. Symptoms of depression as a prospective risk factor for stroke. Psychosomatic Medicine 2000; 62(4):463–472.

92. Ostir GV, Markides KS, Peek MK, Goodwin JS. The association between emotional well-being and the incidence of stroke in older adults. Psychosomatic Medicine 2001; 63:210–215.

93. Banerjee S, Shamash K, Macdonald AJDM, Mann AH. Randomised controlled trial of effect of intervention by psychogeriatric team on depression in frail elderly people at home. British Medical Journal 1996; 313:1058–1061.

94. Bennett KM. Customary physical activity and gender as precursors for late life personal disturbance. British Journal of Clinical Psychology 1997; 173:4–7.

95. Audit Commission. Forget me not: mental health services for older people. Abingdon: Audit Commission; 2000.

96. McCracken CFM, Boneham MA, Copeland JRM, et al. Prevalence of dementia and depression among elderly people in black and ethnic minorities. British Journal of Psychiatry 1997; 171:269–273.

97. Han H. Depressive symptoms and self-rated health in community dwelling older adults: a longitudinal study. Dissertation abstracts international: The Sciences and Engineering 2000; 61(4b):1863.

98. Beck DA, Koenig HG. Minor depression – a review of the literature. International Journal of Psychiatry in Medicine 1996; 26(2):177–209.

99. Bruce ML. Depression and disability in late life: directions for future research. American Journal of Geriatric Psychiatry 2001; 9(2):102–112.

100. Pearson JL, Brown GK. Suicide prevention in late life: direction for science and practice. Clinical Psychology Review 2000; 20(6):685–705.

101. Ciliska D, Hayward S, Thomas H, et al. A systematic overview of the effectiveness of home visiting as a delivery strategy for public health nursing interventions. Canadian Journal of Public Health 1996; 87(3):193–198.

102. Morrow HN, Becker KS, Judy L. Evaluating an intervention for the elderly at increased risk of suicide. Research on Social Work Practice 1998; 8(1):28.

103. Fiske A, Arbore P. Future directions in late life suicide prevention. Omega: Journal of Death and Dying 2000; 42(1):37–53.

104. Okun MA, Stock WA, Haring MJ, Witter RA. The social activity/subjective well-being relation: a quantitative synthesis. Research on Aging 1984; 6(1):45–65.

105. Cooper H, Arber S, Fee L, Ginn J. The influence of social support and social capital on health. London: Health Education Authority; 1999.

106. Brugha TS, Wing JK, Brewin CR, et al. The relationship of social network deficits in social functioning in long term psychiatric disorders. Social Psychiatry and Psychiatric Epidemiology 1993; 28:218–224.

107. Cohen S, ed. Measuring stress: a guide for health and social scientists. Oxford: Oxford University Press; 1997.

108. Oxman TE, et al. Social support and depressive symptoms in the elderly. American Journal of Epidemiology 1992; 135:356–368.

109. Health Development Agency. Pre-retirement health checks and plans: literature review. London: Health Development Agency; 2002.

110. Cattan M, White M. Developing evidence based health promotion for older people: a systematic review and survey of health promotion interventions targeting social isolation and loneliness among older people. Internet Journal of Health Promotion 1998 (URL: http://www.rhpeo.org/ijhp-articles/1998/13/index.htm).

111. Wheeler FA, Gorey KM, Greenblatt B. The beneficial effects of volunteering for older volunteers and the people they serve: a meta-analysis. International Journal of Aging and Human Development 1998; 47(1):69–79.

112. May N, et al. The review and synthesis of qualitative and quantitative evidence. London: SDO (NHS Service and Delivery Organisation); In press.

113. Lavis J, et al. Towards syntheses that inform health-care management and health policy making. London: SDO (NHS Service and Delivery Organisation); In press.

114. Crisp AH. The tendency to stigmatise. British Journal of Psychiatry 2001; (178):197–199.

115. Health Development Agency. Promoting mental health, a review of reviews. Evidence briefing. London: HDA (forthcoming). Online. Available: http://www.hda.nhs.uk/evidence

116. Gowman N, Coote A. Evidence and public health: towards a common framework. London: Kings Fund; 1999.

Chapter **13**

Tackling inequalities in health

David Evans

SUMMARY OVERVIEW AND LINKS TO OTHER TOPICS

In previous chapters, we saw that (with a few rare exceptions such as breast cancer) diseases and behaviours which put health at risk are more prevalent in people from poorer socio-economic groups, and many are more prevalent in particular population groups such as black and minority ethnic groups. This chapter considers the nature, causes and extent of these inequalities in health and what can be done about them.

A massive amount of research has shown that health inequalities exist; the reasons are complex, but it is largely due to the direct effects of poverty and associated behavioural and cultural factors. Health inequalities are getting worse: although overall population health has improved, the gap between the health of rich and poor has been widening in recent decades.

Tackling inequalities has been a focus of national policy since the late 1990s, with *Tackling Health Inequalities: A Programme for Action*[1] in 2003 aiming to support and engage with people with high health needs, prevent illness and provide effective treatment and care, and address the underlying determinants of health such as poor housing and unemployment. However, policy implementation is beset with contradictions and limitations.

What should we be doing about inequalities – what works? We can address the fundamental causes through national social and economic policy and/or work directly with poorer individuals and communities to tackle their immediate problems. We can focus on ensuring that everyone receives the same standard of service and/or we can selectively target benefits and services at those who most need them.

In practical terms, there is evidence to suggest that there are five ways that public health practitioners can tackle inequalities effectively: lobbying; working in partnerships; supporting community development; promoting healthy behaviours; and improving access to health care.

Clearly this chapter is relevant to all others; also, it complements Chapter 14 'Helping individuals to change behaviour', which addresses an important way of working with people with high health needs.

WHAT ARE INEQUALITIES IN HEALTH?

The last century has witnessed remarkable improvements in health in the UK and internationally. In developing countries, infant, child and maternal mortality have fallen dramatically. In the UK, Europe and the rest of the developed world mortality from the major killer diseases (coronary heart disease [CHD] and cancer) has been falling. Despite these general improvements, the health of some individuals and communities is systematically worse than others. This is often referred to as a health gap or more commonly as inequalities in health.

Inequalities in health have been defined as 'the virtually universal phenomenon of variation in health indicators (infant and maternal mortality rates, mortality and incidence rates of many diseases, etc) associated with socio-economic status'.[2] For almost every indicator, there is a clear positive relationship between health and wealth: in general, the wealthier people are, the better their health; the poorer, the worse their health and the greater their risk of dying prematurely. For example, Figure 13.1 shows that in 1997–1999 male life expectancy at birth was 71.1 years for unskilled manual workers compared to 78.5 years for professionals, a gap of 7.4 years.[3]

The concept of inequalities in health has also been used to describe the relatively worse health experience of black and minority ethnic groups in the UK.[4] For example, mortality from CHD is relatively high among people of South Asian origin, whilst people of West African and Caribbean

Figure 13.1   Life expectancy by social class, males. Width is proportionate to population in each category. (Reproduced with permission from Wanless 2003.[3] Crown copyright material is reproduced with the permission of the controller of HMSO and the Queen's Printer for Scotland.)

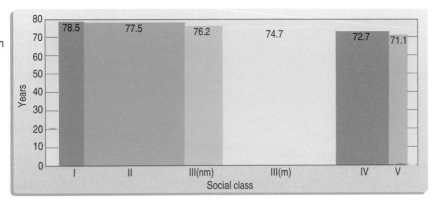

origin have relatively high mortality from stroke. Inequalities also exist between geographical areas and between women and men. A number of groups also experience worse health than the rest of the population, including looked after children, prisoners, travellers and rough sleepers.

WHAT IS THE EVIDENCE FOR SOCIO-ECONOMIC INEQUALITIES IN HEALTH?

Health inequalities have been documented in the UK since the ground-breaking work of William Farr on vital statistics first published in 1837; subsequently, health inequalities were identified by Rowntree (1901), Booth (1902–03), Boyd Orr (1936), Titmuss (1943) and Tudor Hart (1971) amongst many others.[5] In 1977 the Labour government commissioned Sir Douglas Black to lead a review of the evidence on inequalities in health and make policy recommendations.[6] Black concluded that:

> Most recent data show marked differences in mortality rates between the occupational classes, for both sexes and at all ages. At birth and in the first month of life, twice as many babies of 'unskilled manual' parents (class V) die as do babies of professional class parents (class I) and in the next eleven months nearly three times as many boys and more than three times as many girls ... A class gradient can be observed for most causes of death, being particularly steep in the case of diseases of the respiratory system.[6]

The rejection of the Black Report in 1980 by the incoming Conservative government stimulated additional studies, the vast majority of which confirmed the fundamental link between inequalities in health and wealth. Nearly 20 years later the Labour government elected in 1997 commissioned Sir Donald Acheson to chair an *Independent Inquiry into Inequalities in Health*.[7] Acheson not only confirmed the existence of the inequalities identified in the Black Report, but concluded that in the intervening period the differences in the rates had widened:

> For example, in the early 1970s, the mortality rate among men of working age was almost twice as high for those in class V (unskilled) as for those in

class I (professional). By the early 1990s, it was almost three times higher. This increasing differential is because, although rates fell overall, they fell more among the high social classes than the low social classes. Between the early 1970s and the early 1990s, rates fell by about 40 per cent for classes I and II, about 30 per cent for classes IIIN, IIIM and IV, but by only 10 per cent for class V. So not only did the differential between the top and bottom increase, the increase happened across the whole spectrum of social classes.[7]

WHY ARE INEQUALITIES IN HEALTH IMPORTANT?

Fundamentally, the importance of inequalities is a value judgement. Most people working in public health think it is not right that poorer people die younger and experience worse health than the affluent. By contrast, in general younger people experience better health than older people, but these differences are not usually regarded as unfair, or defined as inequalities.

Thus when commentators discuss inequalities in health, they often mean *inequities*: that is, those inequalities that are perceived to be unfair. As Baggot points out, concepts of equity and inequity are value based, and refer to 'what should be'.[8] There is much controversy about whether certain inequalities are actually inequitable and what should be done about them. Are we concerned simply with inequality of outcome as measured by health indicators? Or are we also seeking to ensure equity of access to services (which may or may not lead to equitable outcomes) or equity of opportunity for people to attain their full health potential (which may require shifting resources towards poorer individuals and communities)?

WHAT ARE THE CAUSES OF INEQUALITY IN HEALTH?

There is a considerable literature seeking to explain the causes of health inequalities. This is a complex field, beset with conceptual and methodological difficulties in measuring inequality and in demonstrating cause and effect. Following a discussion in the Black Report, five major potential causes of the observed inequalities generally have been considered:[9]

- *artefact* – observed inequalities are not genuine but due to how we measure;
- *social selection* – health determines socio-economic position rather than socio-economic position determining health;
- *behavioural/cultural* – including the impact of unhealthy behaviours such as smoking;
- *psychosocial* – for example, the stress of low status jobs with little control or autonomy at work;
- *material* – the direct effects of poverty.

Although these debates are unresolved (and possibly unresolvable as the different explanations are not necessarily mutually exclusive), most researchers and policy analysts accept that artefact and social selection account for relatively little of the observed differences in health between rich and poor. There is more continuing debate on the relative importance of material, behavioural/cultural and psychosocial factors.

What is notable about this literature, however, is how much of it is concerned with documenting and explaining inequalities of health and how little focuses on evaluating interventions to reduce inequalities.[10] This chapter is intended to help redress the balance by primarily focusing on what the evidence tells us works in reducing inequalities in health, particularly from the practitioner perspective.

Some of the excess mortality and morbidity associated with poverty can be explained by recognized behavioural risk factors, in particular smoking, but also poor diet, high alcohol consumption and lack of physical exercise (see also Chs 4, 5, 10 and 6 respectively). Such risk factors explain some of the inequality in health, particularly for cardiovascular disease where risk factors such as smoking, high blood cholesterol levels and high blood pressure play a part (see Ch. 2). But they explain less than half of the socio-economic differences in mortality.[10] Some commentators have sought to explain this finding through the psychological effects of income inequality,[11] while others have stressed the cumulative impact of inequality over the life course.[12]

The debates between these various schools of thought can be highly technical. They are important because understanding the causal pathways leading to inequalities in health should help us plan interventions to reduce inequalities. But such understanding is advantageous rather than essential. The causal pathways are clearly complex and likely to be multifactorial. Recent research, for example, has demonstrated that there is significant variation in the association between socio-economic position and mortality for particular causes of ill health and death, with some risk factors having differing impacts at different stages of the life course.[12] Nonetheless, there is clear evidence to support some policy interventions to reduce inequalities in health whether their specific causal pathways are fully understood or not.

ARE INEQUALITIES IN HEALTH GETTING BETTER OR WORSE?

Although the overall health of the population has been improving, socio-economic inequalities in health remain and are increasing between socio-economic groups, geographical areas and ethnic communities. Inequalities in health are as obvious in the UK today as 100 years ago, despite the creation of the Welfare State and the virtual abolition of absolute poverty. The health of the poorest has improved over time, but not as fast as for the rest of the population; thus the health gap between rich and poor has widened (see Fig. 13.2).[1] This gap in health is, of course, only one aspect of the widening socio-economic gap between rich and

Figure 13.2   The widening mortality gap between social classes. England and Wales. Men of working age (varies according to year, either aged 15 or 20 to age 64 or 65). (Source: Office for National Statistics, Decennial Supplements. Reproduced with permission from Department of Health 2003.[1] Crown copyright material is reproduced with the permission of the Controller of HMSO and the Queen's Printer for Scotland.)

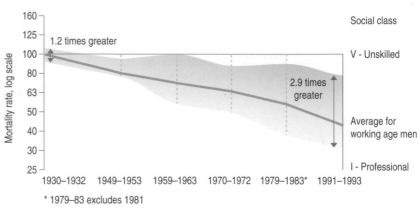

poor which can also be seen in income, housing, education and other aspects of social life.

Health inequalities are much greater in some countries than in others; for example inequalities in health are markedly smaller in absolute terms in Sweden (which for many years has pursued equality-oriented social and labour-market policies) than in the UK, thus suggesting that social policy can impact on health inequalities.

HOW ARE INEQUALITIES IN HEALTH ADDRESSED IN NATIONAL POLICY?

The Labour government elected in 1997 launched a range of initiatives to tackle social exclusion, including a specific focus on inequalities in health. As well as commissioning the Acheson inquiry, the government accepted its recommendations. Acheson laid out three priorities:

- All policies likely to have an impact on health should be evaluated in terms of their impact on health inequalities.

- A high priority should be given to the health of families with children.

- Further steps should be taken to reduce income inequalities and improve the living standards of the poor.[7]

The new government came to power recognizing that inequalities needed to be tackled through 'joined-up thinking' across both central government and local partnerships. Thus the Prime Minister established a Social Exclusion Unit reporting directly to his office with a remit to work across departmental boundaries. Local authorities and other agencies were required to establish local strategic partnerships and community strategies, with a range of national targets and performance indicators relating to inequalities.

In England, the government published a public health strategy *Saving Lives: Our Healthier Nation*[13] with the accompanying *Reducing Health Inequalities: An Action Report*,[14] which laid out the range of government policies that addressed inequalities. Similar strategies were published in the other UK countries. *The NHS Plan*[15] set out more concrete action and established two new national targets to reduce inequalities in life expectancy and infant mortality by 10% by 2010. The action needed to tackle health inequalities was restated in a Treasury-led review[16] and in the Treasury commissioned report on the future of the NHS led by Derek Wanless.[17] Most recently, in 2003 the government published *Tackling Health Inequalities: A Programme for Action*[1] which sets out a detailed 3 year plan to tackle inequalities in health. The programme is organized around four themes:

- supporting families, mothers and children – to ensure the best possible start in life and break the intergenerational cycle of poor health;
- engaging communities and individuals – to ensure relevance, responsiveness and sustainability;
- preventing illness and providing effective treatment and care – making certain that the NHS provides leadership and makes the contribution to reducing inequalities that is expected of it;
- addressing the underlying determinants of health – dealing with the long term underlying causes of health inequalities.

A range of initiatives have been put in place to address these themes as illustrated in Box 13.1. In addition, *Tackling Health Inequalities: A Programme for Action* identifies further action that needs to be taken at national, regional and local levels.

HOW EFFECTIVE HAS UK POLICY BEEN IN REDUCING INEQUALITIES IN HEALTH?

What then is the evidence of the effectiveness of UK policy in tackling inequalities in health? Given the complexity and the long term cumulative impact of health inequalities, it is unsurprising that definitive answers are not yet available.[19]

For many commentators, the key question is whether the government is successfully tackling poverty by redistributing income from rich to poor. Early evidence on this is mixed. Shaw and colleagues argue that although most families gained from the first three Labour budgets, overall the poorest did not improve their relative position.[20] Writing slightly later, the same research group found that relative income inequality continued to rise in 1996–1997 and 1998–1999, that is, into the third year of the new government.[21] By contrast, Benzeval and colleagues found that the government had been successful in redistributing from rich to poor, with the poorest tenth of the population seeing almost 10% increase in disposable income whilst the richest tenth experienced a small decrease.[22]

Shaw and colleagues also point to direct evidence that health inequalities are continuing to increase.[21] They found that the poverty gradient for premature mortality (defined as death before 75 in this study) increased over the period 1990–1999, including between 1996–1997 and 1998–1999. As it may take many years for changes in policy to impact upon health, more data over a longer period will be necessary before a definitive judgement can be made on the impact of government policy changes since 1997 on health inequalities.

Box 13.1   Government commitments to tackle inequalities in health 2003–2006[1]

Supporting families, mothers and children

- Improving access to maternity services
- Increase take up and duration of breast feeding
- Ensure low income families access to a healthy diet
- Develop multidisciplinary family support schemes
- Learning from Sure Start to be applied to mainstream children's services
- Narrow the gap in educational attainment
- Strengthen teaching of personal, social and sex education
- Reduce truancy and improve learning opportunities
- Develop sports facilities through the New Opportunities Programme
- Assess health needs and provide health promotion to young people in prison
- Clear guidance on arrangements for homeless families and children
- Early antenatal booking and smoking cessation for teenage mothers
- Sure Start Plus for teenage parents and pregnant teenagers.

Engaging communities and individuals

- National strategy on neighbourhood renewal
- Greater use of school facilities, e.g. through Creative Partnerships
- Sustainable communities action plan
- Support local enterprise and community entrepreneurship through Regional Development Agencies
- Improve access to and use of drug and alcohol services
- Improve access to mental health services
- Good practice in care of asylum seekers and refugees

- Implement *Valuing People*[18] White Paper for people with learning disabilities
- Improve access to services by improving transport.

Preventing illness and providing effective treatment and care

- National Service Frameworks to raise service quality
- More smoking prevention and cessation services for low income groups
- Improve nutrition of families and children through 5 a day programme
- Raise levels of physical activity
- Reduce illness and death by accidental injury
- Improve access to and quality of primary care services
- Tackle the 'inverse care law' by matching need with high quality services
- Prevent falls in older people through national guidelines.

Addressing the underlying determinants of health

- Reduce number of children in low income households
- Ensure all social housing meets the decent housing standard by 2010
- Improve basic skills and workforce training
- Improve employment prospects in the worst areas
- Improve job prospects of black and minority ethnic groups
- Develop consistent transport and land use policies
- Integrated and sustainable approach to regional economic development.

ARE THERE CONTROVERSIAL ISSUES IN TACKLING INEQUALITIES IN HEALTH?

A number of commentators have analysed policy on tackling health inequalities and concluded that it is beset with limitations and contradictions.

- The Acheson Report itself has been criticized for a lack of prioritization, a weak evidence base and being uncosted.[23,24]

- The government's focus on area-based initiatives has been criticized because most poor people live outside the specified areas of deprivation. Even within targeted areas, the resources allocated to tackling inequality are relatively small compared to mainstream spend in public services. Thus the government has emphasized the need to 'bend mainstream services'. However, there is little evidence of effective practice in doing this.

- Different local agencies continue to receive differing 'must do's' from central government.

- Other aspects of government policy, particularly the short timescales within which regeneration funds must be spent, often work against coherent interagency planning for long term service change.

Within the NHS, the major central policy drivers focus on improving access (for example, reducing hospital waiting times) and service quality rather than on tackling the wider determinants of health inequalities.

Despite the government's stated commitment to tackling inequalities in health, it has been suggested that there has been a '*de facto* relegation of health inequalities' in central priorities, resource allocation and performance management decisions.[23] As Exworthy and colleagues conclude, tackling health inequalities is a policy priority for the government, but locally 'implementation is hampered by deficiencies in performance management, insufficient integration between policy sectors and contradictions between health inequalities and other policy imperatives'.[23]

It is too early to assess what the impact of these contradictions will be on the health gap between rich and poor.

WHAT CHOICES DO WE FACE IN TRYING TO REDUCE INEQUALITIES IN HEALTH?

Two fundamental choices in approaches to tackling inequality are summarized in Figure 13.3. Interventions to reduce inequalities can be categorized as *upstream* (tackling the fundamental causes through national social and economic policy) or *downstream* (working directly with poor individuals and communities to tackle their immediate problems). A second

Figure 13.3   Approaches to reducing inequalities in health.

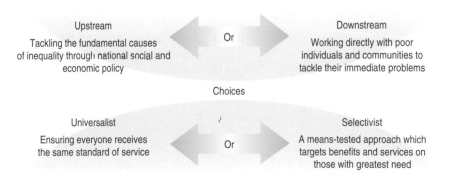

Upstream
Tackling the fundamental causes of inequality through national social and economic policy

Or

Downstream
Working directly with poor individuals and communities to tackle their immediate problems

Choices

Universalist
Ensuring everyone receives the same standard of service

Or

Selectivist
A means-tested approach which targets benefits and services on those with greatest need

important distinction is between policies which are *universalist* (ensuring everyone receives the same standard of service) and *selectivist* (a means-tested approach which targets benefits and services on those with greatest need).

For some commentators, the solution to health inequalities is upstream and universalist:

> There is one central and fundamental policy that should be pursued: the reduction of income inequality and consequently the elimination of poverty. Ending poverty is the key to ending inequalities in health ... Any child can tell you how this can be achieved: the poor have too little money so the solution to ending their poverty is to give them more money. Poverty reduction really is something that can be achieved by 'throwing money at the problem'.[24]

Other commentators have suggested that while there is good evidence for such downstream interventions as smoking cessation, there is a lack of good quality studies of 'upstream' interventions.[25] Davey Smith and colleagues, however, have countered that such analysis inappropriately focuses on individual level determinants of health while ignoring more important national level determinants: 'The *Cochrane Library* is unlikely ever to contain systematic reviews or trials of the effects of redistributive national fiscal policies, or of economic investment leading to reductions in unemployment, on health'.[16] A different type of evidence is needed to support national economic interventions to tackle poverty, an evidence base that Davey Smith and colleagues have sought to provide in numerous publications.[20,21,24,26]

WHAT CAN YOU DO AS A PRACTITIONER ABOUT INEQUALITIES IN HEALTH?

Such debates leave one with a dilemma: if the only fundamental way to tackle health inequalities is through national economic policy, what can the practitioner working at the local level do? The choice is either to do nothing about inequalities, which for most of us is ethically unacceptable, or to identify what can usefully be done locally.

WHAT WORKS? THE EVIDENCE BASE

Fortunately, there is an increasing body of evidence to guide such decisions including reviews by Arblaster and colleagues,[27,28] the Acheson Report,[7] Roberts' work on what works in reducing inequalities in child health[29] and Mackenbach and Bakker's[10] European survey, as well as the ever growing literature available online via the National Electronic Library for Health (www.NELH.nhs.uk).

Essentially, there are five options for the individual practitioner: lobbying, partnership working, community development, promoting healthy behaviours and improving access to health care, summarized in Figure 13.4.

LOBBYING

You can seek to influence how national policy addresses the upstream determinants of inequalities by lobbying ministers, members of parliament

Figure 13.4   What you can do about inequalities in health: evidence-based options.

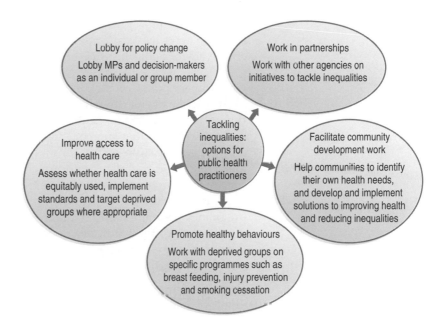

(MPs), regulatory bodies and other decision makers. Lobbying can be done:

- on an individual basis (such as letters to ministers and MPs); or
- through membership of national non-statutory organizations, for example, the Child Poverty Action Group or the UK Public Health Association (UKPHA), professional organizations (such as the Community Practitioners and Health Visitors Association or the Faculty of Public Health), trade unions or political parties.

The media can be an effective tool for public health lobbying.[30] Lobbying national decision makers has the potential advantage of allowing you to address the 'upstream' determinants of health and those who shape policies. At a local level you can act as an advocate for tackling inequalities within your own organization and across local partnerships.

It can be very difficult, however, to assess whether one is having an impact as a lobbyist or advocate. There has been little evaluative research on the impact of practitioners in lobbying for public health action to tackle health inequalities.

However, an assessment of its value can be gleaned by examining the shifting national policy on health inequalities. Throughout the 1980s and early 1990s, the Conservative government studiously ignored continued lobbying from the public health field on health inequalities. Most notably, the *Health of the Nation* White Paper[31] did not address health inequalities despite this being the most common issue raised by those who responded to the preceding consultative Green Paper. However, a number of commentators are confident that the lobbying of the public health field was important in finally bringing the government to acknowledge and begin to address health 'variations', and for the new Labour government to have it as high up its list of priorities as it did.[8] Practical advice on how to lobby effectively for public health is given by Muir Gray.[32]

PARTNERSHIPS WORKING

Government policy on tackling inequality emphasizes intersectoral and multidisciplinary partnership between local agencies and communities through the formation of *local strategic partnerships*. There is an increasing body of evidence that such partnership is an important prerequisite for effective local action on health inequalities. Arblaster and colleagues identify a multidisciplinary approach as an important characteristic of successful interventions to improve the health of disadvantaged groups in areas including injury prevention, reducing smoking and CHD risk, pregnancy prevention and sexual health.[27] Gillies has reviewed studies of partnerships for health promotion and concluded there is strong evidence for their effectiveness.[33]

You can contribute to partnership working on inequalities by:

- representing your agency on relevant partnership groups (such as local strategic partnerships, neighbourhood partnerships, healthy living centres); and
- facilitating partnership action on specific health-related issues (for example, promoting healthy eating, physical activity, tobacco control and so on).

Within such partnerships you can act as an advocate for:

- evidence-based universalist initiatives and services to tackle inequalities (such as universal pre-school education, affordable high quality day care,[29] vehicle speed reduction);[34] and
- targeted services where appropriate (for example, advice services to increase benefit uptake by disadvantaged groups).[27]

Important as partnership working undoubtedly is, there are opportunity costs in the time necessary to make partnerships work. There has been little robust evaluation of the relative benefits and costs of different models of partnership working or comparisons of their impact on inequalities. Published evaluations often focus on process issues and give practitioners only partial guidance on how to prioritize their time between the range of potential initiatives to tackle health inequalities.

COMMUNITY DEVELOPMENT

Community development has been defined as 'a process by which people are involved in collectively defining and taking action on issues that affect their lives.'[35]

For public health practitioners, it involves facilitating local communities:

- to identify their own health needs and agenda, and
- to develop and implement their own solutions to improving health and reducing inequalities.

Community development approaches have a long history in tackling inequalities and are often advocated.[36] There is a substantial, diverse and mainly qualitative literature describing it,[37,38] which is methodologically very different from the experimental studies that make up most of the reviews of interventions to tackle inequalities in health. The term 'community development' does not even feature in the indexes of two major recent collections on tackling inequalities in health.[10,39] Health sector led community development projects have been reported to be critical catalysts for regeneration in a number of deprived communities.[35,40–42]

PROMOTING HEALTHY BEHAVIOURS

There is an expanding literature on the effectiveness of health promotion programmes (such as smoking cessation, injury prevention, breast feeding) specifically targeted on individuals in lower socio-economic groups who are at higher risk of health damaging behaviours. The majority of the studies in Arblaster et al,[28] Roberts[29] and other reviews are experimental evaluations of these types of intervention. For example:

- Connett and Stamler have shown that interventions can be successfully carried out to reduce the incidence of smoking in deprived groups.[43] A recent NHS report from the North West region provides additional evidence that smoking cessation services can effectively reach and help smokers from deprived communities.[44]

- Colver and colleagues showed that pre-arranged home visits to identify specific targets for change in families living in a deprived area encouraged them to make changes in their homes that would be expected to reduce the risk of childhood accidents.[45]

- Oakley and colleagues demonstrated the effectiveness, appropriateness and safety of social support provided by midwives to women with high risk pregnancies.[46]

- A recent review suggests that small group informal discussions appear to be the most effective way to encourage breast feeding.[47]

Smoking accounts for over half of the health gap between more affluent and poorer men, so smoking cessation is potentially the single most important behavioural intervention to reduce inequalities in health.[48] (See also Ch. 4 'Smoking' and Ch. 14 'Helping individuals to change behaviour'.)

IMPROVING ACCESS TO HEALTH CARE

Access to the NHS is mainly free at the point of service and in principle universally accessible to everyone. In primary care, recent studies have found that lower income groups were more likely than others to use GP services, and that this higher usage broadly reflected need.[49] There is also a strong positive relationship between levels of deprivation and hospital outpatient and admission rates. There is, however, convincing evidence of socio-economic differences in the likelihood of receiving some specialist services and in survival. Several studies have found that men living in more affluent areas were more likely to receive a certain type of heart surgery (coronary revascularization) than men from poorer areas, despite having less need as measured by mortality rates.[50,51]

You can pursue more equitable access to health care through:

- universalist initiatives, including explicit referral guidelines and standards, such as maximum 2-week waits for cancer referrals; or
- selectivist approaches targeted on more deprived groups, such as home visiting for families in areas of deprivation.

Paterson and Judge identify 36 interventions either aimed at lower income groups or which report separate results for them.[49] Just over half (19) report interventions aimed at lower income groups which were judged effective. These studies were mainly from the USA and included interventions for cancer screening, treating health risks such as hypertension or substance misuse, and improving maternal health and child health. The interventions were diverse and included hospital-based education programmes, community outreach activities and home visiting.

As a service provider, the first step is to consider whether the services you provide are promoting equity and contributing to achieving health inequalities targets. The Department of Health has recently developed a basket of local indicators which can be used in local needs assessment, performance monitoring and equity audit.[1] Further guidance on equity audit is available at www.phel.gov.uk.

WHAT QUESTIONS STILL NEED ANSWERING?

As indicated above, there is a large and growing research base on the existence and causes of inequalities in health; the evidence on what works in reducing inequalities in health at either a national or local level is still relatively sparse. In particular:

- The government has invested huge sums in area-based initiatives such as Sure Start and healthy living centres. We need to know whether these interventions are effective either in improving the health of their populations or in 'bending' mainstream services.

- Similarly, we need to know if the effort required to make local partnerships work does deliver more effective local services which improve the health of the communities they serve.

CONCLUSION

The five options outlined above (Fig. 13.4) for practitioners to consider in tackling inequalities in health are not mutually exclusive and many practitioners adopt several or all of these approaches in different contexts. Unfortunately, there is no evidence base on which to decide what level of effort it is sensible to put into each; or indeed whether one should simply focus on universal health improvement and not seek specifically to tackle inequalities at all. The evidence base for the last two options is the largest and easiest to interpret, simply because they are more amenable to traditional methods of evaluation.

There are a number of constructive responses to this uncertainty. First, practitioners can seek to incorporate into their work Arblaster and colleagues' characteristics of successful interventions to reduce inequalities in health:

- systematic and intensive approaches
- improvements in access and prompts to encourage the use of services
- multifaceted interventions
- multidisciplinary approaches
- ensuring interventions meet identified need of the target population
- involvement of peers in the delivery of interventions.[28]

In addition, there are a small number of interventions which have a particularly strong evidence base for their effectiveness in tackling health inequalities, including:

- smoking cessation
- breast feeding support
- early years day care
- education and social support
- traffic speed reductions.

Thus you can usefully begin by considering whether such interventions are in operation in your patch, and if not, working to put them in place.

Key sources of further information and help

The first steps in any initiative to tackle inequalities in health are to identify the nature and extent of the inequality and then to search the literature to establish if any intervention has been shown to reduce it effectively. With the rapid expansion of internet-based knowledge sources, evidence of effective interventions will increasingly be most accessible online. Key sources of knowledge on tackling inequalities are listed below:

- **Department of Health:** www.dh.gov.uk. The DOH inequalities in health website pages can be found by following links from the DOH home page to a–z site index, health inequalities.
- **Department of Health:** *Independent inquiry into inequalities in health (Acheson report).*[7] See website www.doh.gov.uk/ih/ih.htm
- **Department of Health:** *Tackling health inequalities – a programme for action.*[1] See website www.doh.gov.uk/healthinequalities/programmeforaction.
- **Health Action Zones:** www.haznet.org.uk. HAZnet provides examples of good practice from the

Health Action Zone initiative for tackling health inequalities in England and Northern Ireland.

- **Health Development Agency:** www.hda-online.org.uk. The national authority on what works to improve people's health and reduce health inequalities. It gathers evidence and produces advice for policy makers, professionals and practitioners, working alongside them to get evidence into practice.
- **Health equity audit:** www.phel.gov.uk. PHEL is the Public Health Electronic Library which aims to provide knowledge and know-how to promote health, prevent disease and reduce health inequalities.
- **Health Equity Network:** www.ukhen.org.uk. This site is a resource for all those interested in equity and inequality in health, aiming to provide relevant information and links.
- **National Electronic Library for Health:** www.NELH.nhs.uk. A digital library for NHS staff, patients and the public.

References

1. Department of Health. Tackling health inequalities: a programme for action. London: Department of Health; 2003.

2. Last J. A dictionary of epidemiology. Oxford: Oxford University Press; 1995.

3. Wanless D. Securing good health for the whole population. London: HMSO; 2003.

4. Davey Smith G, Chaturvedi N, Harding S, et al. Ethnic inequalities in health: a review of UK epidemiological evidence. Critical Public Health 2000; 10(4):375–408.

5. Davey Smith G, Dorling D, Shaw M, eds. Poverty, inequality and health in Britain: a reader. Bristol: The Policy Press; 2001.

6. Department of Health and Social Security. Inequalities in health: report of a research working party (the Black report). London: DHSS; 1980.

7. Department of Health. Independent inquiry into inequalities in health (the Acheson report). London: The Stationery Office; 1998.

8. Baggot R. Public health: policy and politics. Basingstoke: Macmillan Press; 2000.

9. Macintyre S. The Black report and beyond: what are the issues? Social Science and Medicine 1997; 44(6):723–745.

10. Mackenbach J, Bakker M, eds. Reducing inequalities in health: a European perspective. London: Routledge; 2002.

11. Wilkinson R. Unhealthy societies: the afflictions of inequality. London: Routledge; 1996.

12. Davey Smith G, Gunnell D, Ben-Shlomo Y. Life-course approaches to socio-economic differentials in cause-specific adult mortality. In: Leon D, Walt G, eds. Poverty, inequality and health. Oxford: Oxford University Press; 2001.

13. Secretary of State for Health. Saving lives: our healthier nation. Cm 4386. London: The Stationery Office; 1999.

14. Department of Health. Reducing health inequalities: an action report. London: Department of Health; 1999.

15. Department of Health. The NHS plan: a plan for investment, a plan for reform. London: The Stationery Office; 2000.

16. HM Treasury/Department of Health. Tackling inequalities: summary of the 2002 cross cutting review. London: HM Treasury; 2002.

17. Wanless D. Securing our future health: taking a long term view. London: HM Treasury; 2002.

18. Secretary of State for Health. Valuing people: a new strategy for learning disability for the 21st century. Cm 5086. London: Stationery Office; 2001.

19. Exworthy M, Stuart M, Blane D, Marmot M. Tackling health inequalities since the Acheson report. Bristol: Policy Press; 2003.

20. Shaw M, Dorling D, Gordon D, Davey Smith G. The widening gap: health inequalities and policy in Britain. Bristol: Policy Press; 1999.

21. Davey Smith G, Dorling D, Mitchell R, Shaw M. Health inequalities in Britain: continuing increases up to the end of the 20th century. Journal of Epidemiology and Community Health 2002; 56(6):434–435.

22. Benzeval M, Taylor J, Judge K. Evidence on the relationship between low income and poor health: is the government doing enough? Fiscal Studies 2000; 21(3):375–399.

23. Exworthy M, Berney L, Powell M. 'How great expectations in Westminster may be dashed locally': the local implementation of national policy on health inequalities. Policy and Politics 2002; 30(1):79–96.

24. Davey Smith G, Dorling D, Gordon D, Shaw M. The widening health gap: what are the solutions? Critical Public Health 1999; 9(2):151–170.

25. Macintyre S, Chalmers I, Horton R, Smith R. Using evidence to inform health policy: case study. British Medical Journal 2001; 322(1280):222–225.

26. Davey Smith G, Ebrahim S, Frankel S. How policy informs the evidence: 'Evidence based' thinking can lead to debased policy making. British Medical Journal 2001; 322:184–185.

27. Arblaster L, Entwistle V, Lambert M, et al. Review of the research on the effectiveness of health service interventions to reduce variations in health. CRD Report 3. York: NHS Centre for Reviews and Dissemination; 1995.

28. Arblaster L, Lambert M, Entwistle V, et al. A systematic review of the effectiveness of health service interventions aimed at reducing inequalities in health. Journal of Health Services Research and Policy 1996; 1(2):93–103.

29. Roberts H. What works in reducing inequalities in child health. Barkingside: Barnardo's; 2000.

30. Chapman S. Using media advocacy to shape policy. In: Pencheon D, Gust C, Melzer D, Muir Gray J, eds. Oxford handbook of public health practice. Oxford: Oxford University Press; 2001.

31. Secretary of State for Health. The health of the nation. Cm 1986. London: HMSO; 1992.

32. Muir Gray J. The public health professional as political activist. In: Pencheon D, Gust C, Melzer D, Muir Gray J, eds. Oxford handbook of public health practice. Oxford: Oxford University Press; 2001.

33. Gillies P. Effectiveness of alliances and partnerships for health promotion. Health Promotion International 1998; 13:99–120.

34. Towner E, Dowswell T, Jarvis S. The effectiveness of health promotion interventions in the prevention of unintentional childhood injury: a review of the literature. London: Health Education Authority; 1993.

35. Radford G, Lapthorne D, Boot N, Maconachie M. Community development and social deprivation. In: Scally G, ed. Progress in public health. London: FT Healthcare; 1997.

36. Benzeval M, Judge K, Whitehead M, eds. Tackling inequalities in health: an agenda for action. London: King's Fund; 1995.

37. Beattie A. Success and failure in community development initiatives in National Health Service settings: eight case studies. Milton Keynes: Open University Press; 1991.

38. Stewart-Brown S, Prothero D. Evaluation in community development. Health Education Journal 1998; 47(4):156–161.

39. Leon D, Walt G, eds. Poverty, inequality and health. Oxford: Oxford University Press; 2001.

40. Hunt S. Evaluating a community development project. British Journal of Social Work 1987; 17(6):661–667.

41. Smithies J, Adams L. Community participation in health promotion. London: Health Education Authority; 1990.

42. Whitehead M. Tackling inequalities: a review of policy initiatives. In: Benzeval M, Judge K, Whitehead M, eds. Tackling inequalities in health: an agenda for action. London: King's Fund; 1995.

43. Connett J, Stamler J. Responses of black and white males to the special intervention programme of the Multiple Risk Factor Intervention Trial. American Heart Journal 1984; 108:839–849.

44. Lowey H, Fullard B, Tocque K, Bellis M. Are smoking cessation services reducing inequalities in health? Liverpool: North West Public Health Observatory; 2002.

45. Colver A, Hutchinson P, Judson E. Promoting children's home safety. British Medical Journal 1982; 285:1177–1180.

46. Oakley A, Rajan L, Grant A. Social support and pregnancy outcome. British Journal of Obstetrics and Gynaecology 1990; 97:155–162.

47. NHS Centre for Reviews and Dissemination. Promoting the initiation of breastfeeding. Effective Healthcare Bulletin 2000; 6(2):1–12.

48. Richardson K, Crosier A. Smoking and health inequalities. London: ASH/Health Development Agency; 2001.

49. Paterson I, Judge K. Equality of access to healthcare. In: Mackenbach J, Bakker M, eds. Reducing inequalities in health: a European perspective. London: Routledge; 2002.

50. Ben-Shlomo Y, Chaturvedi N. Assessing equity in access to health care provision in the UK: does where you live affect your chances of getting a coronary artery bypass graft? Journal of Epidemiology and Community Health 1995; 49:200–204.

51. Payne N, Saul C. Variations in use of cardiology services in a health authority: comparison of coronary artery revascularisation rates with prevalence of angina and coronary mortality. British Medical Journal 1997; 314:257–261.

Chapter 14

Helping individuals to change behaviour

Pip Mason

SUMMARY OVERVIEW AND LINKS TO OTHER TOPICS

Chapters 1 to 12 have shown that individuals' health-related behaviours make a major contribution to their own, and in some cases other people's, health. A common frustration expressed by health professionals is that their patients or clients do not make the behaviour changes expected of them.

The health professional's role is not to 'victim blame' or nag, but to adopt a patient-centred approach to empower individuals to make their own informed, well considered choices and carry them through into action as far as is possible in their current circumstances.

Many theoretical models address the process of changing health behaviours. One of the most useful and popular is the 'Stages of Change' model[1] in which people are seen to progress through a cycle of stages from contemplation through preparation and action to maintenance of a new behaviour.

Other models offer practical help for practitioners working with clients. Motivational interviewing is a counselling style that uses person-centred skills within a flexible structure for helping people to explore the pros and cons of change and to prepare for action. Rollnick et al's useful client consultation framework[2] identifies the important tasks of: establishing rapport and setting the agenda;

exchanging information; assessing importance, confidence and readiness to change; and building confidence, exploring importance and reducing resistance. Finally, this chapter looks at techniques for behaviour modification.

Is working with individuals effective in achieving behaviour change? This complex question is unpacked, and the conclusion is that the evidence is encouraging and that the patient-centred approach is beneficial for both client and professional.

Clearly this chapter is relevant to all others where health-related behaviour plays a part in the causation and management of health problems. It complements Chapter 13 'Tackling inequalities in health', which discusses how to change the conditions of living which shape and constrain individual health choices and behaviours.

WHY IS BEHAVIOUR CHANGE IMPORTANT?

Chapters 1 to 12 have shown that individuals' choices about how they live their lives make a major contribution to their own, and in some cases other people's, health. Individuals can increase their chances of living long, healthy lives by changing their eating, drinking, smoking, exercise and sexual behaviour and their use of medication and other drugs. Most medical and public health interventions rely on some level of active participation or at least cooperation by individuals.

A wide range of healthcare practitioners are engaged in helping people make lifestyle changes. These include, for example, doctors, nurses, pharmacists, podiatrists, dentists, accident and emergency staff, physiotherapists and dietitians.

IS FOCUSING ON BEHAVIOUR CHANGE VICTIM BLAMING?

A major frustration expressed by health professionals is that their patients or clients do not make the changes expected of them:

If only these people would help themselves sometimes.
How many times do we have to tell them?
That man is his own worst enemy!

Isn't this attitude just 'victim blaming' when we know that poverty and social inequalities play such an important part?

It can be. The picture is complex. Individuals make their choices within the context of their family, social and economic situations. Healthy choices are made easier or harder for them by external factors. However, some socially advantaged people make very unhealthy choices and some disadvantaged people choose healthily. Not all poor people smoke; not all professional people are physically active.

In this chapter we are not looking at blaming anyone. Neither are we looking at controlling or restricting choice. We are looking at *empowerment*: how to ensure that people are making informed, well considered choices and living the lives they really want to live, as far as is possible in their current situation. Health professionals cannot make people change but they have a role in facilitating people's decision making.

WHAT IS THE HEALTH PROFESSIONAL'S ROLE?

A PATIENT-CENTRED APPROACH

While health professionals have a clear public health agenda, the people consulting them may have several agendas competing for attention. There is increasing interest and research into patient- or person-centred approaches to consultations about health which respect and take account of the patient's viewpoint.[3,4]

These have developed out of the wish to improve on the success rates gained by simply giving people advice and information. Brief interventions to promote change in behaviours such as smoking and drinking, though cost-effective, only bring about change in a small minority of people. Also, clinicians have consistently shown reluctance to deliver such brief advice in a systematic way outside of a research project. In primary care particularly, where health professionals have long term relationships with their patients, the quality of the interaction and a holistic understanding of the family and social context are valued highly. Neither patients nor practitioners want consultations to become opportunities for the hapless patients to be harangued about what they could be doing to improve their health.

A RANGE OF ROLES AND TASKS

Health professionals are accustomed to taking different roles to meet the demands of the situation. Paramedics and intensive care staff take complete control over a person's life for a period because the patient is (usually temporarily) unable to regulate their own body functions in the normal way. Decisions are made for the person about their breathing, fluid intake, medication, whether relatives can be in attendance and so on. As the sick person recovers, control is given back gradually and the healthcare staff move more into a role of offering help, drinks, food, pain control, elective surgery and so on. In some scenarios the health carer takes on an educational role to help the patient manage a new situation, teaching them, for example, how to administer an insulin injection or do exercises to regain function in a damaged limb.

Moving from one role to another is demanding. The author found this a challenge on the first ward she worked on as a student nurse. All the patients had experienced strokes but were in different stages of recovery. Some needed a high level of care with basic functions and were unable to make their own decisions as yet. Some would be able to go home once they regained their independence but were demoralized by their illness and needed a vast amount of encouragement to get dressed and feed themselves. It was easier for busy nurses to feed and dress everyone, but the quality nursing care came from judging how much function each person had regained and encouraging them to push themselves to their limits in the interests of their longer term independence.

So what is the appropriate role to take in health promotion work? In a consultation about behaviour change there are three levels of task.

● The first is to ensure the person has, and understands, all relevant information about what impact the behaviour has on their health and what change would entail. (This is the health professional's agenda.)

- The second level is to assist them to make a decision whether or not to change. (This is the patient or client's agenda.)

- If they decide to change, the third level is to help them work out how to do it, build their confidence and support them through the process. (This is joint problem-solving.)

It is interesting to see how easy it is to move from level one to level three and miss out the crucial decision-making stage:

'You need to lose weight. The pain in your back and knees is made much worse by carrying that extra couple of stones. You know that don't you? Now I want you to look at this diet sheet. If you follow it you should lose a couple of pounds a week. It would be good to do a bit of exercise too. We can give you free membership of an exercise class on prescription under a new scheme. They do a yoga class and that would be a good place to start. I'd like you to come back in a week's time to see how you're getting on. We'll give you all the help we can.'

Because level two is missing this consultation comes over as rather 'bossy' although constructive help is being offered. How would you respond if you were the patient?

WHAT MODELS DO WE HAVE FOR UNDERSTANDING HEALTH BEHAVIOUR CHANGE?

Several models have been put forward to explain the process of changing health behaviours and to predict it. Some focus mainly on the decision to change. For example:

- Self-efficacy theory focuses on perceptions of self-efficacy and outcome expectations, i.e. do I believe I can master this behaviour change and do I believe it will lead to the outcomes I desire?[5]

- Janis and Mann use the concept of a decisional balance to describe how ambivalence is explored and resolved in the process of making a decision.[6]

- The theory of reasoned action model focuses on attitudes and intention and takes account of normative values.[7,8]

- The theory of planned behaviour[9] is an extension of the theory of reasoned action to include those behaviours where the person does not feel entirely in control of or able to perform the behaviour.

- Behavioural choice theory addresses the question of how individuals decide between various options.[10]

KEY THEMES

There are some key threads running through these models, seen from the client's perspective:

- What information do I have about the impact this behaviour has on health?
- Do I believe this information?
- Do I consider it relevant to me?

- Do I see my health as a priority at the moment?
- What do I like about the way I live now and am I willing to give that up?
- Do I believe this behaviour is potentially within my control?
- If so do I have faith in my ability to make changes?

So, an obese person advised repeatedly to lose weight may not do so because of one or more of the following:

- He does not fully understand the connection between obesity and health.

- He understands what the doctor is saying but believes that 'you go when your time has come'. His father was thin and died young. His mother was fat and lived well into her retirement.

- He finds going to the pub for a few pints of beer and having fish and chips on the way home a great way to unwind at the end of the day. With the life he's living at the moment he feels he deserves a pint and a decent supper.

- He has always been on the heavy side and is not aware of any deterioration in his health other than that which he attributes to the normal ageing process.

- At present he is very stressed at work and also busy helping a daughter whose marriage has broken up, leaving her with a young family and money problems. His own weight is the least of his worries.

- He believes he inherited his body shape and his large appetite from his mother. His sister is the same. She's always going on diets and it doesn't seem to make much difference to her. In a month or two she reverts to her normal eating pattern and the weight all goes back on again. 'You are what you are.'

- Even if changing his eating and being more active would lead to weight loss, he can't imagine himself eating salads and going to the gym. He's 'not that sort of person'.

THE 'STAGES OF CHANGE' MODEL

Another model, which has become very popular, describes the stages people go through in making a change and helps us to understand why various interventions are effective. Prochaska and DiClemente's 'Stages of Change' model[1] is transtheoretical (meaning that it draws from a range of psychological theories). It was originally developed from research into smoking cessation but has since been found applicable to a range of other health and social behaviours. The model describes people moving from 'precontemplation' into four stages of change:

- contemplation
- preparation (or 'determination')
- action
- maintenance,

and the regular occurrence of 'relapse' when the person reverts back to old ways. This cycle is illustrated in Figure 14.1.

Figure 14.1   Prochaska and DiClemente's Stages of Change model.[1]

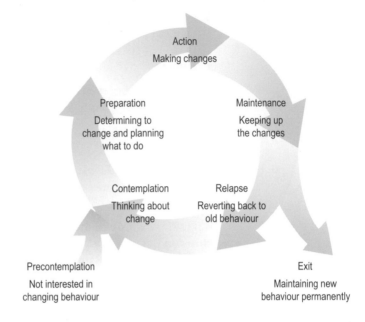

At each stage people are engaged in different activities and mental processes. These are described as:

- consciousness-raising (becoming aware there is an issue to address);
- social liberation (social changes making healthier choices easier);
- emotional arousal (a major emotional experience triggered by an event relevant to the problem);
- self re-evaluation (wondering 'Who am I? Who do I want to be and how does this behaviour fit into that?');
- commitment (making a robust decision to change);
- countering (doing other things instead, for example going to the swimming pool instead of the pub after work, having cereal for breakfast instead of a bacon sandwich);
- environment control (taking charge of one's surroundings);
- rewards (making it more worthwhile and appreciating the intrinsic benefits of change);
- helping relationship (engaging with support offered).

The 'Stages of Change' model can help in the following ways.

- Health professionals can see that their role is to support natural processes of change. Intervention to promote health behaviour change might be better seen as supported self-help rather than treatment.

- It can help health professionals to see what sort of help is appropriate: for example, it is unhelpful to discuss how a person might try to stop smoking (appropriate for the 'preparation' stage) if they have not yet decided whether to do so (because they are at the 'contemplation' stage).

- It can also help clients and practitioners to see that 'relapse' is not a disastrous failure, but part of a normal cycle of behaviour change. It can provide an opportunity for clients to work out why they lapsed and find strategies to help prevent it happening again.

(For a critique of this model see Miller and Heather.[11])

WHAT MODELS DO WE HAVE FOR PRACTICAL WORK WITH INDIVIDUALS?

When working with individuals it is not possible or helpful to separate social and psychological factors. Advice and information clearly have a part to play but the real impetus for individual change comes from the way people receive and make sense of what health professionals tell them in the context of their own life experiences and values. We have seen that there are models that help us to understand behaviour change: now we consider models and guidelines for practical work with individuals.

MOTIVATIONAL INTERVIEWING

In the area of the addictions much work has been done developing approaches that facilitate people in making robust decisions to change.[12] It has long been recognized, when trying to help people dependent on alcohol or drugs, that a person's ambivalence about change is not just an obstacle to solving the problem; it is a *major part of* the problem. Any approach that does not engage and work with the ambivalence is missing the point. Miller and Rollnick's motivational interviewing is a counselling style that uses person-centred skills within a flexible structure for helping people to explore the pros and cons of change and to prepare for action. It has been defined as: 'a client-centred, directive method for enhancing intrinsic motivation to change by exploring and resolving ambivalence'.[13]

Below is a brief overview of motivational interviewing and it will be clear that the key themes outlined in the section above on behaviour change models run through it. We examine motivational interviewing by looking at:

- how to engage constructively with a client's feelings of *ambivalence* and *resistance*;
- how to deal with the key issues of the *importance* of the change for the client, and their *confidence* in making it.

Ambivalence

Ambivalence about change is normal. When we consider a change we can see advantages and disadvantages of the way things are now, and we can see advantages and disadvantages of the change. The decision hangs in the balance until something tips it in one or other direction. For example, a woman in her thirties considering giving up smoking might see it as described in Box 14.1.

How does all this balance up for the woman? We cannot tell just by looking at it because it depends on her value system and her current life situation. If she feels reasonably healthy at the moment, apart from some minor problems which she puts down to stress, the health gain of quitting will not weigh heavily but the fact that she feels smoking helps her cope with stress will be a real plus in favour of continuing to smoke. If

---

Box 14.1   Client's views on the pros and cons of smoking

Pros of smoking

- I really enjoy a cigarette with a drink
- It seems to help me unwind when stressed
- It gives me something to do with my hands
- It helps me keep my weight down.

Cons of smoking

- It's bad for my health
- It's expensive
- I get nicotine stains on hands and teeth
- It makes the house smell
- It's bad for my skin
- It's socially unacceptable.

Pros of quitting

- It'll reduce risks to my health
- It'll save money eventually
- I'll have a clean skin
- I'll have a clean house
- If I start a family it's better for a baby.

Cons of quitting

- Withdrawal symptoms – irritability
- Withdrawal – poor concentration
- How will I cope with stress?
- I'll put on weight
- Nicotine patches cost ££.

---

she is in a happy relationship and considering a family the possibility of gaining a bit of weight may be something she feels she can cope with, but the impact on a future pregnancy will be important. If she's single and actively looking for a partner the issues around appearance and social acceptability may take a higher priority.

So the task is not to explore *what are the pros and cons about smoking and quitting?* but *what are the pros and cons of smoking and quitting for you, at the moment?*

It can take weeks, months, years or a lifetime for the ambivalence to be resolved. People's perceptions of the pros and cons change as they move through Prochaska and DiClemente's stages of change (see Fig. 14.1).[1] 'Contemplators' are highly ambivalent. The temptation for the health professional is to try and hurry this process by emphasizing how bad the current behaviour is and how beneficial change would be. It is also tempting to minimize or even argue with the benefits of the current behaviour and the disadvantages of change. Then the tendency is to move swiftly into suggesting solutions:

'Smoking doesn't really help you cope with stress; nicotine is a stimulant and the stress you experience is really withdrawal and a craving for the next cigarette. That would go away in time if you were to stop. Meanwhile perhaps you could try some aromatherapy or some relaxation tapes? Putting on a few pounds is not a serious health risk compared to smoking. I wouldn't worry about that too much and think of how much better your skin and teeth will be! The withdrawal symptoms can be a nuisance but not everybody has really bad symptoms and we can give you some patches or gum to help with that. We can give it on prescription now to save you money. It's best to give up smoking before you get pregnant because we're not so keen on people using nicotine replacement once

they're pregnant. Shall I tell you about the groups that have started running on Thursday nights?'

This is where resistance can come in.

Resistance

People who have more or less made up their mind to quit and have come for advice on how to do it might find the above advice helpful and supportive but what might go through the ambivalent contemplator's mind?

'I don't know about that; I feel much better when I've had a fag break. Even the first drag calms me down. I can't exactly put on relaxation tapes at work can I? It's all right for you to say don't worry about a few pounds. Look at how slim you are! My skin and teeth aren't that bad, if you don't mind, but my husband can't bear fat women. No chance of getting pregnant if I start piling on the weight! I don't fancy those patches. My friend tried them and they gave her a horrible skin rash and I'm certainly not going to group therapy! Sitting around with a lot of strangers moaning about how hard it is ...'

So what's going on here? The health professional took on one side of the ambivalence and began promoting change. The ambivalent smoker then found herself supporting the other side and rehearsing the arguments against change. (This may have been a mental process only, if the smoker is polite and wants to appear compliant, or it might result in a confrontational verbal exchange.) The outcome is that the smoker becomes more aware and attached to the arguments for continuing smoking and defends herself against the well-meaning and potentially useful advice given.

What the health professional needs to do is to act as a sounding board for the smoker, allowing her to express and explore all the views she has about smoking, providing information in a way that will facilitate an informed decision without eliciting more resistance. So how can this be done?

Importance and confidence

It can be helpful to think about this work in terms of an enquiry or exploration rather than an intervention. If we ask someone how they feel about a behaviour change and express genuine interest and curiosity they tend to become more curious themselves and look more deeply into their own attitudes. We are thus encouraging and supporting the important stage of contemplation. The complex mesh of beliefs and attitudes that contribute to change can be explored under the umbrella of two key concepts: importance and confidence. The importance to a person of making the change and the confidence they have that an attempt would be successful are two very different aspects of their beliefs about it. When there is a high level of importance and a lot of confidence this becomes a powerful cocktail and becomes readiness to do it.

In brief consultations it is helpful to have an element of structure to keep this enquiry focused. The use of scaling questions (adapted from those originally formulated by de Shazer and colleagues)[12] has been found helpful as a starting point. In Box 14.2 is an example of how they might be used by a nurse with an overweight male patient.

Box 14.2   Enquiring about importance and confidence using scaling questions

Nurse: *One of the things that is making your knee problems worse is the extra weight you're carrying. I think we've discussed this before.*

Patient: Yes, I know it doesn't help but I don't really know what I can do about it.

Nurse: *Is losing weight something that's important to you?*

Patient: Well, I'd like to do something to make me a bit more mobile and ease the trouble in my knees but I've never been one for all those weird diets.

Nurse: *So, in some ways you'd like to lose weight but you don't much fancy the idea of going on a diet. Can I try asking you like this? If there's a scale from 1 to 10 and 1 is 'It's not at all important to me to lose weight' and 10 is 'Doing something to help me lose weight is the most important thing to me in my life at the moment' what number would you give it at the moment?*

Patient: Well, if you had a magic wand and I didn't have to put any effort in I'd go for 10 straight away but realistically probably about half way. Say 5 or 6.

Nurse: *So around halfway or a bit more. Why is it a 5 or 6 rather than lower? Tell me about the part of you that would like to do it.*

Patient: Well, I already said about my back and knees. I hate not being able to move in other ways too. It's a struggle to put my shoes on or pick things up off the floor or even to get in and out of the car, and I have to go to special shops to get my clothes these days.

Nurse: *That sounds expensive!*

Patient: It is. I can't get the bargains off the market any more; they don't fit.

Nurse: *So, being overweight makes a difference to your life in other ways apart from your health.*

Patient: I do worry about the health side too. I know you're more likely to get diabetes if you're big, and heart attacks and although it sounds like I'm having a moan today I'm not ready to go yet!

Nurse: *So there's your health, not being very agile, and the problems you have buying clothes all making it up to a 5 or 6. What would need to happen to make it important enough to do it?*

Patient: Actually the more I talk about it the more I realize it bugs me. Perhaps it's not so much that I don't want to do it but I don't know if I could.

Nurse: *So perhaps the importance is even higher than a 6. What do you think you'd have to do to lose enough weight to make a difference to you?*

Patient: Eat less! That's the trouble. I eat all the wrong things and lots of it! I like a beer too and I know that's fattening. If I lost a bit I might be able to do a bit more exercise which would help, but I don't know what I could manage with my knees and I've never been the sporty type.

Nurse: *So you don't need me to tell you what you'd have to do but you're not all that optimistic. If I ask you about another scale about your confidence where 1 is 'I could never stick to a diet and lose weight' and 10 is 'I could do it any time I liked if I chose to' what number would you give yourself for confidence?*

Patient: Quite low. 2 or 3.

Nurse: *Hmm. So the confidence isn't so high. But I'm interested that you didn't say 1! I thought you might. Is there a bit of you that thinks it's not completely hopeless then?*

Patient: Oh! I wonder why I said that! I suppose there's a bit of me that's quite stubborn and if I make my mind up to do something I do tend to give it my best shot. I'm not like my sister who starts a diet and can't keep to it for 5 minutes. I'd need to set myself really clear rules and then I'd stick to them against all odds to show everybody. But they'd have to be realistic and I can't imagine quite what would work for me.

Nurse: *So, you're quite high up the scale in terms of wanting to lose weight, for a lot of reasons, not just because of the joint problems we've been discussing earlier. You're less positive about whether you could do it. Although you know you're the sort of person who would stick to a plan once you made your mind up you can't see just now what sort of plan would be realistic, for you, in your life. So where does this leave you now?*

Patient: Not sure. I need to have a real think about what I could do and whether I really want to give it a go. The other nurse gave me some leaflets a while back and my sister's got loads of books on diets but I'm not sure they're all particularly healthy. Would you be able to help me here at all with weighing and so on?

You can see in this example how the patient is encouraged to explore and elaborate on his concerns about his weight and his beliefs about the possibilities of change by a few brief but well chosen interventions by the nurse.

Most of the nurse's interventions are open questions and reflections of what the patient has said himself. The scaling questions help focus. Asking why the numbers given are as high as they are encourages him to express (and hear back when it is reflected) what motivation and faith in himself he has. By the end of this exchange he is actively seeking information and support, and talking in terms of taking some control over his eating because that is what he wants to do, rather than just to be compliant. He has not, however, embarked on a change plan and it may be some time before he is ready to 'give it his best shot' as he puts it. The nurse does not push him prematurely into such a commitment and thus elicits no real resistance.

It is, of course, possible he will ultimately be unable to find a plan that he believes in and is willing to stick to. If so, the nurse will not have failed. She too will have 'given it her best shot' and given him the support to explore it thoroughly. There are no magic tricks to make people want to change or to make it easy for them to do so.

This example is intended merely to give a flavour of the sort of approach that is currently finding favour in working with individuals around health behaviour change. There has been much interest in training health practitioners to use motivational interviewing in health promotion consultations as it has been found so useful in specialist addictions work. However, as a counselling approach it does require a high level of skill in reflective listening and lengthier consultations than most health professionals have available to them. Consequently, the model has been adapted to be more appropriate to a public health or primary care setting.[2]

This style was originally developed in the context of one-to-one consultations but the spirit of it and key concepts are also being used in group work such as smoking cessation courses.

A CLIENT CONSULTATION FRAMEWORK

A useful framework for thinking about what is involved in a consultation about behaviour change in a public health setting was developed by Rollnick, Mason and Butler and is set out in Figure 14.2.[2]

This framework identifies tasks which are not necessarily carried out in a tidy step-by-step way, but which provide a set of optional strategies for practitioners to choose from.

● The tasks of *establishing rapport* and *setting the agenda* are about making introductions and deciding the focus of the discussion in a non-confrontational, non-threatening way. With some clients the agenda is obvious because they come with a single issue to address, but others may have a range of health behaviours they are considering changing so that it is necessary to agree which to focus on.

● The task of *exchanging information* is likely to happen at any stage of the consultation. It is an *exchange*: the client is the expert on his own

Figure 14.2   Key tasks in consultations about behaviour change. (Reproduced with permission from Rollnick et al 1999.[2])

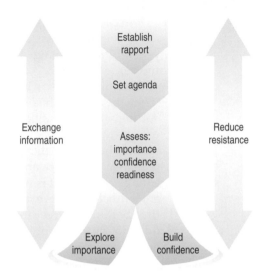

knowledge, feelings and circumstances; the practitioner has expertise on the health issue under discussion. If the client already knows what 'should' be done, the practitioner may not give any information at all.

● The tasks of *assessing importance, confidence and readiness* are crucial. Assessing readiness to change can be helped by bearing in mind the 'Stages of Change' model we have already discussed (Fig. 14.1).

● *Building confidence, exploring importance and reducing resistance* were all discussed in more detail above when we looked at motivational interviewing.

TECHNIQUES OF BEHAVIOUR MODIFICATION

If clients are ready to change, see the change as important, and are reasonably confident about it, what further help is there?

Techniques of behaviour modification have been developed to help people adopt a healthier pattern of, for example, eating or activity, and have been shown to be effective.[14]

They are rooted in cognitive behavioural therapy, which:

● Helps people to challenge and change unhelpful thoughts and beliefs that underlie their behaviour (e.g. I'm a fat person so I'm not worth helping);

● Finds ways of changing unhelpful established behaviour patterns (e.g. a habit of buying cigarettes with the morning newspaper on the way to work).

Box 14.3[15] summarizes some techniques which practitioners may find useful when helping people to change eating behaviour, but many can appropriately be adapted to use with other behaviours. People will, of course, only be interested in these ideas if they are committed to change and at the stage of preparing to take action.

Box 14.3   Techniques of behaviour modification for weight management (Reproduced with permission from Thomas 2001[15])

Stimulus control

- Shopping: don't go food shopping when you're hungry; only buy what's on the shopping list; only carry enough money for the foods on the list.
- Planning meals: plan what you'll eat for meals and snacks; eat at scheduled times; don't accept food offered by others.
- Availability of food: remove inappropriate foods from your home or at least put them out of sight; keep healthier food visible; eat all food in the same place.
- Serving food: use smaller plates; avoid being the person who serves out the food; leave the table immediately after eating; save leftovers for another meal instead of finishing them off.
- Holidays and parties: prepare in advance what you'll do; practise polite ways to decline food and drink.

Eating behaviour

- Eat slowly and chew thoroughly.
- Pause in the middle of a meal to assess hunger.
- Do nothing else while eating except enjoy the food.

Physical activity

- Plan how to increase activity in everyday life, such as walking and climbing stairs more.
- Keep a record of frequency, intensity and duration of activities such as walking.
- Start a mild exercise programme and keep a record of it.

Social support

- Ask family and friends to help by: showing interest and encouragement; not giving you food presents (e.g. chocolates) or offering second helpings; not pressing you to eat or drink when you say 'no thanks'.

Rewards

- Ask family and friends to help with praise and material rewards.
- Keep records to monitor your behaviour as a basis for rewarding yourself.
- Plan specific rewards for specific behaviour.
- Gradually make rewards more difficult to achieve.

Cognitive restructuring

- Set achievable, realistic weight loss and behaviour change goals.
- Focus on progress not shortcomings.
- Avoid imperatives such as 'never' (e.g. I'll never eat chocolate again) or 'always' (e.g. I'll always exercise every day).
- Challenge and counter self-defeating thoughts with positive thoughts.

Relapse management

- Learn to see lapses as opportunities to learn more about your behaviour change.
- Identify triggers to lapses.
- Plan in advance how to prevent lapses.
- Generate a list of coping strategies for high risk situations.
- Distinguish hunger from cravings.
- Make a list of things to do which make it impossible to give in to cravings.
- Confront or ignore cravings.
- Outlast urges to eat.

IS WORKING WITH INDIVIDUALS EFFECTIVE?

There are a number or research questions here. At present we have better answers to some than others.

DOES INDIVIDUAL BEHAVIOUR CHANGE IMPROVE HEALTH?

It is a core assumption that if people change their behaviour in particular ways they will experience better health or be at reduced risk of poor health. The evidence for this in relation to each topic has been discussed in previous chapters.

IS IT WORTH TALKING TO INDIVIDUALS ABOUT BEHAVIOUR CHANGE AT ALL?

Is it worth it – as opposed to fiscal measures, legislation, reduction of social inequalities and so on?

The answer to this seems to be 'yes'. In earlier chapters, such as those on smoking and alcohol, the extensive research into the effectiveness of counselling and brief interventions in primary care has been mentioned. A small percentage of people who receive brief advice from a respected health professional do make changes. This small percentage would add up to a huge public health gain if such interventions were used widely and consistently, but we still have the challenge of achieving widespread implementation.

Brief interventions by health professionals are, of course, only credible against a backcloth of population and other measures. For example, patients would be more cynical about health service professionals' advice to give up smoking if nothing were being done to restrict advertising and if nicotine replacement therapy were not available on prescription with support available to would-be quitters.

DOES A MORE PATIENT–CENTRED APPROACH WORK BETTER THAN AN ADVICE-GIVING STYLE?

This is a complex research area and fraught with methodological problems. However, the evidence we do have suggests it does, at least slightly. And perhaps more importantly, health professionals prefer it because it fits in with the way they see their relationships with patients or clients and does not feel like 'nagging', so they may be more likely to continue doing it. (For a review of the research on this see Rollnick et al[2] and Miller and Rollnick.[13])

WHAT ABOUT BRIEF AS OPPOSED TO LONGER INTERVENTIONS?

This is a complex question. It depends what you mean by brief, who intervenes and what sort of people are the recipients. For GPs, brief advice might take a couple of minutes and they would need patients to make special appointments in order to be able to spend as much as 15 minutes on health promotion. For people severely dependent on alcohol 6 hours' counselling would be considered a brief form of treatment, whereas for people dependent on nicotine intensive treatment it might be six half-hour sessions. There is not always a clear line between 'health promotion' and 'treatment'.

All sorts of interventions seem to help all sorts of people and it is necessary to look at the literature on each topic area to see how much understanding we have gained so far about matching people to briefer or longer interventions.

Key sources of further information and help

Further reading

- Hunt P, Hillsden M. Changing eating and exercise behaviour. Oxford: Blackwell; 1996.
- Miller W, Rollnick S. Motivational interviewing. New York: Guilford; 2002.
- Rollnick S, Mason P, Butler C. Health behavior change. Edinburgh: Churchill Livingstone; 1999.

Research reports and training

- **www.motivationalinterview.org:** the official motivational interviewing website, providing information about the approach, as well as links, training resources, and information on reprints and recent research.

References

1. Prochaska JO, DiClemente CC. Stages and processes of self-change of smoking: Towards an integrated model of change. Journal of Consulting and Clinical Psychology 1983; 51:390–395.
2. Rollnick S, Mason P, Butler C. Health behavior change, a guide for practitioners. Edinburgh: Churchill Livingstone; 1999.
3. Stewart M, Stewart M, Bellebrown J, et al. Patient-centred medicine. Transforming the clinical method. Thousand Oaks: Sage; 1995.
4. Stott NCH, Rees M, Rollnick S, Pill R, Hackett P. Professional responses to innovation in clinical method: diabetes care and negotiation skills. Patient Education and Counselling 1996; 29:67–73.
5. Bandura A. Self-efficacy: toward a unifying theory of behavioural change. Psychological Review 1977; 84:191–215.
6. Janis IL, Mann L. Decision making: a psychological analysis of conflict, choice and commitment. New York: Collier Macmillan; 1977.
7. Ajzen I, Fishbein M. Understanding attitudes and predicting social behaviour. Englewood Cliffs, NJ: Prentice Hall; 1980.
8. Fishbein M, Ajzen I. Belief, attitude, intention and behaviour. New York: Wiley; 1975.
9. Ajzen I. Attitudes, personality and behaviour. Milton Keynes. Open University Press; 1988.
10. Marcus BH, Forsyth LA. Motivating people to be physically active. Champaign, IL: Human Kinetics; 2003.
11. Miller WR, Heather N, eds. Treating addictive behaviours. 2nd edn. New York: Plenum; 1998.
12. De Shazer S, Berg I, Lipchick E, et al. Brief therapy: a focused solution development. Family Process 1986; 25:207–222.
13. Miller W, Rollnick S. Motivational interviewing. New York: Guilford; 2002.
14. Scottish Intercollegiate Guidelines Network. Obesity in Scotland: integrating prevention with weight management. Edinburgh: SIGN; 1996.
15. Thomas B, ed, in conjunction with the British Dietetic Association. Manual of dietetic practice. Oxford: Blackwell; 2001.

Glossary

Aetiology	The cause of diseases and disorders.
Age adjusted rate	A way of comparing rates in which allowances have been made for the different age structures of populations. This means that fair comparisons can be made between populations with, for example, different proportions of children or older people.
Angina	Chest pain caused by heart disease.
Antimicrobial	A drug or other substance that kills or suppresses microorganisms.
Antiretroviral	A drug or other substance that kills or suppresses retroviruses such as HIV.
Body mass index (BMI)	A measure of a person's relative weight for height, calculated by dividing weight in kilograms by height in metres squared (kg/m^2).
Brief interventions	Providing advice and feedback to people in a short space of time such as 5 or 10 minutes. For example, may be used by GPs in advising people to stop smoking or cut down on alcohol intake.
Carcinogen	Substance that, when exposed to living tissue, may cause the production of cancer.
Cardiorespiratory	To do with heart and lung function.
Cardiovascular	To do with the heart and blood circulation.
Cardiovascular disease	Diseases of the heart and the body's circulatory system; includes coronary heart disease and stroke.
Chemotherapy	Treatment of disease with chemicals such as cancer destroying drugs.

Cognitive behavioural models	Approaches to psychotherapy focused on changing ways a person thinks and behaves.
Cohort study	A research study that examines a whole group of people over a period of time.
Community development	Working with people to identify their concerns, and support them in collective action for the good of the community as a whole.
Community Safety Partnerships	Partnerships drawing members from a range of agencies working together to create safer places for people to live and work in, tackling issues such as crime, violence, accidents and injuries.
Computerized tomography (CT scans)	Specialized form of X-ray examination producing cross-sectional images; can be used to detect tumours.
Congenital	A condition present since birth, whether inherited or caused by environmental factors.
Connexions	Government-funded local partnership in England designed to provide help, support, advice and guidance for all young people aged 13–19. Connexions Access Points are centres where young people can get advice and help on issues such as education and training, and housing.
Coronary heart disease (CHD)	Heart disease caused by poor circulation of blood to the heart muscle because the blood vessels have become blocked. This may show up as a heart attack or chest pain (angina).
Drug Action Team	Multidisciplinary, cross-agency groups working together to reduce drug misuse in the community; includes social services, education, health services and the police.
Drug Treatment and Testing Orders (DTTO) scheme	Scheme whereby people can opt to enter a drug misuse treatment programme and undergo regular drug testing as opposed to having a custodial sentence.
Ectopic pregnancy	Development of a fetus at a site other than in the uterus.
Environment Agency	The leading public body for protecting and improving the environment in England and Wales. Its job is to make sure that air, land and water are looked after by everyone in today's society, so that tomorrow's generations inherit a cleaner, healthier world.
Epidemic	An outbreak of disease where the number of people affected is clearly in excess of what is normally expected. The term 'epidemic proportions' is often applied to health problems (such as obesity) which are not communicable diseases, but which become prevalent in the population.

Epidemiology	The study of the distribution, determinants and control of disease in populations.
Evidence based	Based on reliable research evidence that an intervention (such as a medical treatment or a public health programme) works.
Food Standards Agency	An independent food safety watchdog set up by an Act of Parliament in 2000 to protect the public's health and consumer interests in relation to food.
Genotype	The genetic constitution of an individual or group, as determined by the particular set of genes it possesses.
Gestational	During pregnancy.
Green Paper	A government policy document issued for consultation; it becomes a White Paper when it is finalized and formally agreed as government policy.
Health Action Zones	Areas of high health need selected by the government for special funding and health programmes run by partnerships of NHS, local authority and other agencies.
Health and Safety Executive	Public body responsible for the regulation of almost all the risks to health and safety arising from work activity in the UK. Its mission is to protect people's health and safety by ensuring risks in the changing workplace are properly controlled.
Health Development Agency (HDA)	The national authority for England on what works to improve people's health and reduce health inequalities. It gathers evidence and produces advice for policy makers, professionals and practitioners, working alongside them to get evidence into practice. There are comparable bodies in Scotland (the Health Education Board for Scotland), Wales (the Health Promotion Division of the National Assembly for Wales), and Northern Ireland (the Health Promotion Agency for Northern Ireland).
Health promoting schools	Networks of schools committed to a 'whole school approach' to promoting health with programmes of social, personal and health education for the pupils and a wider focus on the way the school is run and the health and well-being of staff, parents and the local community who have contact with the school.
Health promotion	The process of enabling people to increase control over, and to improve, their health.
Health Protection Agency (HPA)	A national organization for England and Wales, established in 2003, dedicated to protecting people's health and reducing the impact of infectious diseases, chemical hazards, poisons and radiation hazards. It brings together the expertise of health and scientific professionals working in

public health, communicable disease, emergency planning, infection control, laboratories, poisons, chemical and radiation hazards.

Health–related behaviour   What people habitually do in their daily life which affects their health: usually refers to issues such as whether they smoke, whether they take exercise, what they eat, their sexual behaviour, how much alcohol they drink, and drug use. Sometimes simply called 'health behaviour'.

Helicobacter pylori   A bacterium found in the stomach. It can cause inflammation and ulcers; it is implicated in some forms of stomach cancer.

High risk approach   Public health approach which prioritizes people particularly at risk of ill health. (Compare with *whole population* approach.)

Hypoglycaemia   Low level of glucose in the bloodstream, causing faintness, mental confusion and sweating; may be called a 'hypo'.

ICD–10 Classification   WHO International Statistical Classification of Diseases and Related Health Problems. An internationally recognized way of classifying diseases.

Incidence   The number of new episodes of illness arising in a population over a specified period of time. (Compare with *prevalence*.)

Inequalities in health   The gap between the health of different population groups, such as better off and more deprived communities, or people with different ethnic backgrounds.

Invasive procedures   Medical procedures which involve getting into the body, e.g. through surgery or insertion of an instrument into an orifice.

Key stage   Broad stage of learning when children must be taught specified parts of the National Curriculum. At Key Stage 1 children are ages 5–7; at Key Stage 2 ages 7–11; at Key Stage 3 ages 11–14; at Key Stage 4 ages 14–16.

Lifestyle   The particular way of life of a person or group, often referring to health-related behaviour such as smoking, drinking, diet and exercise.

Local Strategic Partnerships (LSP)   Local authority, health services and other agencies working together to develop and implement local strategy for improving economic, social and environmental well-being.

Locus of control   Psychological concept about the centre of responsibility for a person's behaviour. People with an *internal* locus of control tend to believe that they can control events related to their life, whereas people with an *external* locus of control tend to believe that forces outside themselves determine their lives.

Longitudinal study	A prospective research study which follows up subjects at intervals over a long period of time, with the aim of identifying patterns of disease and associated factors. (See also *prospective study*.)
Looked after children	Children in the care of the local authority. Also known as 'children in care'.
Maculopathy	Abnormality of the macula (a part of the retina at the back of the eye).
Meta–analysis	A systematic review which analyses and aggregates the results of many research studies on the same topic.
Metastasize	The spread of malignant tumours (cancer).
Morbidity/morbidity rate	Illness/incidence of illness in a population in a given period.
Mortality/mortality rate	Death/incidence of death in a population in a given period.
Motivational interviewing	A counselling style that uses person-centred skills within a flexible structure for helping people to explore the pros and cons of change (their motivation) and to prepare for action.
Musculoskeletal	To do with muscle and bone.
National Institute for Clinical Excellence (NICE)	An NHS organization responsible for producing guidance for both the NHS and patients on medicines, medical equipment, diagnostic tests, and clinical and surgical procedures and where they should be used.
National Service Framework (NSF)	National document which sets out the pattern and level of service (standards) which should be provided for a major care area or disease group such as mental health or heart disease.
Needle exchange	A scheme whereby drug users can return needles they have used for injecting drugs and receive sterile ones; the aim is to reduce infection caused by injecting with dirty needles.
Neighbourhood renewal	Tackling social and economic conditions in the most deprived local authority areas.
Neoplasm	Any new and abnormal growth, benign or malignant.
New Opportunities Programme	Lottery-funded programmes across the UK that are designed to improve the quality of life for people and communities, address disadvantage, encourage community participation and complement government strategies.
NHS trust	An independent body within the NHS which provides health services in hospitals. Some NHS trusts provide specialized services such as ambulance services or mental health services.

Office for Standards in Education (OFSTED)	The national government body which sets and monitors standards in education.
Opportunistic screening	Screening when an opportunity arises, e.g. when a patient goes to the doctor with an unrelated condition.
Perinatal	Relating to the period variably defined as from the 20th to 28th week of pregnancy, including the birth and up to 28 days later.
Personal, social and health education (PSHE)	That part of the school curriculum dealing with relationships (including sex education) and health.
Precautionary principle	An ethical principle which considers that if an activity raises threats of harm to human health or the environment, precautionary measures should be taken even if some cause and effect relationships are not fully established scientifically.
Premature mortality/ premature death	Death under 65 years of age. High rates of premature death in a population indicate poor health overall.
Prevalence	Measure of how much illness there is in a population at a particular point in time or over a specified period of time. (Compare with *incidence*.)
Primary care	Services which are people's first point of contact with the NHS, e.g. services provided by GPs, practice nurses, district nurses and health visitors. (As distinct from *secondary care* provided in hospitals.)
Primary care trust (PCT)	An NHS body whose main tasks are to assess local health needs, develop and implement plans to improve the health of the local population, provide primary care services and ensure that secondary care services are provided by local hospitals and specialized services.
Primary prevention	Stopping ill health arising in the first place. For example, eating a healthy diet, not smoking and taking enough exercise are factors in the primary prevention of heart disease. (Compare with *secondary* and *tertiary* prevention.)
Prospective study	Research study which gathers new information over a future period, e.g. to observe emerging patterns of disease and aetiological factors in a healthy population over a period of time. This includes longitudinal studies. (Compare with *retrospective* studies using data relating to the past, to compare exposures of people who already have disease with those who do not.)
PSA testing	Testing to detect prostate cancer. PSA stands for 'prostate-specific antigen'.
Public health	Preventing disease, prolonging life and promoting health through work focused on the population as a whole.

Radiotherapy	Treating disease (e.g. destroying cancer cells) with penetrating radiation.
Randomized controlled trials (RCT)	An experimental method whereby subjects are allocated randomly between an experimental group which receives an intervention and a control group which does not, so that the two groups can be fairly compared to see the effect of the intervention.
Regional Development Agencies	Nine public bodies in England under the government Department of Trade and Industry (DTI) which aim to further economic development and regeneration; promote businesses, employment and the skills needed; and contribute to sustainable development.
Retinopathy	Disorders of the retina (the light sensitive layer which lines the interior of the eye) resulting in impairment or loss of vision.
Risk factor	An attribute, such as a habit (e.g. smoking) or exposure to an environmental hazard (e.g. asbestos) that leads to a greater likelihood of developing an illness.
Screening	The application of a special test for everyone at risk of a particular disease to detect whether the disease is present at an early stage. It is used for diseases where early detection makes treatment more successful.
Secondary care	Specialized healthcare services provided by hospital inpatient and outpatient services.
Secondary prevention	Avoiding or alleviating consequences of disease by early detection and action, e.g. preventing cancer spreading to other sites in the body by detecting and treating it at an early stage. (Compare with *primary* and *tertiary* prevention.)
Sex and relationship education (SRE)	That part of the school curriculum dealing with sex education and personal relationships.
Sexually transmitted infection (STI)	Disease which is passed to other people through sexual contact: not only penetrative heterosexual sex, but also oral and anal sex.
Social capital	Investment in the social fabric of society, so that communities have characteristics such as high levels of trust, and supportive networks for the exchange of information, ideas and practical help.
Social Exclusion Unit (SEU)	Unit set up in 1997 by the Prime Minister to help improve government action to reduce social exclusion by producing 'joined-up solutions to joined-up problems' on policy areas such as truancy and school exclusion; rough sleeping; teenage pregnancy; 16–18 year olds not in education, employment or training; neighbourhood renewal; and reducing re-offending by ex-prisoners.

Social inclusion/exclusion	A sense of belonging to/feeling alienated from the community in which a person lives. Social exclusion is a shorthand term for what can happen when people or areas suffer from a combination of linked problems such as unemployment, poor skills, low incomes, poor housing, high crime environments, bad health and family breakdown.
Standardized	(E.g. as in 'standardized mortality rates') A way of comparing rates in which allowances have been made for different population characteristics, most commonly age and sex. This means that fair comparisons can be made between populations with, for example, different proportions of children or older people.
Strategy Unit	Government unit with four main roles: undertaking long term strategic reviews of major areas of policy; undertaking studies of cross-cutting policy issues; working with departments to promote strategic thinking and improve policy making across Whitehall; and provide strategic leadership to social research across government. Reports to the Prime Minister through the Cabinet Secretary.
Sure Start	Government schemes in areas of high health need, which aim to support parents and children under four.
Sure Start Plus	Sure Start programme which focuses on providing support to pregnant teenagers and teenage parents.
Survival rates	The percentage of people still alive 1, 3, 5 and 10 years after they have been diagnosed with cancer. The 5 year survival rate is often quoted.
Tertiary prevention	Preventing avoidable complications of established disease or disability (e.g. coronary rehabilitation programmes aiming to help patients who have had heart attacks to reduce the risk of further attacks.) (Compare with *primary* and *secondary* prevention.)
White Paper	Government policy often accompanied by legislation. Usually follows a Green Paper.
Whole population approach	Public health approach which focuses on a whole community rather than on individuals identified as being in particular need. (Compare with *high risk* approach.)
World Health Organization (WHO)	An inter-governmental organization within the United Nations system whose purpose is to help all people attain the highest possible level of health through public health programmes. Its headquarters are in Geneva, Switzerland.

Index